Pain Control

Editor

JANET L. ABRAHM

HEMATOLOGY/ONCOLOGY CLINICS OF NORTH AMERICA

www.hemonc.theclinics.com

Consulting Editors
GEORGE P. CANELLOS
H. FRANKLIN BUNN

June 2018 • Volume 32 • Number 3

ELSEVIER

1600 John F. Kennedy Boulevard • Suite 1800 • Philadelphia, Pennsylvania, 19103-2899

http://www.theclinics.com

HEMATOLOGY/ONCOLOGY CLINICS OF NORTH AMERICA Volume 32, Number 3
June 2018 ISSN 0889-8588, ISBN 13: 978-0-323-61056-8

Editor: Stacy Eastman
Developmental Editor: Kristen Helm

Hematology/Oncology Clinics (ISSN 0889-8588) is published bimonthly by Elsevier Inc., 360 Park Avenue South, New York, NY 10010-1710. Months of issue are February, April, June, August, October, and December. Business and Editorial Offices: 1600 John F. Kennedy Blvd., Ste. 1800, Philadelphia, PA 19103–2899. Customer Service Office: 3251 Riverport Lane, Maryland Heights, MO 63043. Periodicals postage paid at New York, NY and at additional mailing offices. Subscription prices are $413.00 per year (domestic individuals), $787.00 per year (domestic institutions), $100.00 per year (domestic students/residents), $471.00 per year (Canadian individuals), $974.00 per year (Canadian institutions) $536.00 per year (international individuals), $974.00 per year (international institutions), and $255.00 per year (international and Canadian students/residents). International air speed delivery is included in all *Clinics* subscription prices. All prices are subject to change without notice. **POSTMASTER:** Send address changes to *Hematology/Oncology Clinics of North America*, Elsevier Health Sciences Division, Subscription Customer Service, 3251 Riverport Lane, Maryland Heights, MO 63043. Customer Service (orders, claims, online, change of address): Elsevier Health Sciences Division, Subscription **Customer Service, 3251 Riverport Lane, Maryland Heights, MO 63043. Tel: 1-800-654-2452 (U.S. and Canada); 314-447-8871 (outside U.S. and Canada). Fax: 314-447-8029. E-mail: journalscustomerservice-usa@elsevier.com (for print support); journalsonlinesupport-usa@elsevier.com (for online support).**

Reprints. For copies of 100 or more, of articles in this publication, please contact the Commercial Reprints Department, Elsevier Inc., 360 Park Avenue South, New York, New York 10010-1710; Tel.: 212-633-3874, Fax: 212-633-3820, E-mail: reprints@elsevier.com.

Hematology/Oncology Clinics of North America is covered in *MEDLINE/PubMed (Index Medicus), EMBASE/ Excerpta Medica, and BIOSIS.*

Contributors

CONSULTING EDITORS

GEORGE P. CANELLOS, MD
William Rosenberg Professor of Medicine, Department of Medical Oncology, Dana-Farber Cancer Institute, Boston, Massachusetts

H. FRANKLIN BUNN, MD
Professor of Medicine, Division of Hematology, Brigham and Women's Hospital, Harvard Medical School, Boston, Massachusetts

EDITOR

JANET L. ABRAHM, MD, FACP, FAAHPM
Professor of Medicine, Division of Adult Palliative Care, Department of Psychosocial Oncology and Palliative Care, Dana-Farber Cancer Institute, Harvard Medical School, Boston, Massachusetts

AUTHORS

EBTESAM AHMED, PharmD, MS
Director, Pharmacy Internship, MJHS Institute for Innovation in Palliative Care, Clinical Professor of Pharmacy, St. John's University College of Pharmacy and Health Sciences, New York, New York

JOSEPH ARTHUR, MD
Assistant Professor, Department of Palliative Care, Rehabilitation and Integrative Medicine, The University of Texas MD Anderson Cancer Center, Houston, Texas

JEFFREY R. BASFORD, MD, PhD
Professor, Department of Physical Medicine and Rehabilitation, Mayo Clinic, Rochester, Minnesota

AMANDA M. BRANDOW, DO, MS
Associate Professor, Department of Pediatrics, Section of Pediatric Hematology/Oncology, Medical College of Wisconsin, MFRC, Milwaukee, Wisconsin

JEANNINE M. BRANT, PhD, APRN, FAAN
Oncology Clinical Nurse Specialist, Nurse Scientist, Department of Collaborative Science and Innovation, Billings Clinic, Billings, Montana

BRENDA BURSCH, PhD
Professor of Clinical Psychiatry and Biobehavioral Sciences, Professor of Clinical Pediatrics, Clinical Director, Pediatric Psychiatry Consultation Liaison Service, David Geffen School of Medicine at UCLA, Los Angeles, California

HOLLY CARESKEY, MD, MPH
Clinical Fellow in Pain Medicine, Department of Anesthesiology, Perioperative and Pain Medicine, Brigham and Women's Hospital, Harvard Medical School, Boston, Massachusetts

ANDREA L. CHEVILLE, MD, MSCE
Professor, Department of Physical Medicine and Rehabilitation, Mayo Clinic, Rochester, Minnesota

RYAN C. COSTANTINO, PharmD, BCPS, BCGP
PGY2 Pharmacy Practice Resident, Pain Management/Palliative Care, University of Maryland School of Pharmacy, Baltimore, Maryland

MELLAR P. DAVIS, MD, FCCP, FAAHPM
Geisinger Medical Center, Danville, Pennsylvania

MICHAEL R. DeBAUN, MD, MPH
Professor of Pediatrics and Medicine, Vice Chair for Clinical Research, Department of Pediatrics, Vanderbilt University School of Medicine, Vanderbilt University Medical Center, Nashville, Tennessee

AREEJ R. EL-JAWAHRI, MD
Division of Hematology/Oncology, Bone Marrow Transplant, Massachusetts General Hospital, Boston, Massachusetts

BETTY R. FERRELL, RN, PhD, MA, FAAN, FPCN, CHPN
Director and Professor, Division of Nursing Research and Education, Department of Population Sciences, City of Hope Medical Center, Duarte, California

NICHOLAS FIGURA, MD
Resident, Department of Radiation Oncology, Moffitt Cancer Center, Tampa, Florida

REGINA M. FINK, PhD, APRN, FAAN
Associate Professor, Co-Director, Interprofessional Master of Science, General Internal Medicine, University of Colorado Anschutz Medical Campus School of Medicine, College of Nursing, Aurora, Colorado

DENISE HESS, MDiv, LMFT
Executive Director, Supportive Care Coalition, Providence St. Joseph Health, Hillsboro, Oregon

DAVID HUI, MD, MSc
Associate Professor, Departments of Palliative Care, Rehabilitation and Integrative Medicine and General Oncology, The University of Texas MD Anderson Cancer Center, Houston, Texas

STEPHEN D.W. KING, PhD
Manager, Chaplaincy, Child Life, Clinical Patient Navigator, Seattle Cancer Care Alliance, Seattle, Washington

MONICA KRISHNAN, MD
Clinical Assistant Professor, Department of Radiation Oncology, Dana-Farber Cancer Institute, Brigham and Women's Cancer Center, Boston, Massachusetts

THOMAS W. LeBLANC, MD, MA, MHS
Division of Hematologic Malignancies and Cellular Therapy, Duke University School of Medicine, Durham, North Carolina

WEIDONG LU, MB, MPH, PhD
Leonard P. Zakim Center for Integrative Therapies and Healthy Living, Dana-Farber Cancer Institute, Harvard Medical School, Boston, Massachusetts

JOSEPH D. MA, PharmD
Division of Clinical Pharmacy, UC San Diego Skaggs School of Pharmacy and Pharmaceutical Sciences, La Jolla, California

ALEXANDRA L. McPHERSON, PharmD, MPH
PGY2 Pharmacy Practice Resident, Pain Management/Palliative Care, University of Maryland School of Pharmacy, Baltimore, Maryland

MARY LYNN McPHERSON, PharmD, MA, MDE, BCPS, CPE
Executive Director, Advanced Post-Graduate Education in Palliative Care, Program Director, Online Master of Science and Graduate Certificates in Palliative Care, Professor, University of Maryland School of Pharmacy, Baltimore, Maryland

SANJEET NARANG, MD
Assistant Professor in Anaesthesia, Department of Anesthesiology, Perioperative and Pain Medicine, Brigham and Women's Hospital, Harvard Medical School, Boston, Massachusetts

RUSSELL K. PORTENOY, MD
Executive Director, MJHS Institute for Innovation in Palliative Care, Chief Medical Officer, MJHS Hospice and Palliative Care, New York, New York; Professor of Neurology and Family and Social Medicine, Albert Einstein College of Medicine, Bronx, New York

CHRISTINA M. PUCHALSKI, MD, OCDS, FACP, FAAHPM
Professor, Department of Medicine and Health Sciences, Professor, Health Leadership and Management, Director, The George Washington Institute for Spirituality & Health, The George Washington University School of Medicine & Health Sciences, The George Washington University School of Public Health, Co-Director, MFA-GWU Supportive and Palliative Care Clinic, Washington, DC

ERIC J. ROELAND, MD
Department of Medicine, UC San Diego Moores Cancer Center, La Jolla, California

DAVID S. ROSENTHAL, MD
Leonard P. Zakim Center for Integrative Therapies and Healthy Living, Dana-Farber Cancer Institute, Harvard Medical School, Boston, Massachusetts

RON SHILOH, MD
Clinical Instructor, Department of Radiation Oncology, Dana-Farber Cancer Institute, Brigham and Women's Cancer Center, Boston, Massachusetts

JOSHUA SMITH, MD
Professor, Department of Supportive Care Medicine, Moffitt Cancer Center, Tampa, Florida

SEAN R. SMITH, MD
Assistant Professor, Department of Physical Medicine and Rehabilitation, University of Michigan, University of Michigan Health System, Ann Arbor, Michigan

THOMAS B. STROUSE, MD
Maddie Katz Professor, Medical Director, Resnick Neuropsychiatric Hospital at UCLA, Vice Chair for Clinical Affairs, UCLA Department of Psychiatry, David Geffen School of Medicine, Los Angeles, California

HSIANG-HSUAN MICHAEL YU, MD, ScM
Professor, Department of Radiation Oncology, Moffitt Cancer Center, Tampa, Florida

Contents

> Pain is widespread, multidimensional, and one of the most distressing symptoms patients with cancer face. Pain assessment is the foundation to optimal pain management. Despite evidence-based practice guidelines, inadequate pain assessment is a barrier. Patients should be routinely screened for pain at each encounter. If new, worsening, or persistent pain is present, a comprehensive pain assessment and reassessment should be regularly performed and documented to communicate the pain problem. Patient self-report of pain is the gold standard even in those who are nonverbal or cognitively impaired. Clinicians should follow the Hierarchy of Pain Assessment Framework to guide pain assessment approaches.

> Patients with cancer experience many acute and chronic pain syndromes, the identification of which may be helpful in the assessment and treatment of pain. Syndromes are defined by the relationship with the cancer, the pain pathophysiology, and the clinical characteristics of the pain. The most common pain syndromes are directly related to the tumor; bone pain syndromes are most common. Neuropathic pain syndromes may involve cancer-related injury at any level of the peripheral nervous system. Treatment-related pain syndromes may follow any type of antineoplastic therapy. This article reviews the phenomenology of common acute and chronic cancer pain syndromes.

> Opioids are highly effective for cancer pain but are associated with multiple adverse effects and risk of addiction. This article provides a synopsis on the management of various opioid-related adverse effects and strategies to minimize aberrant opioid use in patients who have cancer. Many adverse effects can be effectively managed. Some patients on chronic opioid therapy may demonstrate aberrant behaviors suggestive of opioid misuse or diversion. Through intensive education, longitudinal monitoring, early identification, and timely management, clinicians can optimize the risk to benefit ratio to support safe opioid use.

> Methadone is a valuable opioid in the management of patients who have cancer with pain. Methadone is a mu-, kappa-, and delta-opioid agonist and an N-methyl-D-aspartate receptor antagonist. These mechanisms of action make methadone an attractive option for complex pain syndromes. It is critically important that providers consider a patient's risk status before beginning administration of methadone. Careful consideration must be given to dosing methadone in both opioid-naive and opioid-tolerant patients, with vigilant monitoring for therapeutic effectiveness and potential toxicity until the patient achieves steady state.

> Neuropathic pain is the result of neuroplastic and neuroinflammatory changes from trauma or diseases that damage the somatosensory system. Cancer-related neuropathic pain is caused by treatment, cancer, or paraneoplastic reactions to cancer. Approximately 30% of patients with cancer have neuropathic pain, mostly mixed nociceptive and neuropathic pain. History, physical examination, quantitative sensory testing, skin punch biopsies, and functional MRIs help to divide pain into phenotypes that may facilitate analgesic choices. Guidelines for treating cancer-related neuropathic pain are not consistent and are highly dependent on trials in patients without cancer. Combinations of analgesics are promising, whereas evidence for cannabinoids is meager.

> This article reviews anesthetic interventional approaches to the management of pain in hematology and oncology patients. It includes a discussion of single interventions, including peripheral nerve blocks, plexus injections, and sympathetic nerve neurolysis, and continuous infusion therapy through implantable devices, such as intrathecal pumps, epidural port-a-caths, and tunneled catheters. The primary objective is to inform members of hematology and oncology care teams regarding the variety of interventional options for patients with cancer-related pain for whom medical pain management methods have not been effective.

> Metastatic bone pain is a complex, poorly understood process. Understanding the unique mechanisms causing cancer-induced bone pain may lead to potential therapeutic targets. This article discusses the effects of osteoclast overstimulation within the tumor microenvironment; the role of inflammatory factors at the tumor-nociceptor interface; the development of structural instability, causing mechanical nerve damage; and,

ultimately, the neuroplastic changes in the setting of sustained pain. Several adjuvant therapies are available to attenuate metastatic bone pain. This article discusses the role of pharmacologic therapies, surgery, kyphoplasty, vertebroplasty, and radiofrequency ablation.

Several variables may be considered when deciding on the optimal modality of radiation therapy for each patient with cancer with bone pain, including prognosis, tumor histology, location and extent of metastases, and association with cord compression. Hypofractionated external beam radiation therapy is as effective as a multiple fraction radiotherapy course in most cases, although retreatment rates are higher after a single dose of radiation. Stereotactic body radiation may be used in cases of oligometastatic disease, repeat irradiation, and radiation-resistant tumors. Radiopharmaceuticals may be used for pain from diffuse bone metastases and have an overall survival benefit in patients with castrate-resistant prostate cancer.

Rehabilitation medicine offers strategies that reduce musculoskeletal pain, targeted approaches to alleviate movement-related pain, and interventions to optimize patients' function despite the persistence of pain. These approaches fall into four categories: modulating nociception, stabilizing and unloading painful structures, influencing pain perception, and alleviating soft tissue musculotendinous pain. Incorporating these interventions into individualized, comprehensive pain management programs offers the potential to empower patients and limit pain associated with mobility and required daily activities. Rehabilitative approach may be particularly helpful for patients with refractory movement-associated pain and functional vulnerability and for those who do not wish for, or cannot, tolerate pharmacoanalgesia.

Psychological approaches to pain management have been demonstrated to be effective for individuals newly diagnosed with cancer, in remission, and/or with progressive or terminal disease. Modalities that have been demonstrated to be most effective are cognitive behavioral approaches that include relaxation skills and/or hypnotherapy.

Pain is a reality for approximately half of all patients with cancer and can negatively affect patient cognitive and emotional states, resulting in "total pain." Total pain may not respond to pharmacologic interventions and may pave the way for the onset of suffering, where suffering is defined as physical pain accompanied by negative cognitive interpretations. Mindfulness-based interventions provide an alternate interpretive framework for both pain and suffering and may lessen a patient's experience of pain. Mindfulness-based interventions have the potential to alter a patient's relationship to pain, reducing pain catastrophizing and enhancing patient-reported overall well-being.

Spiritual Considerations   505

Christina M. Puchalski, Stephen D.W. King, and Betty R. Ferrell

Spiritual issues play a prominent role for patients with cancer. Studies have demonstrated a positive connection between a patient's spirituality and health outcomes, including quality of life, depression and anxiety, hopefulness, and the ability to cope with illness. Spiritual or existential distress is prominent in patients with cancer. Models are described that identify ways for clinicians to identify or diagnose spiritual or existential distress and to attend to that distress. It is critical that all clinicians assess for spiritual distress as part of a routine distress assessment, identify appropriate treatment strategies, and work closely with trained spiritual care professionals.

Oncology Acupuncture for Chronic Pain in Cancer Survivors: A Reflection on the American Society of Clinical Oncology Chronic Pain Guideline   519

Weidong Lu and David S. Rosenthal

Chronic pain syndromes associated with cancer treatment are common but difficult to manage. The American Society of Clinical Oncology recently published a practice guideline to address the unmet needs of cancer survivors, *Management of Chronic Pain in Survivors of Adult Cancers*, which stresses the importance of implementing integrative therapies, including acupuncture. This article focuses on randomized clinical trials of acupuncture for chronic pain in cancer survivors, including its use in chemotherapy-induced peripheral neuropathy, aromatase inhibitor–associated arthralgia, and post neck dissection pain, and provides future directions of oncology acupuncture research in cancer survivorship. The features of oncology acupuncture are also discussed.

Key Components of Pain Management for Children and Adults with Sickle Cell Disease   535

Amanda M. Brandow and Michael R. DeBaun

Sickle cell disease pain manifests as severe acute pain episodes and a debilitating chronic pain syndrome. Acute pain episodes are the most common reason for health care use; however, acute pain episodes are also frequently managed at home. Chronic pain syndrome develops in 30% to 40% of individuals with sickle cell disease, with an increasing incidence and severity with age. The authors review the critical aspects of pain management that are integral to the comprehensive approach to sickle cell disease pain and are rooted in the biopsychosocial model. The article focuses on opioid pharmacology and psychosocial comorbidities.

Erratum

In the article on "Emerging Therapies" appearing in the April 2018 issue of *Hematology/Oncology Clinics of North America* (Volume 32, Issue 2), the following errors were made on page 347 in Table 1:

- NCT02633943: This is an observational and long-term follow-up study (instead of an early phase 1 study) after patients have completed studies NCT01745120, NCT02151526, NCT02906202, NCT03207009.
- NCT02453477: This study did not use the LentiGlobin BB305 vector. The following studies did use the LentiGlobin BB305 vector: NCT01745120, NCT02151526, NCT02906202, NCT03207009.

In the article on "Gene Therapy and Genome Editing" in the same issue, the following errors were made:

- In Table 1, on page 334, the Northstar study (NCT01745120) evaluated patients aged 12-35 years of age, instead of 12-17 years of age.
- On page 335 in the third sub-bullet, HGB-207 and HGB-212 studies (instead of HGB-206 and HGB-207 studies) are evaluating patients with non-β^0/β^0 and β^0/β^0 genotypes, respectively.

Sources for all information can be found on clinicaltrials.gov.
These corrections have been made in the online versions of the articles.

Hematol Oncol Clin N Am 32 (2018) xiii
https://doi.org/10.1016/j.hoc.2018.04.009
0889-8588/18/© 2018 Elsevier Inc. All rights reserved.

hemonc.theclinics.com

Preface

Pain, a Complex Challenge

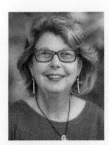

Janet L. Abrahm, MD, FACP, FAAHPM
Editor

Despite the many diagnostic and therapeutic advances in the 26 years since the last *Hematology/Oncology Clinics of North America* issue on Pain, control of pain in our patients remains a complex challenge.

Pain remains prevalent. As of the 2012 National Health Interview Survey, 25 million adults in the United States had daily chronic pain and an additional 23 million experienced severe pain.[1] Thirty to forty percent of patients with cancer experience pain, and this proportion increases to 70% to 90% of patients with advanced disease.[2]

Pain is debilitating, depressing, and the root of much suffering. Pain robs us of aspects of our "personhood," destroying our roles in the family, community, workplace, and place of worship. As Cassell states: "All the aspects of personhood—the lived past, the family's lived past, culture and society, roles, and the instrumental dimension, associations and relationships, the body, the unconscious mind, the political being, the secret life, the perceived future, and the transcendent-being dimension—are susceptible to damage and loss."[3]

Our role, then, as clinicians and healers, is to do our best to prevent or manage this devastating complication of illness in the context of the opioid crisis. We must enable patients once again to become whole, even if they are not cured. The authors in this issue are experts in the many and varied aspects of pain. It is our hope that readers will gain a comprehensive understanding of the state-of-the-art in pain assessment, and in the wide variety of modalities available to their patients in pain. Special articles are devoted to the care of patients with sickle cell diseases, and those undergoing hematopoietic stem cell transplants.

The issue includes:

1. Complex Cancer Pain Assessment, by Regina M. Fink, RN, PhD, AOCN, CHPN, FAAN and Jeannine M. Brant, PhD, APRN-CNS, AOCN, FAAN
2. Cancer Pain Syndromes, by Russell K. Portenoy, MD and Ebtesam Ahmed, PharmD, MS
3. Safe Opioid Use: Management of Opioid-Related Adverse Effects and Aberrant Behaviors, by Joseph Arthur, MD and David Hui, MD, MSc

Hematol Oncol Clin N Am 32 (2018) xv–xvi
https://doi.org/10.1016/j.hoc.2018.02.002
0889-8588/18/© 2018 Published by Elsevier Inc.

hemonc.theclinics.com

Janet L. Abrahm, MD, FACP, FAAHPM
Division of Adult Palliative Care
Department of Psychosocial Oncology and
Palliative Care
Dana-Farber Cancer Institute
Harvard Medical School
D 2010
450 Brookline Avenue
Boston, MA 02215, USA

E-mail address:
jabrahm@partners.org

REFERENCES

1. Nahin RL. Estimates of pain prevalence and severity in adults: United States 2012. J Pain 2015;16:769–80.
2. Levy MH, Chwistek M, Mehta RS. Management of chronic pain in cancer survivors. Cancer J 2008;14:401–9.
3. Cassell EJ. The nature of suffering and the goals of medicine. 2nd edition. Oxford (United Kingdom): Oxford University Press, Inc; 2004. p. 42.

Complex Cancer Pain Assessment

Regina M. Fink, PhD, APRN[a],*, Jeannine M. Brant, PhD, APRN[b]

KEYWORDS

- Cancer pain • Pain assessment • Breakthrough pain • Pain syndromes • Barriers
- Pain behaviors

KEY POINTS

- Approximately 40% of all cancer patients report moderate to severe pain (defined as ≥ 5 on a 0-10 numeric rating scale).
- 60% of patients with cancer experience breakthrough cancer pain.
- Patients must be routinely screened for pain at each time of contact.
- If new, worsening, or persistent pain is present, a comprehensive pain assessment and reassessment should be performed, occurring at regular intervals, individualized, and documented.
- For patients unable to self-report, clinicians should follow the hierarchy of pain assessment framework to guide pain assessment approaches.

INTRODUCTION

Cancer pain is widespread, multidimensional, and not adequately managed despite the availability of evidence-based practice guidelines and multiple position papers.[1–3] Barriers to optimal pain management exist; inadequate pain assessment is one of the most important barriers identified. Pain assessment is the foundation to optimal pain management. This article reviews cancer pain epidemiology; pain definitions, types, and syndromes; pain assessment parameters for patients who can self-report and those who are nonverbal and/or cognitively impaired; populations requiring special consideration; and barriers to pain assessment.

Disclosure Statement: R.M. Fink reports no commercial or financial conflicts of interest. J.M. Brant is on speaker's bureaus for Insys and Genentech. The authors alone are responsible for the content and writing of this article.
[a] General Internal Medicine, University of Colorado Anschutz Medical Campus School of Medicine, College of Nursing, 12631 East 17th Avenue, B-180, Aurora, CO 80045, USA;
[b] Department of Collaborative Science and Innovation, Billings Clinic, 2800 Tenth Avenue North, Billings, MT 59101, USA
* Corresponding author.
E-mail address: regina.fink@ucdenver.edu

Hematol Oncol Clin N Am 32 (2018) 353–369
https://doi.org/10.1016/j.hoc.2018.01.001
0889-8588/18/© 2018 Elsevier Inc. All rights reserved.

EPIDEMIOLOGY OF PAIN

Pain is one of the most common and most distressing symptoms described by patients with cancer. A recent systematic review and meta-analysis of 122 articles published since 2005 found that pain prevalence rates are 39.3% after curative treatment; 55% during anticancer treatment; 66.4% in advanced, metastatic, or terminal disease; and 50.7% in all cancer stages.[4] Approximately 40% of all patients with cancer report moderate to severe pain (defined as ≥5 on a 0–10 numeric rating scale). Lower pain prevalence rates (52%) are documented in urogenital cancers (prostate, bladder) compared with head and neck (70%), gynecologic (60%), gastrointestinal (59%), lung (55%), and breast (54%) cancers. Therefore, pain in persons with cancer remains a major problem.

PAIN DEFINITIONS

According to the International Association for the Study of Pain, pain is "a sensory and emotional experience associated with actual or potential tissue damage or described in terms of such damage."[5] This definition not only encompasses the physical aspect of pain but also acknowledges the emotional experience associated with the experience. The definition reinforces the need for health care professionals to conduct a comprehensive assessment that includes all aspects of the pain experience.

Consistent nomenclature is essential in the assessment and diagnosis of pain. How pain is classified (eg, acute vs chronic) and described (eg, allodynia) provides information about the cause of the pain and aids in an appropriate pain management plan. In addition, substance use disorders have skyrocketed in the last few years. Confusion still exists around definitions, such as opioid misuse, abuse, diversion, and addiction. Misinterpretation of these terms can lead to inaccurate assessment, misdiagnosis, and undertreatment of pain. A list of pain assessment–related terms and their definitions is included in **Table 1**[2,5–8] (also see Joseph Arthur and David Hui's article, "Safe Opioid Use: Management of Opioid-Related Adverse Effects and Aberrant Behaviors," in this issue).

TYPES OF PAIN SYNDROMES

Cancer pain can be classified as acute or chronic. Acute pain is self-limiting and usually resolves within 3 months. Examples of acute pain include postsurgical pain and mucositis. Most cancer pain is chronic, persisting for greater than 3 months, and may be related to cancer treatment or the disease itself. Patients with cancer can also experience chronic noncancer pain, such as pain related to arthritis or another comorbid condition.[4,9]

Breakthrough cancer pain (BTCP) is also common among patients with cancer. BTCP is defined as an exacerbation of pain in the presence of well-controlled background pain. It is usually described as severe peaks within 1 to 10 minutes and lasts between 15 and 60 minutes. A systematic review of 19 studies found that approximately 60% of patients with cancer experience BTCP.[10] Of those, 44% report it related to an incident, 41.5% complained of insidious pain, and 14.5% had a combination of both.[11] BTCP is often underrecognized and underreported. The assessment requires a detailed patient interview to differentiate BTCP from uncontrolled background pain. Studies have shown that using a specific tool to measure BTCP is essential in its identification and management.[12–14]

ASSESSMENT

Pain is not only a physical experience, it is also multidimensional. To describe the all-encompassing nature of pain within a "whole person" framework, Dame Cicely

Table 1
Pain assessment-related definitions

Aberrant behavior	Behaviors indicative of prescription drug abuse, some of which are more indicative of abuse or addiction
Abuse	Use of a drug for nontherapeutic purposes to obtain psychotropic effects
Acute pain	Short-term pain usually lasting <3–6 mo that dissipates with normal tissue healing; considered a normal physiologic response to tissue damage; may occur on top of chronic pain
Addiction	A primary, chronic, neurobiologic disease, with genetic, psychosocial, and environmental factors influencing its development and manifestations. It is characterized by behaviors that include one or more of the following: impaired control over drug use, compulsive use, continued use despite harm, and craving
Allodynia	Pain due to a stimulus that normally does not produce pain
Breakthrough pain	A transient exacerbation of pain that occurs either spontaneously or in relation to a specific predictable or unpredictable trigger, despite relatively stable and adequately controlled background pain
Chronic pain	Longer-term pain lasting >3–6 mo that persists beyond the expected period of tissue healing; considered a condition or disease in and of itself
Dysesthesia	An abnormal, unpleasant sensation usually associated with neuropathic pain
End of dose failure	Pain that occurs before the next dose of a long-acting analgesic
Hyperalgesia	Increased pain from a stimulus that normally causes pain
Hyperesthesia	Heightened pain sensitivity to a stimulus
Hypoalgesia	Diminished pain response from a stimulus that normally causes pain
Incident pain	Pain that is associated with movement or activity; a type of breakthrough pain
Idiopathic pain	An unexpected episode of nonincident pain; a type of breakthrough pain
Misuse	Use of a prescription drug without a prescription or in a manner that is not prescribed
Neuralgia	Pain that runs along nerve distribution
Neuropathic pain • Centrally mediated • Peripherally mediated	Pain that is initiated in the central somatosensory nervous system Pain that is initiated in the peripheral somatosensory nervous system
Nociception	The process by which the nervous system codes noxious stimuli, which includes autonomic and behavioral responses to pain
Nociceptive pain	Pain arising from the activation of nociceptors due to actual or potential damage of nonneural tissue
Paresthesia	An abnormal sensation, either spontaneous or provoked, that manifests as numbness, tingling, or increased sensitivity
Physical dependence	A state of adaptation manifested by a drug class–specific withdrawal syndrome that can be produced by abrupt cessation, rapid dose reduction, decreasing blood level of the drug, and/or administration of an antagonist

(continued on next page)

Table 1 (continued)	
Pseudoaddiction	Pattern of drug-seeking behavior in patients with pain who are receiving inadequate pain management; can be mistaken for addiction
Somatic pain	A type of nociceptive pain arising from ligaments, tendons, bones, blood vessels, fasciae, and muscles
Substance use disorder	A cluster of cognitive, behavioral, and physiologic symptoms indicating that an individual continues to use the substance despite significant substance-related problems
Tolerance	A state of adaptation in which exposure to a drug induces changes that result in a diminution of one or more of the drug's effects over time
Visceral pain	A type of nociceptive pain arising from the activation of nociceptors of the thoracic, pelvic, or abdominal viscera (organs)

Adapted from Brant JM. Pain. In: Yarbro CH, Wujcik D, Gobel BH, editors. Cancer symptom management. 4th edition. Burlington (NJ): Jones & Bartlett Learning; 2013. p. 70; with permission.

Saunders created the concept of "total pain" and suggested the interplay of physical, psychological, social, and spiritual components.[15] Suffering encompasses all of a person's struggles; the contribution of each domain is specific to each individual and his or her situation. **Table 2** outlines the 4 domains of total pain and accompanying pain assessment components.

A patient's self-report of pain is the most valuable component of a comprehensive pain assessment because pain is typically managed accordingly. Patients must be routinely screened for pain at each encounter.[3] If new, worsening, or persistent pain is present, a comprehensive pain assessment and reassessment should be performed, occurring at regular intervals, individualized, and documented so that all involved in the patient's care will have an understanding of the pain problem. Multiple mnemonics are available to assist the clinician in the key aspects of a pain assessment (review **Table 2**). The WILDA approach incorporates 5 key components and begins with an open-ended question, "Tell me about your pain." This question facilitates the patient to tell his or her story, including the aspects of the pain experience most problematic.[16]

Words

Asking patients to describe their pain using descriptors will guide clinicians to appropriate pharmacologic and nonpharmacologic interventions for specific pain types. **Table 3** lists pain types and word descriptors. For example, if the patient complains of numbness or tingling in fingers or toes following taxane therapy, the clinician assumes peripheral neuropathy and may use an anticonvulsant.

Intensity

Quantifying the pain using a pain intensity scale assists in communication among the patient, family caregiver, and health care team and can measure the patient's response to both pharmacologic and nonpharmacologic interventions. Timely reassessment may inform the pain management regimen. When patients are unable to

Table 2	
Total pain domains	
Domain	**Pain Assessment Components**
Physical domain	
WILDA	• *W*ords used to describe the pain • *I*ntensity: On a scale of 0–10, what is your pain now, at rest, with movement, worst pain possible in the past 24 h? What is your comfort/function goal? • *L*ocation: Where is your pain? • *D*uration: Is the pain constant? Does the pain come and go? Do you have both types of pain (one that is constant and one that comes and goes)? • *A*ggravating/Alleviating factors: What makes the pain worse? What makes the pain better?
PQRST	• *P*rovocation/Palliation: What caused it? What relieves it? • *Q*uality: What does it feel like? • *R*egion/Radiation: Where is the pain located? Does the pain radiate? • *S*everity: How severe is the pain on a 0–10 scale? • *T*iming: Constant or intermittent?
OLDCART	• *O*nset: When did the pain start? • *L*ocation: Where is the pain located? Is there more than one location? • *D*uration: How often does the pain occur? Is it constant or intermittent? How long does the pain last? • *C*haracteristics: How does the pain feel (intensity)? What words would you use to describe the pain? (Descriptors can aid in diagnosing the pain syndrome). • *A*ggravating factors: What makes your pain worse? • *R*elieving factors: What makes your pain better? • *T*reatment: What treatments (pharmacologic and/or nonpharmacologic) have you tried to control the pain? How are they working? How do the treatments affect the pain intensity?
Psychological domain	• The meaning of pain to the patient and family • History of anxiety, depression, or other psychological illness • Cognition, including confusion or delirium • Usual coping strategies in response to pain • Psychological responses to pain and illness, such as depression, anxiety, and fear • Past pain experience • Beliefs about opioids, addiction, and other concerns • Willingness to try complementary modalities, such as cognitive behavioral therapy
Social domain	• Functional assessment: Interference of pain on daily living, including physical or social withdrawal from activity • Family caregiver communication and response to illness • Support system • Economic impact of the pain and its treatment (eg, ability to afford analgesics)
Spiritual/existential domain	• Spiritual beliefs related to pain and illness • Presence of a spiritual community and its role related to pain and illness • Influence of religion or spirituality on coping with pain • Influence of suffering on the pain experience • Use of traditional medicine in healing

Data from Refs.[15,16,48,49]

Table 3 Pain types and word descriptors	
Pain Type Potential Cause	Word Descriptors
Neuropathic Nerve involvement by tumor, postherpetic neuralgia, diabetic or peripheral neuropathies, HIV-associated neuropathy, chemotherapy-induced neuropathy, phantom limb pain	Burning, shooting, tingling, numb, radiating, "firelike," electrical, pins and needles
Somatic Bone or spine metastasis, fractures, injury to deep musculoskeletal structures or superficial cutaneous tissues, arthritis, osteoporosis, fractures	Aching, throbbing, dull, sharp, sore, well localized
Visceral Bowel obstruction, venous occlusion, ascites, liver metastasis, postabdominal or thoracic surgery, thrombosis	Squeezing, pressure, crampy, distention, deep, stretching, bloated-feeling, poorly localized

Adapted from Montgomery RK, Lyda C, Hornick L, et al. Analgesic reference guide. Aurora (CO): University of Colorado Health; 2013; with permission.

provide a "0 to 10" response using the numeric rating scale, it is important to have other assessment tools available (verbal descriptor scale, vertical pain thermometer, and Faces scales). A nonverbal pain assessment scale should be used for patients who cannot provide a self-assessment of pain. Having culturally tailored pain assessment scales in multiple languages is crucial. Refer to **Table 4** for a review of common pain assessment instruments.

Note: Although pain intensity assessment is a very important component of pain care, clinical decision making should be based on a *total* patient pain assessment rather than relying only on a severity rating score. The practice of prescribing and dosing opioid analgesics based solely on a patient's pain intensity should not be encouraged because it disregards the relevance of other vital elements of an assessment and may contribute to untoward patient outcomes.[17]

Location

Information should be gathered for each pain location. Most patients have 2 or more sites of pain. Thus, it is important to ask patients, "Where is your pain?" or "Do you have pain in more than one area?" The patient may actually be referring to a different pain than the clinician is talking about. Having the patient point to his or her painful area or areas can be more specific.

Duration

Patients should be queried, "Is your pain always there (persistent)?," "Does it come and go (breakthrough pain)?," and "Do you have both types of pain?" Pain duration can determine whether controlled release and/or immediate release opioids should be prescribed.

Aggravating and Alleviating Factors

What makes the pain worse or better informs the pain management plan of care. If a patient complains of pain with activities of daily living or pain is interfering with

Table 4
Common pain assessment tools

Assessment Tool	Description	Guidelines for Use
Verbal Pain Intensity Tools		
Numeric rating scale	• "0–10" scale with "0" being no pain and "10" being pain as bad as it can be or worst pain possible • 0–5, 0–6, 0–20, and 0–100 scales also available	• Gold standard to assess pain intensity in the adult population • Children who are developmentally able to report pain (7 y and older) can use this scale
Verbal descriptor scale (VDS)	• None, mild, moderate, severe, very severe	• Preferred in adults with cognitive impairment and the elderly
Vertical pain thermometer	• Visual vertical thermometer with pain descriptors alongside • Slight pain, mild pain, moderate pain, severe pain, very severe pain, most intense pain imaginable	• Evidence exists to support its use in patients with cognitive impairment
Present pain inventory	0 = no pain 1 = mild 2 = discomforting 3 = distressing 4 = horrible 5 = excruciating	• Adults • Less evidence exists for use in cognitive impairment compared with VDS and pain thermometer
Nonverbal/Preverbal/Cognitively Impaired Pain Assessment Tools		
Faces Pain Scale (FPS)–Revised	• Six elongated cartoon pain faces	• May be preferred by those with language barriers • Caution: May measure other constructs (eg, distress, depression, sadness) • Linear relationship of this scale with the VAS for children ages 6–16
Wong-Baker Faces	• Six round cartoon faces with expressions suggestive of pain	• Less evidence exists compared with FPS for use in older adults with cognitive impairment • Caution: Presence of tears may introduce cultural bias when used by patients from cultures where crying is not approved in response to pain

Faces, Legs, Arms, Cry, Consolability Scale–Revised (FLACC-r)	• Five criteria scored from 0-2
	  ○ Face
	  ○ Legs
	  ○ Activity
	  ○ Cry
	  ○ Consolability
	• Total score 0–10
		• Commonly used in preverbal children
		• Validated in critically ill adults

Checklist of Nonverbal Pain Indicators	• Six behaviors rated with movement and at rest • Total score 0–12	• Valid in acute and long-term care settings • Useful in nonverbal adult population

(continued on next page)

Table 4 (continued)		
Assessment Tool	**Description**	**Guidelines for Use**

Critical Care Pain Observation Tool	• Four domains scored on 3 behaviors from 0 to 2
	  ○ Facial expression
	  ○ Body movements
	  ○ Compliance with the ventilator (intubated patients) or vocalization (extubated patients)
	  ○ Muscle tension
	Total score 0–8
		• Valid in critically ill patients who are unable to self-report
		• Presence of pain is suspected at scores >2 or when the score increases by 2 or more

Pain Assessment in Advanced Dementia	Five domains scored from 0–2 • Breathing (independent of vocalization) • Negative vocalization • Facial expression • Body language • Consolability Total score 0–10	• Valid in patients with advanced dementia • Derived from the behaviors and categories of the FLACC • Intended to measure pain in noncommunicative patients/residents
Pain Assessment Behavioral Scale	Five items scored from 0–10 • Face • Restlessness • Muscle tone • Vocalization • Consolability Total score 0–10	• Valid in cognitively impaired and nonverbal patients in acute care and long-term care settings • Patients/residents observed at rest and with movement • Two scores generated; the higher score is documented
Comprehensive Pain Assessment Tools		
Brief Pain Inventory Short Form	• Fifteen items • Worst, least, average pain intensity rated and relief from current regimen • Includes 7 items that rate impact of pain on function • Body diagram on tool for patient to mark pain locations	• Note: A longer form exists but authors recommend Short Form use • Commonly used in research
McGill Pain Questionnaire (MPQ)	• Three classes of words (total of 78) that describe the sensory, affective, and evaluative aspects of pain • Scoring involves ranking adjectives according to increasing intensity	• Adult population • Developed for chronic pain; useful to help diagnose various pain syndromes
MPQ Short Form (MPQ-SF)	• Two subscales from the original: 11 sensory words to describe pain and 4 affective words	• Shorter version of adjectives • Now commonly replaced by version 2 of the SF
MPQ-SF-2	• Revised tool includes 22 pain descriptors	• New version encompasses additional neuropathic descriptors • Validated in younger and older populations

Data from Refs.[41,50–60]

function, oral analgesics should be provided at least an hour before the activity to achieve comfort. Other nonpharmacologic approaches (massage, relaxation, mindfulness, music therapy, biofeedback, heat or cold therapies) and blocks are additional interventions that may relieve the pain and should be considered to alleviate the pain or before the aggravating activity.

Inquiring about the presence or absence of changes in mood, appetite, activity, sleep, relationships, sexual functioning, and decreased ability to concentrate will help the clinician to understand the pain experience for each individual. Other things to learn in the pain assessment are presence of contributing symptoms or side effects associated with pain and its treatment. These side effects include nausea/vomiting, constipation, drowsiness, urinary retention, itching, sleepiness, and/or dizziness. Some patients may tolerate these symptoms without specific treatment; others may decide to stop taking analgesics or adjuvant medications because of side-effect intolerance. Adjustment of the dosing frequency, change of agent, addition of therapy to treat the side effect (eg, laxatives for constipation), or titration of the analgesics or adjuvants may be all that is necessary.

HISTORY AND PHYSICAL EXAMINATION

The patient's past history and review of symptoms identify events leading up to the present illness, key medical comorbidities (including medication use), and psychological, social, spiritual, or existential concerns that may contribute to pain and/or impact response to treatment. How pain is perceived by the patient and his/her family caregiver, what has worked in the past and what does not work to help the pain, and patient satisfaction with pain relief should also be discerned.[18]

Although patient history is the foundation of pain assessment, a comprehensive physical examination can provide additional information. The examination includes inspection of the affected painful areas and evaluation of the musculoskeletal and sensory systems. Pain often clusters with depression; therefore, a psychological examination or psychosocial assessment should accompany the physical assessment.[19]

Visual observation of a painful area can reveal inflammation, possible infection, or sympathetic nervous system dysfunction. Changes in skin integrity can occur with some pain syndromes, such as herpes zoster. Sympathetic nervous system dysfunction can be indicated by changes in skin pigmentation and color, abnormal or asymmetric sweating, hair and nail changes, and edema. Signs of neuropathy include poor healing and cold skin and piloerection or gooseflesh.[20]

Musculoskeletal symptoms such low back pain or knee pain with complaints of aching, spasm, and increased pain with movement or activity warrant a musculoskeletal examination. Structures that affect the area are tested for range of motion and mobility. Splinting or an abnormal gait used to splint pain can exacerbate the pain problem.[21]

The sensory examination can diagnose nerve injury or nervous system dysfunction. Abnormal responses to touch, heat, or cold should be noted. Abnormal pain responses should be documented according to the nomenclature in **Table 4**.[20,21]

Pain does not often occur in isolation but can often cluster with other symptoms. Pain and depression cooccur in approximately 36.5% of all patients.[22] Distress screening should be used in all oncology settings and can screen for the cooccurrence of these problems.[23] A more in-depth psychosocial assessment should follow for patients with high distress, depression, or other psychological concerns. Patients should also be assessed for aberrancy and medication diversion before prescribing opioids, as recommended by the National Cancer Comprehensive Network.[24]

DIAGNOSTIC STUDIES

The patient interview is the most valuable tool for the assessment of pain, but, in addition to the physical examination, diagnostic studies can be helpful to identify the cause of the pain. Understanding the cause of the pain can also aid in consideration of management options, such as cancer-directed therapies, or nerve blocks and other procedural interventions. Radiographic techniques are the most common diagnostic tool. Computed tomography is helpful in identifying bone and joint disease; MRI is superior in neurologic evaluation. Nerve blocks can be helpful in the differential diagnosis of some pain syndromes, such as centrally mediated or peripheral neuropathic pain.[20]

Findings from the comprehensive pain assessment, the history and physical examination, and the psychological examination can be concurrently considered in the differential diagnosis and treatment plan. Physiologic findings may be lacking so reliance on the patient report and description of pain is important. Differentiating between somatic, visceral, or neuropathic pain is most important so that appropriate treatment can be tailored to the specific pain syndrome.[2]

SPECIAL POPULATIONS
Older Adults

More than 65% of all cancers are diagnosed in persons older than 65.[25] Because aging is so heterogeneous, older adults require a personalized assessment of pain that considers overall health and function, sensory ability, and mental processing.[26] Assessment should include functional status and ability to tolerate potentially sedating medications. Sensory impairments, such as vision and hearing loss and loss of fine motor skills, may be present, limiting ability to open medication bottles and read medication dosages and instructions. Dementia is also common problem in the elderly. Patients with dementia are a population at risk for underassessment and mismanagement of pain. Inability to communicate and loss of language over time make pain assessment challenging. Although a variety of tools are available to assess pain in patients with dementia, validity and reliability are lacking to recommend one particular tool for use. Most important is to use the 5-step hierarchy of pain assessment beginning with self-report as described in later discussion. Clinicians should also recognize that most older adults suffer from some type of chronic pain syndrome along with the pain caused from the cancer.[27]

Patients with Substance Use Disorders

Substance use is common and should be assessed in all patients with cancer. The use of nicotine, cannabis, alcohol, opioids, and other substances can all influence the management plan. For example, smokers were found to use more opioids and have a harder time stopping opioid therapy.[28,29] Alcohol can contribute to pain expression and an increase in opioid use. The CAGE (Cut down, Annoyed, Guilt, Eye opener) can be used to assess alcohol risk. A recent study indicated that 17% of patients with advanced cancer were CAGE positive, which can indicate a higher expression of pain and increased opioid use.[30] Opioid misuse and abuse are discussed in detail in Joseph Arthur and David Hui's article, "Safe Opioid Use: Management of Opioid-Related Adverse Effects and Aberrant Behaviors," in this issue.

The prevalence of substance use disorders in patients with chronic pain is estimated at 15% to 20%,[31] but the incidence in the cancer population is unknown. One recent study found that 10% of patients with advanced cancer deviated from prescribed doses, which was more frequent in men and nonwhites.[32] On the other hand, pain is grossly undermanaged and so balancing risks of misuse or abuse and benefits of pain management is imperative. Clinicians may be fearful of misuse, abuse, and diversion, which could lead to suboptimal pain management. Joseph Arthur and David Hui's article, "Safe Opioid Use: Management of Opioid-Related Adverse Effects and Aberrant Behaviors," in this issue includes a thorough discussion of several risk assessment tools, including the CAGE and the Opioid Risk Tool.[33] Universal precautions are a potential solution to consistently assess patients in primary care, but this assessment strategy has not been consistently translated to the oncology setting. The strategy aims to use opioid risk as a routine part of care, thereby reducing stigma and yet recognizing risk of opioid misuse and abuse. Universal precautions are included in **Table 5**.[34] A more practical strategy may be to routinely use the 5 A's, which assess analgesia, activities of daily living and affects, adverse events, aberrancy, and adjuvants (see **Table 5**).[35] Studies are needed that examine the use of opioid and substance use risk in patients with cancer.

Culturally Diverse Populations

Patients from diverse ethnic populations are at high risk for undertreatment of pain. Communicating pain with providers has been noted as a significant challenge.[36] A large meta-analysis of cultural differences between Asian and Western patients found that Asian patients had more concerns about cancer progression, drug tolerance, fatalism, and barriers interfering with pain management.[37] In another systematic review, patients reported suboptimal pain management, and clinicians were found to underestimate pain in 75% of African Americans and 64% of Hispanics.[38] Clinicians should be aware that these challenges exist. Studies are needed to evaluate best methods to communicate with culturally diverse groups.

Patients Who Are Nonverbal or Cognitively Impaired

A patient's self-report is the gold standard even in some nonverbal or cognitively impaired patients. However, for patients unable to self-report (eg, patients with dementia, those who are unconscious or intubated), it is recommended that clinicians follow the hierarchy of pain assessment framework to guide assessment approaches[39-41]:

1. Establish a procedure for pain assessment
   a. Attempt to obtain self-report of pain from all patients
   b. Search for potential causes or pathologies of pain
   c. Look for pain behaviors and consider use of evidence-based, valid, and reliable behavioral pain instruments for special populations
   d. Obtain proxy or surrogate pain reports from family, unlicensed, and professional caregivers
   e. Consider and attempt an analgesic trial if potential benefits outweigh the risks
2. Use behavioral assessment tools as appropriate
3. Minimize the emphasis on physiologic indicators
4. Reassess and document

Observing a patient's behavior or nonverbal cues, understanding the meaning of the pain experience to the patient, and collaborating with family caregivers to determine how the patient usually exhibits pain and their interpretation of the patient's pain are all part of the assessment process. Patients may exhibit any of the following nonverbal pain behaviors[42]:

- Verbalizations (saying "Ouch," "Don't touch me," "Stop hurting me") during activity such as positioning, movement, or bathing

Table 5
Universal precautions

Universal Precaution	Elements of Precaution
1. Make a pain diagnosis	• Physical examination • Status of cancer • History including past medical history records • Refer to other resources as needed, for example, anesthesia
2. Conduct a psychological and risk assessment	• Be sensitive and respectful during the conversation • Conduct a mental health assessment; include a depression index such as the Beck or CES-D • Use an opioid risk assessment tool to screen for misuse, abuse, or diversion • Consider urine drug testing • Refer to the statewide prescription drug monitoring program to review past use of opioids and controlled substances
3. Provide informed consent on the proposed treatment	• Discuss the risks and benefits of opioid treatment • Set therapeutic expectations using the 5 A's (see later)
4. Complete a treatment agreement	• Sets behavioral expectations of the patient and the provider • Provides a platform for discussion
5. Conduct a preintervention assessment of pain and function	• Baseline assessment will be used to determine the effectiveness of the opioid intervention • Goal of treatment will be to improve pain and function
6. Initiate an opioid trial	• Discuss the specific opioid treatment, including long-acting opioids and breakthrough pain (BTP) medication • Specify the number of BTP doses that can be given in a day
7. Conduct ongoing reassessment	• Assess pain intensity • Assess function • Urine drug testing as needed
8. Review and assess the 5 A's on an ongoing basis: Analgesia, Activities of daily living, Adverse events, Aberrancy, Adjuvants	• Analgesia: pain should improve with treatment plan • Activities: physical function and psychological affect may or may not improve (depends on cancer stage, response to treatment); monitor according to patient condition • Adverse events: side effects should be minimized • Aberrancy: early refills, lost prescriptions, early requests for prescriptions, lack of approval for dose escalation, and other red flags should be noted • Adjuvants: adjuvants should be maximized and titrated upward to decrease opioid requirements as able
9. Periodically review the diagnosis, comorbidities, and treatment plan	• Note disease progression that may warrant increased dose • Assess for comorbidities that increase pain, such as anxiety and depression • A diagnosis of addiction should be made if indicated
10. Document the process	• Document treatment plan, adherence to the regimen • Note education provided • Document outcomes

Adapted from Gourlay DL, Heit HA. Universal precautions revisited: managing the inherited pain patient. Pain Med 2009;10(2):S116; with permission.

Table 6
Barriers to pain assessment

Type of Barrier	Barriers

Patient and family caregiver–related	• Patient's failure to report pain
	  ○ Lack of a common language to describe pain
	  ○ Cultural and age-related influences regarding need to be stoic
	  ○ Fear that pain is the result of progressive disease
	  ○ Not wanting to "bother" staff
	• Fear of addiction and tolerance
	• Belief that pain is an inevitable component of cancer
	• Difficulty distinguishing between physical pain and emotional/spiritual suffering
	• Lack of knowledge regarding how to report pain
	• Patient and family caregiver misuse, abuse, and/or diversion
	  ○ Patients may be in denial or protect caregiver

Health care team–related	• Failure to consistently assess pain • Failure to use validated pain assessment tools • Observation of behaviors and vital signs to solely determine patients' pain levels • Fear of addiction/opiophobia • Fear regarding patient and family caregiver misuse, abuse, and diversion • Lack of continuity of care • Failure to believe the patients' reports of pain or do not take reports seriously • Use of personal pain experiences to assess and manage pain • Bias in working with patients • Inability to empathize or establish rapport with patient and family caregiver
System-related	• Limited time and resources to conduct a comprehensive pain assessment • Lack of systems that use ongoing pain assessment and surveillance, resulting in high risk for emergent visits for pain • Hierarchy within the health care system, for example, nurse's concerns about pain not always acknowledged • Lack of electronic tools that assist in measuring patient-reported outcomes about pain and consistent surveillance • Lack of availability of culturally sensitive instruments for pain assessment in health care settings

Adapted from Brant JM. Pain. In: Yarbro CH, Wujcik D, Gobel BH, editors. Cancer symptom management. 4th edition. Burlington (NJ): Jones & Bartlett Learning; 2013. p. 783; and Fink RM, Gates RA, Montgomery RK. Pain assessment. In: Ferrell BR, Coyle N, Paice JA, editors. Oxford textbook of palliative nursing. 4th edition. Oxford (United Kingdom): Oxford University Press; 2015. p. 136; with permission.

- Vocalizations (moaning, groaning, crying, screaming, shouting, sighing)
- Facial expressions (frowning, closing eyes, wrinkled or furrowed brow, tight jaw, clenched teeth)
- Changes in movement or activity (posturing, splinting, bracing, guarding a body part, rubbing a painful area, pacing, rocking, lying still in bed)
- Mental status changes (restlessness, agitation, distress, confusion)

When patients are no longer able to verbally communicate about their pain, attempt to elicit feedback from the patient, for example, ask patient to nod head, squeeze hand, move eyes up or down, or raise fingers to signal pain presence or absence. The best approach is to assume that the patient's underlying disease is still painful and continue with pain management interventions if prescribed or there is evidence that an individual in a similar condition would experience pain.[43]

BARRIERS TO PAIN ASSESSMENT

A multitude of barriers interfere with the assessment of cancer pain.[44–46] Barriers can be classified as patient and caregiver related, health care related, and system related (Table 6). Pain assessment lacks priority in overall clinic responsibilities; diagnosing and treating disease is often the priority. Lack of pain assessment results in lack of identification of the problem; simply assessing pain consistently improves the quality of its management.[47] Professionals also lack knowledge about pain assessment and do not use standardized tools to routinely assess pain. A significant barrier is fear of addiction, which has heightened with the current opioid crisis.

Patients and caregivers also fear addiction and may be reluctant to take opioids. They may also fail to report pain, because acknowledging the pain is associated with fear of disease progression. Patients and families may also fear that pain is inevitable with cancer, and therefore, lack reporting it. Finally, health care systems are more conducive to the treatment of cancer, and infrastructure is lacking for global assessments and the use of patient-reported outcomes. Unfortunately, these barriers have existed for more than 20 years, have persisted, and have not been adequately addressed.[45,46] Concerted efforts to address these barriers and adequately address pain assessment are warranted, especially in this current environment when pain assessment and management are challenging.

SUMMARY

Quality pain management for patients with cancer is dependent on an accurate and continuous pain assessment taking into account the whole person and the physical, psychological, social, and spiritual components of their pain experience. Being knowledgeable about evidence-based pain assessment practices is key. Documentation of pain assessment and the effectiveness of interventions are essential to facilitate communication among health care providers about the current status of the patient's pain and responses to the plan of care. Application of evidence-based approaches involves ongoing commitment and advocacy for patient comfort and well-being.

REFERENCES

1. Oncology Nursing Society. Putting evidence into practice. 2017. Available at: https://www.ons.org/practice-resources/pep. Accessed August 27, 2017.
2. American Pain Society. Principles of analgesic use in the treatment of acute pain and cancer pain. 6th edition. Glenview (IL): APS Press; 2017.
3. National Comprehensive Cancer Network. Adult cancer pain v.2. NCCN clinical practice guidelines in oncology 2017. Available at: http://www.nccn.org/professionals/physician_gls/PDF/pain.pdf. Accessed September 25, 2017.
4. van den Beuken-van Everdingen MH, Hochstenbach LM, Joosten EA, et al. Update on prevalence of pain in patients with cancer: systematic review and meta-analysis. J Pain Symptom Manage 2016;51(6):1070–90.e9.
5. International Association for the Study of Pain. Definition of pain. In: Merskey H, Bogduk N, editors. Taxonomy. Seattle: IASP Press; 1994. p. 209–14.
6. Smith SM, Dart RC, Katz NP, et al. Classification and definition of misuse, abuse, and related events in clinical trials: ACTTION systematic review and recommendations. Pain 2013;154(11):2287–96.

7. Federation of State Medical Boards of the United States. Model guidelines for the use of controlled substances for the treatment of pain. Euless (TX): Federation of State Medical Boards; 2013.
8. Mercadante S. Breakthrough pain in cancer patients: prevalence, mechanisms and treatment options. Curr Opin Anaesthesiol 2015;28(5):559–64.
9. Institute of Medicine. Relieving pain in America. Washington, DC: Institute of Medicine; 2011.
10. Deandrea S, Corli O, Consonni D, et al. Prevalence of breakthrough cancer pain: a systematic review and a pooled analysis of published literature. J Pain Symptom Manage 2014;47(1):57–76.
11. Davies A, Buchanan A, Zeppetella G, et al. Breakthrough cancer pain: an observational study of 1000 European oncology patients. J Pain Symptom Manage 2013;46(5):619–28.
12. Rustoen T, Geerling JI, Pappa T, et al. How nurses assess breakthrough cancer pain, and the impact of this pain on patients' daily lives–results of a European survey. Eur J Oncol Nurs 2013;17(4):402–7.
13. Webber K. Development of the breakthrough pain assessment tool (BAT) in cancer patients. Int J Palliat Nurs 2014;20(9):424.
14. Davies AN, Webber K. Breakthrough Pain Assessment Tool (BAT). 2009. Available at: http://www.cfp.ca/content/cfp/suppl/2014/12/09/60.12.1111.DC1/Breakthrough_pain.pdf. Accessed November 11, 2017.
15. Saunders CM. The management of terminal malignant disease, 1st edition. London: Edward Arnold; 1978.
16. Fink R. Pain assessment: the cornerstone to optimal pain management. Proc (Bayl Univ Med Cent) 2000;13(3):236–9.
17. Pasero C, Quinlan-Colwell A, Rae D, et al. American Society for Pain Management Nursing Position Statement: prescribing and administering opioid doses based solely on pain intensity. Pain Manag Nurs 2016;17(3):170–80.
18. Pasero C, Gordon DB, McCaffery M, et al. JCAHO on assessing and managing pain. Am J Nurs 1999;99(7):22.
19. Syrjala KL, Jensen MP, Mendoza ME, et al. Psychological and behavioral approaches to cancer pain management. J Clin Oncol 2014;32(16):1703–11.
20. Fitzgibbon DR, Loeser JD. Cancer pain: assessment, diagnosis, and management. Philadelphia: Lippincott Williams & Wilkins; 2010.
21. McGee SR. Evidence-based physical diagnosis. Philadelphia: Elsevier/Saunders; 2012.
22. Laird BJ, Boyd AC, Colvin LA, et al. Are cancer pain and depression interdependent? A systematic review. Psychooncology 2009;18(5):459–64.
23. National Comprehensive Cancer Network. Distress management. 2017. Available at: http://www.nccn.org/professionals/physician_gls/pdf/distress.pdf. Accessed May 15, 2017.
24. Swarm RA, Abernethy AP, Anghelescu DL, et al. Adult cancer pain. J Natl Compr Canc Netw 2013;11(8):992–1022.
25. American Cancer Society. Cancer facts and figures 2017. Available at: https://www.cancer.org/research/cancer-facts-statistics/all-cancer-facts-figures/cancer-facts-figures-2017.html. Accessed October 12, 2017.
26. Wedding U, Stauder R. Cancer and ageism. Ecancermedicalscience 2014;8:ed39.
27. Lichtner V, Dowding D, Esterhuizen P, et al. Pain assessment for people with dementia: a systematic review of systematic reviews of pain assessment tools. BMC Geriatr 2014;14:138.

28. Hooten WM, Townsend CO, Bruce BK, et al. The effects of smoking status on opioid tapering among patients with chronic pain. Anesth Analg 2009;108(1): 308–15.

29. John U, Alte D, Hanke M, et al. Tobacco smoking in relation to analgesic drug use in a national adult population sample. Drug Alcohol Depend 2006;85(1):49–55.

30. Parsons HA, Delgado-Guay MO, El Osta B, et al. Alcoholism screening in patients with advanced cancer: impact on symptom burden and opioid use. J Palliat Med 2008;11(7):964–8.

31. Hojsted J, Ekholm O, Kurita GP, et al. Addictive behaviors related to opioid use for chronic pain: a population-based study. Pain 2013;154(12):2677–83.

32. Nguyen LM, Rhondali W, De la Cruz M, et al. Frequency and predictors of patient deviation from prescribed opioids and barriers to opioid pain management in patients with advanced cancer. J Pain Symptom Manage 2013;45(3):506–16.

33. Barclay JS, Owens JE, Blackhall LJ. Screening for substance abuse risk in cancer patients using the Opioid Risk Tool and urine drug screen. Support Care Cancer 2014;22(7):1883–8.

34. Gourlay DL, Heit HA. Universal precautions: it's not about the molecule! J Pain 2011;12(6):722 [author reply: 723–4].

35. Passik SD, Weinreb HJ. Managing chronic nonmalignant pain: overcoming obstacles to the use of opioids. Adv Ther 2000;17(2):70–83.

36. Im EO, Lee SH, Liu Y, et al. A national online forum on ethnic differences in cancer pain experience. Nurs Res 2009;58(2):86–94.

37. Chen CH, Tang ST, Chen CH. Meta-analysis of cultural differences in Western and Asian patient-perceived barriers to managing cancer pain. Palliat Med 2012; 26(3):206–21.

38. Kwok W, Bhuvanakrishna T. The relationship between ethnicity and the pain experience of cancer patients: a systematic review. Indian J Palliat Care 2014;20(3): 194–200.

39. Herr K. Pain assessment strategies in older patients. J Pain 2011;12(3 Suppl 1): S3–13.

40. Hadjistavropoulos T, Herr K, Turk DC, et al. An interdisciplinary expert consensus statement on assessment of pain in older persons. Clin J Pain 2007;23(1 Suppl): S1–43.

41. Herr K, Coyne PJ, McCaffery M, et al. Pain assessment in the patient unable to self-report: position statement with clinical practice recommendations. Pain Manag Nurs 2011;12(4):230–50.

42. American Geriatrics Society Panel. Pharmacological management of persistent pain in older persons. Pain Med 2009;10(6):1062–83.

43. Herr K, Coyne PJ, Key T, et al. Pain assessment in the nonverbal patient: position statement with clinical practice recommendations. Pain Manag Nurs 2006;7(2): 44–52.

44. Kwon JH. Overcoming barriers in cancer pain management. J Clin Oncol 2014; 32(16):1727–33.

45. Kwon JH, Hui D, Chisholm G, et al. Experience of barriers to pain management in patients receiving outpatient palliative care. J Palliat Med 2013;16(8):908–14.

46. Kwon JH, Oh SY, Chisholm G, et al. Predictors of high score patient-reported barriers to controlling cancer pain: a preliminary report. Support Care Cancer 2013; 21(4):1175–83.

47. Porche RA, editor. Approaches to pain management: an essential guide for clinical leaders. Oakbrook Terrace (IL): Joint Commission; 2010.

48. Brant JM. Strategies to manage pain in palliative care. In: O'Connor M, Lee S, Aranda S, editors. Palliative care nursing: a guide to practice. 3rd edition. Victoria (Australia): Ausmed; 2012. p. 93–113.
49. Bates B. OLDCART: a pocket guide to physical examination and history taking. Philadelphia: Lippincott; 1995. PQRST: Available at: http://www.crozerkeystone. org/healthcare-professionals/nursing/pqrst-pain-assessment-method.
50. Cleeland CS, Ryan KM. Pain assessment: global use of the brief pain inventory. Ann Acad Med Singapore 1994;23(2):129–38.
51. Dworkin RH, Turk DC, Revicki DA, et al. Development and initial validation of an expanded and revised version of the Short-form McGill Pain Questionnaire (SF MPQ-2). Pain 2009;144(1–2):35–42.
52. Feldt KS. The checklist of nonverbal pain indicators (CNPI). Pain Manag Nurs 2000;1:13–21.
53. Fink RM, Gates RA, Montgomery RK. Pain assessment. In: Ferrell BR, Coyle N, Paice JA, editors. Oxford textbook of palliative nursing. 4th edition. Oxford (United Kingdom): Oxford University Press; 2015. p. 113–34.
54. Gauthier LR, Young A, Dworkin RH, et al. Validation of the short-form McGill pain questionnaire-2 in younger and older people with cancer pain. J Pain 2014;15(7): 756–70.
55. Gelinas C, Johnston C. Pain assessment in the critically ill ventilated adult: validation of the critical care pain observation tool and physiologic indicators. Clin J Pain 2007;23:497–505.
56. Hicks CL, von Baeyer CL, Spafford P, et al. The faces scale-revised: toward a common metric in pediatric pain measurement. Pain 2001;93:173–83.
57. Voepel-Lewis T, Zanotti J, Dammeyer JA. Reliability and validity of the faces, legs, activity, cry, consolability behavioral tool in assessing acute pain in critically ill patients. Amer J Crit Care 2010;19(1):55–62.
58. Wong DL, Baker CM. Pain in children: a comparison of assessment scales. Pediatr Nurs 1988;14:9–17.
59. Warden V, Hurley AC, Volicer L. Development and psychometric evaluation of the Pain Assessment in Advanced Dementia (PAINAD) scale. J Am Med Dir Assoc 2003;4(1):9–15.
60. Campbell M. Psychometric testing of a new Pain Assessment Behavior Scale (PABS). Abstract presented at the 29th Annual MNRS Research Conference. Cincinnati Ohio, April 3, 2005.

Cancer Pain Syndromes

Russell K. Portenoy, MD*, Ebtesam Ahmed, PharmD, MS

KEYWORDS

- Cancer pain • Cancer pain syndromes • Bone pain • Cancer-related syndrome
- Cancer-related neuropathic pain • Mucositis
- Chemotherapy-induced peripheral neuropathy • Malignant bowel obstruction

KEY POINTS

- Cancer pain syndromes are defined by the relationship to the tumor, the inferred pathophysiology of the pain, and pain characteristics such as temporal features and quality of pain.
- Most cancer pain syndromes are related directly to the tumor and the most common types are bone pain syndromes and neuropathic pain syndromes.
- All types of cancer therapy may be associated with the development of chronic pain syndromes.

INTRODUCTION

Cancer pain is prevalent and heterogeneous,[1] and effective treatment begins with assessment (see Regina M. Fink and Jeannine M. Brants' article, "Complex Cancer Pain Assessment," in this issue). Assessment, in turn, must characterize the symptom, clarify the etiology of the pain, and identify the syndrome. Syndrome identification can direct the diagnostic evaluation to specific etiologies, clarify the prognosis for the pain or the disease itself, and guide therapeutic interventions. The prompt and efficient evaluation and treatment of cancer pain, therefore, requires an appreciation of well-described pain syndromes. These syndromes can be broadly divided into those associated with acute pain—pain with a proximate onset and a duration typically anticipated to be no longer than a few weeks—and those associated with chronic pain.

ACUTE PAIN SYNDROMES

Acute pain syndromes may be related directly to the cancer or to antineoplastic therapy, or to diagnostic or therapeutic interventions. The latter etiologies far are more likely to be the cause of acute pain syndromes than chronic pain syndromes.

Disclosures: Dr R.K. Portenoy has a relationship with AstraZeneca Pharmaceuticals LP and Tabula Rasa for organizational research support. Dr E. Ahmed reports no relevant relationships.
MJHS Institute for Innovation in Palliative Care, 39 Broadway, 3rd Floor, New York, NY 10006, USA
* Corresponding author.
E-mail address: rporteno@mjhs.org

Hematol Oncol Clin N Am 32 (2018) 371–386
https://doi.org/10.1016/j.hoc.2018.01.002
0889-8588/18/© 2018 Elsevier Inc. All rights reserved.

Acute Pain Syndromes Directly Related to the Cancer

When an acute pain syndrome is directly related to the tumor, assessment may lead to a change in primary treatment. Syndromes are identified by the context and pain characteristics.

Pathologic fracture

Pathologic fracture is most likely to occur in patients with breast, lung, or prostate cancer and in patients with multiple myeloma. The diagnosis is usually straightforward and is suggested by the sudden onset of focal aching pain. After radiography confirms the diagnosis, the treatment strategy often combines analgesics with selected surgical, radiation-based, interventional pain, and pharmacologic therapies that aim to augment pain control, restore function, and prevent further bone complications (see also Nicholas Figura and colleagues' article, "Mechanisms of and Adjuvants for Bone Pain," and Ron Shiloh and Monica Krishnan's article, "Radiation for Treatment of Painful Bone Metastases," in this issue).[2]

Obstruction or perforation of a hollow viscus

The characteristics of the pain from obstruction or perforation of a hollow viscus by a tumor mass and its associated features vary with the site (eg, bile duct, ureter, intestine, or bowel) and pathology, and the constellation of symptoms and signs usually pose little challenge in diagnosis. For example, the patient with gastric cancer who develops epigastric pain that worsens over days and is associated with early satiety and postprandial vomiting may be quickly recognized as having an evolving gastric outlet obstruction. This diagnosis, once confirmed, may suggest the usefulness of stenting in combination with symptom control therapies.[3] Syndrome identification may encourage earlier intervention and increase the likelihood of a favorable outcome.

Intratumoral hemorrhage

Hemorrhage into a tumor mass typically presents with acute pain; imaging confirms the diagnosis. Bleeding may become life threatening and syndrome recognition may expedite treatment with transfusions and interventions to stem bleeding. For example, the patient with hepatocellular carcinoma who experiences the sudden onset of severe right upper quadrant pain that worsens with inspiration and is associated with local tenderness may be considered presumptively to have an intratumoral hemorrhage, and is at risk for a life-threatening event; early effective intervention may avert a catastrophic outcome, as well as provide symptom relief.[4]

Superior vena cava obstruction

Superior vena cava obstruction from primary or metastatic tumors in the mediastinum usually presents with dyspnea, facial and neck swelling, and dilated neck and chest wall veins. In some cases, however, acute neck pain or headache is a prominent symptom.[5] If effectively treated with vascular stenting or radiation therapy, the pain quickly resolves.

Pain owing to acute thrombosis

Cancer frequently produces a prothrombotic state and deep vein thrombosis is a common complication.[6] Acute thrombosis usually is accompanied by pain. When an extremity is affected, pain and swelling suggest the diagnosis. Given the high prevalence of these disorders, the onset of acute pain in an extremity often suggests a diagnostic evaluation for venous occlusion, even if associated with minimal swelling.

Acute Pain Syndromes Related to Antineoplastic Treatments

Acute pain syndromes have been described with all types of antineoplastic therapy (**Table 1**).

Chemotherapy-induced acute pain syndromes

Oral mucositis Mucositis is the most common acute painful complication associated with systemic chemotherapy (**Box 1**).[7,8] The incidence of this disorder varies with the drug regimen, concurrent therapies, and host factors; it is virtually universal among patients with hematologic cancer undergoing myeloablative chemotherapy before bone marrow transplantation. The chemotherapeutic agents most strongly associated include methotrexate, 5-fluorouracil, and doxorubicin.

Chemotherapy-induced mucositis typically occurs within 1 or 2 weeks after treatment. It affects the mucosa throughout the entire gastrointestinal tract, and oral pain and ulceration often is accompanied by vomiting and diarrhea. Pain may be severe and lead to nutritional compromise. Treatment options are limited, despite numerous clinical trials, and management typically relies on systemic analgesics and meticulous mouth care, and treatment of concurrent problems such as superinfection.[7,8]

Neuropathy Chemotherapy-induced polyneuropathy can present as an acute pain syndrome. It was first described in patients treated with vinca alkaloids, such as vincristine, and subsequently reported with many other agents, including paclitaxel, cisplatin, oxaliplatin, thalidomide, and bortezomib (**Table 2**).[9] The onset of symptoms is temporally associated with administration of the chemotherapy regimen and the pain usually has neuropathic features, such as burning. Other uncomfortable sensations and paresthesias also may be prominent. Depending on the agent and other factors, there may or may not be associated motor or sensory findings, such as weakness or proprioceptive loss. The acute pain may resolve over weeks, or resolve and recur with additional chemotherapy; it sometimes evolves into a chronic neuropathic pain. Many patients experience symptomatic improvement but manifest long-term abnormalities on neurologic examination.

Table 1	
Acute pain syndromes associated with antineoplastic treatments	
Pain Syndrome	**Clinical Presentation**
Chemotherapy-induced headaches	• Common after treatment with intrathecal methotrexate for leukemia, lymphoma, or leptomeningeal carcinomatosis, all-trans-retinoic acid for leukemia • May last for several days or longer
Diffuse bone pain	Common with trans-retinoic acid
Flare syndrome in advanced prostate cancer, after initiation of LHRH agonist	Characterized by increased bone pain, at times associated with added risk of cord compression, bladder outlet obstruction, and hypercoagulability
Palmar-plantar erythrodysesthesia (hand-foot syndrome)	Painful rash on the palms and soles after the administration of specific chemotherapies (particularly liposomal doxorubicin and capecitabine)
Myalgia and arthralgia	Pain in muscles and joints. Reported in 20% of patients treated with paclitaxel
Steroid-induced perineal burning	Perineal burning, reported with rapid administration of intravenous steroids

Abbreviation: LHRH, luteinizing hormone-releasing hormone.

Box 1
Chemotherapy agents associated with mucositis

Medication

Platinum-based agents
- Cisplatin
- Oxaliplatin

Anthracyclines
- Daunorubicin
- Doxorubicin
- Epirubicin
- Idarubicin

Alkylating agents
- Cyclophosphamide
- Ifosfamide
- Thiotepa
- Melphalan
- Cisplatin
- Busulfan

Antimetabolites
- 6-Mercaptopurine
- Cytarabine
- Fluorouracil
- Gemcitabine
- Hydroxyurea
- Methotrexate
- Docetaxel

Taxanes
- Docetaxel
- Paclitaxel

Targeted agents
- Erlotinib
- Everolimus
- Sorafenib
- Sunitinib
- Cetuximab

Table 2
Acute pain syndromes associated with chemotherapy-induced neuropathy

Medication	Mechanism of Peripheral Neuropathy Toxicity
Platinum-based agents • Cisplatin • Oxaliplatin	Binding to DNA may inhibit the transcription of important proteins and impair axonal transport
Vinca Alkaloids • Vincristine • Vinblastine • Vinorelbine	Interference with axonal microtubule assembly, impairment of axonal transport Vinblastine is included for completeness, but the incidence of neuropathy is lower than others listed
Thalidomide	Unknown
Taxanes • Paclitaxel • Docetaxel	Toxic effect to the neuronal cell body, axon, or both

A far less common disorder than polyneuropathy is acute chemotherapy-related mononeuropathy, a syndrome best described with vincristine.[10] Orofacial pain is the most common expression, with multiple sites affected in the distribution of the trigeminal and glossopharyngeal nerves. Other nerves, including the recurrent laryngeal, optic, and auditory nerves, may also be affected.

Arthralgia, myalgia, or bone pain A substantial minority of patients treated with paclitaxel experience acute arthralgia and myalgia, which often occur soon after chemotherapy administration and typically continue for days, and sometimes longer.[11] The mechanism is not known. Patients treated with pegfilgrastim, the pegylated form of the recombinant human granulocyte colony-stimulating factor, often report a transitory flare of bone pain.

Acute arthralgia and myalgia also can complicate abrupt withdrawal or tapering of a glucocorticoid—a syndrome that has been labeled steroid pseudorheumatism. It seems to be more common after high-dose therapy, but this is variable, and both the severity and duration vary as well. Returning to a higher dose and instituting a more gradual taper may mitigate the discomfort. The mechanism is unknown.

Palmar–plantar erythrodysesthesia and other cutaneous toxicities Palmar–plantar erythrodysesthesia syndrome, or hand–foot syndrome, manifests as a painful rash on the palms and soles after the administration of chemotherapy.[12,13] The syndrome has been associated with numerous drugs, including cytarabine, capecitabine, 5-fluourouracil, vinorelbine, docetaxel, and others. The rash may progress to bullous formation and desquamation. Symptomatic treatment, including analgesics, often is required, and if the syndrome is severe, a dose reduction or a change to a different agent may be warranted.

Other types of cutaneous toxicity are common after administration of epidermal growth factor receptor inhibitors, such as erlotinib, sorafenib, and sunitinib. Pain may accompany this toxicity, which most commonly takes the form of papulopustules and xerosis, but also can lead to paronychia, maculopapular rash, mucositis, and hyperpigmentation.[13–15] If the lesions are severe or progressive, or if symptomatic therapy is unable to manage distress, the cutaneous toxicity may lead to dose reduction or discontinuation of treatment.

Chemotherapy-induced headaches Acute headache is common after intrathecal chemotherapy administration with methotrexate, cytarabine, or trans-retinoic acid.[16] The severity and duration vary, and headaches may or may not recur with repeated drug administrations.

The recognition of drug-induced headache may be complicated by the occurrence of dural puncture headache. The latter syndrome results from the leakage of cerebrospinal fluid through the defect in the dural sheath. It is usually holocephalic and distinguished by its positional quality—occurring or worsening with the upright position. The incidence may be reduced by the use of a small-gauge needle and longitudinal insertion of the needle bevel.[17]

5-Fluorouracil–induced angina Both 5-fluorouracil and its prodrug capacitabine are associated with varied types of cardiac toxicity, including an increased risk of painful ischemia.[18] Cardiac ischemic episodes are most likely the result of vasospasm. Pain is relieved by primary treatment of the cardiac event.

Postchemotherapy gynecomastia A syndrome of acute painful gynecomastia has been reported in association with numerous drugs, including some antineoplastic agents such as imatinib.[19] The data are very limited, however. The mechanism is assumed to be related to acute changes in free testosterone or estradiol levels, or both. The problem is usually transitory, and treatment is symptomatic.

Intraperitoneal chemotherapy Intraperitoneal chemotherapy for the treatment of gynecologic tumors commonly causes acute abdominal pain, presumably related to drug-induced chemical serositis.[20] The characteristics of the pain range from a mild uncomfortable heaviness to pain of severe intensity associated with peritoneal signs. Pain also may herald infectious peritonitis, and repeated evaluation of the peritoneal fluid may be required.

Intravesical therapy Transient bladder irritability characterized by frequency and/or painful micturition can be caused by the administration of intravesical bacillus Calmette-Guérin or other local therapies for transitional cell carcinoma of the bladder.[21] Painful cystitis is likely to be an adverse effect associated with all agents used.[22]

Hepatic artery infusion pain Transarterial chemoembolization for patients with hepatocellular cancer or hepatic metastases is often associated with severe abdominal pain that is usually transitory, but continuous infusions can lead to persistent pain.[23] Pain treatment usually relies on systemic analgesics, but intraarterial lidocaine given before and during the procedure may further reduce pain.[24]

Intravenous infusion pain Chemical phlebitis, vesicant extravasation, venous spasm, and anthracycline-associated flares may cause pain at the site of chemotherapy infusion.[25] The onset and course of the pain and associated signs distinguish venous spasm, which is not accompanied by inflammation, from the other conditions. Painful spasm usually is brief and may be reduced by a slower infusion rate. Extravasation is the most serious event and may be accompanied by severe pain and ulceration.[26] The pain from both spasm and phlebitis is usually managed by local compresses and the time-limited use of analgesics.

Anthracyclines like doxorubicin can cause a venous flare reaction, which manifests with local urticaria and pain at the infusion site.[27] Pain is usually short lived and less prominent than local swelling and itch.

Steroid-induced perineal burning Transient perineal burning and shooting pain has been described immediately after the rapid intravenous administration of a glucocorticoid, particularly dexamethasone.[28] The cause of this unusual syndrome is unknown. Patients may benefit from reassurance that it ends quickly and is not associated with any injury.

Radiation therapy-induced acute pain syndromes
Acute pain owing to radiation and radiopharmaceuticals Approximately 30% to 40% of patients receiving palliative radiotherapy for bone metastases can experience a temporary increase in bone pain immediately after radiotherapy.[29,30] In 1 study, pretreatment with a dose of dexamethasone 8 mg was shown to reduce pain severity.[31,32]

Radiopharmaceutical drugs, such as strontium-89 and samarium-153, are systemically administered beta-emitting compounds for malignant bone pain. They are taken up in areas of osteoblastic activity. A flare response after initial treatment occurs in a minority of patients and presents typically as multifocal deep aching pain that worsens with activity.[33,34] Pain usually lasts days and often requires analgesic therapy.

Radiation-induced mucositis When radiation fields overlap mucosa, acute inflammation associated with pain and mucosal injury commonly occurs. Head and neck radiation is a common cause of oral mucositis, the presentation and outcomes of which compare with chemotherapy-induced mucositis.[35,36] Abdominal or pelvic radiation may result in enteritis, proctitis, or cystitis accompanied, in the case of abdominal radiation, by nausea and vomiting, abdominal cramping, diarrhea, and bleeding.[37] Proctitis causes painful tenesmus, and cystitis is heralded by dysuria accompanied by urgency, frequency, and hematuria.

The onset of the acute pain syndromes related to radiation treatment varies, but typically occurs within 1 to 2 weeks. Pain and associated findings usually progress over weeks before gradually resolving. During this prolonged period, intensive treatment for pain and other symptoms may be needed. Newer radiotherapy methods have reduced the incidence and severity of these painful syndromes, but the risk remains whenever the radiation field includes viscera.

Radiation-induced neuropathy An acute, transient painful brachial plexopathy, accompanied by paresthesias and weakness in the upper extremity, has been reported during or immediately after completion of radiation therapy for breast cancer.[38] The syndrome is usually self-limited and has no clear relationship to radiation-induced brachial plexopathy, which typically presents months to years after treatment completion.

CHRONIC PAIN SYNDROMES

Nearly three-quarters of patients with cancer who have chronic pain have nociceptive (somatic and visceral) or neuropathic syndromes that represent direct effects of the neoplasm (**Box 2**). Chronic pain also can result from the therapies administered to treat the cancer (**Table 3**).

Tumor-Related Somatic Pain Syndromes

Tumor involvement of bone, joints, muscle, or connective tissue can cause persistent somatic pain. Bone metastases are the most common cause of chronic pain.

Multifocal bone pain
Bone pain may be focal, multifocal, or generalized.[35] Multifocal bone pain associated with metastases is most common with tumors of breast, prostate, and lung, as well as multiple myeloma. The pain may be due to direct invasion, secondary pathologic fracture, or damage to adjacent structures. It is typically focal, aching, and worsened by movement or weight bearing. Although the factors that convert a painless to a painful bone metastasis are not known, some combination of direct nociceptor activation by tumor, mechanical distortion related to microfracture, local release of growth factors and/or chemical mediators, and activation of sensitized nociceptors may be involved.[37]

Vertebral pain syndromes
The spine is the most common site of bone metastases and referred pain syndromes are common, usually presenting below the site of metastasis. Lesions affecting the odontoid refer to the base of the neck, C7 or T1 vertebra refer pain to the interscapular region, and those of T12 or L1 refer pain to the iliac crest or region of the greater trochanter. Early recognition facilitates prompt treatment of the pain and underlying bone disease,[35] and potentially averts spinal cord or cauda equina compression at the site of a vertebral metastasis.[38]

Pelvic and hip metastases
Pelvic metastases may involve the pubis, ilium, or sacroiliac areas. Pain presents as continuous local aching, hip or inguinal pain when walking, or pain in the knee or

---

Box 2
Chronic pain syndromes directly related to cancer

Nociceptive pain syndromes

Tumor-related bone pain
- Multifocal bone pain
- Bone metastases
- Bone marrow expansion (hematologic malignancies)

Vertebral syndromes

- Sacral syndrome

- Back pain secondary to spinal cord compression

Pain syndromes related to the pelvis and hip

- Pelvic metastases

- Hip joint syndrome

- Malignant piriformis syndrome

Tumor-related soft tissue pain
- Headache and facial pain
- Pleural pain

Tumor-related visceral pain
- Hepatic distention syndrome
- Malignant perineal pain
- Chronic intestinal obstruction
- Adrenal pain syndrome

Neuropathic pain syndromes

Painful cranial neuralgias
- Glossopharyngeal neuralgia
- Trigeminal neuralgia

Plexopathies
- Malignant brachial plexopathy
- Malignant lumbosacral plexopathy
- Cervical plexopathy

Radiculopathies
- Lumbosacral radiculopathy
- Cervical radiculopathy
- Thoracic radiculopathy

Paraneoplastic Sensory Neuropathy

---

thigh.[39,40] Malignant piriformis syndrome presents as pain in the buttock and/or sciatic distribution, often with exacerbation during internal rotation of the hip or a painful plexopathy.

Sacral syndrome

Severe focal pain radiating to buttocks, posterior thighs, or perineum is associated with tumor-related injury of the sacrum and presacral tissues.[39] The pain is often exacerbated by lying or sitting and is relieved by standing or walking. Involvement of the lateral hip rotators makes movement at the hip painful.

Base of skull metastases

Syndromes from locally extensive or metastatic cancer at the base of the skull are defined by the association of pain with other localizing findings.[41] Orbital syndrome

Table 3
Chronic pain syndromes associated with cancer treatment

Hormonal therapy-related pain syndromes	Arthralgias
	Dyspareunia
	Gynecomastia
	Myalgias
	Osteoporotic compression fractures
Radiation-related pain syndromes	Chest wall syndrome
	Cystitis
	Enteritis and proctitis
	Lymphedema
	Myelopathy
	Osteoporosis
	Osteoradionecrosis and fractures
	Painful secondary malignancies
	Peripheral mononeuropathies
	Plexopathies: Brachial, lumbosacral, sacral
Chemotherapy-related pain syndromes	Bony complications of long-term corticosteroids
	Avascular necrosis
	Vertebral compression fractures
	Carpal tunnel syndrome
	Chemotherapy-induced peripheral neuropathy
Surgical pain syndromes	Lymphedema
	Postamputation phantom pain
	Postmastectomy pain
	Postradical neck dissection pain
	Postsurgery pelvic floor pain
	Postthoractomy pain/frozen shoulder

is characterized by retroorbital pain, proptosis, diplopia, visual distortion, and chemosis of the involved eye, ophthalmoparesis, and ipsilateral papilledema. Parasellar syndrome causes retroorbital and frontal pain associated with ophthalmoparesis with diplopia. Middle cranial fossa syndrome is characterized by malar or jaw pain, and in some cases, a painful trigeminal neuropathy. Jugular foramen syndrome is characterized by pain in the ipsilateral ear, neck, or shoulder, at times accompanied by glossopharyngeal neuralgia; the latter syndrome may or may not be associated with syncope. Occipital condyle syndrome is caused by a tumor just lateral to the foramen magnum and presents as unilateral occipital pain, neck stiffness, and head tilt, possibly associated with unilateral tongue atrophy. Clivus lesions produce vertex headache, which is worsened by neck flexion.

Muscle and soft tissue pain
Local pain is common from locally extensive or metastatic soft tissue sarcomas of muscle, fat, or fibrous tissue. Muscle pain may also be due to cramps from neural injury (eg, radiculopathy or plexopathy) or metabolic disturbances (eg, dehydration, hypokalemia, or hypocalcemia).

Tumor-Related Visceral Pain Syndromes

Hepatic distention syndrome
Pain-sensitive structures in the region of the liver include the liver capsule, vessels, diaphragm, and biliary tract. Nociceptive afferents that innervate these structures travel via the celiac plexus, phrenic nerve, and lower right intercostal nerves. Extensive

intrahepatic metastases, a large primary tumor, or gross hepatomegaly associated with cholestasis may produce discomfort in the right subcostal region, and less commonly in the right midback or flank.[42] Pain is usually a dull aching that worsens with positional changes or may be associated with a sharp twinge on deep inspiration. Depending on the related involvement of the diaphragm and biliary tract, the pain also may be referred to the right shoulder or scapular region, respectively.

Peritoneal carcinomatosis and chronic intestinal obstruction

Diffuse abdominal pain may be due to distention, mesenteric tension, or mural ischemia related to peritoneal carcinomatosis or chronic intestinal obstruction.[43–45] Ovarian cancer and colorectal cancer are the most common causes. Pain may be continuous or colicky, and may be referred to the dermatomes represented by the spinal segments supplying the affected viscera. Associated symptoms include nausea, vomiting, and constipation.

Malignant perineal pain

Perineal pain (rectal, genital, or diffuse) is common in tumors of the rectum or colon, female reproductive tract, and distal genitourinary system. The pain usually is aggravated by sitting or standing, with or without a component of tenesmus or tenesmoid pain, or intermittent severe bladder spasms.

Adrenal pain syndrome

Adrenal metastases commonly originate from lung cancer and can produce unilateral flank and abdominal pain, worsened by lying supine.[46] The pain may radiate into the ipsilateral upper and lower quadrants of the abdomen.

Ureteric obstruction

Malignant obstruction of the ureter, which is usually attributable to a gastrointestinal, genitourinary, or gynecologic cancer, may or may not be painful. If pain occurs, it is usually colicky, often superimposed on dull aching, and may be referred to the inguinal region or genitalia. When severe, the colicky pain may be associated with nausea and vomiting. Urinary diversion or stenting can provide symptomatic relief.[47]

Leptomeningeal metastases

Breast and lung cancers, and lymphoma and leukemia are frequent causes of leptomeningeal metastases.[48–50] The most common symptom is aching back or neck pain, or migrainelike or tensionlike headache, which may worsen in the morning and with Valsalva. Some patients experience only radicular cervical or lumbar pain, like that of a herniated disk. Neurologic complications may include cognitive impairment, seizures, hemiparesis, spinal cord syndromes, or any combination of motor or sensory disturbance consistent with a cranial neuropathy or radiculopathy. Given the variety of presentations, clinicians should maintain a high index of suspicious for leptomeningeal disease whenever headache, neck or back pain, or neurologic dysfunction is not explained. The most sensitive approach to diagnosis combines lumbar puncture and contrast-enhanced MRI.[51]

Tumor-Related Neuropathic Pain

About 1 in 3 patients with cancer pain have a neuropathic component.[52]

Cranial neuralgias

Cranial neuralgias can occur from metastases involving the base of the skull or sinuses, the leptomeninges, or the soft tissues of the head or neck. These syndromes may mimic nonmalignant neuralgias.

Glossopharyngeal neuralgia may be part of the jugular foramen syndrome described previously or may occur in isolation. The pain is usually paroxysmal, but can be continuous as well. It is described as severe stabbing in the throat or neck, radiating to the ear or mastoid region, sometimes with syncope. The attacks may be spontaneous or triggered by chewing, swallowing, coughing, speaking, yawning, certain tastes, or touching the neck or external auditory canal.[53]

A painful trigeminal neuropathy may occur as part of the middle cranial fossa syndrome or from tumor involvement of the trigeminal nerve in other locations. In some cases, the pain is episodic and paroxysmal, and mimics idiopathic trigeminal neuralgia; in others, there is a continuous or nonparoxysmal component to the pain. Some patients have neurologic signs, such as sensory disturbance in the trigeminal distribution or weakness of the ipsilateral muscles of mastication.

Plexopathies

Cervical plexopathy Invasion of the cervical plexus by locally advanced or metastatic tumor causes aching or burning pain in the periauricular, postauricular, or anterior regions of the neck or in the lateral aspect of the face, head, or shoulder.

Brachial plexopathy Infiltration of the brachial plexus is most often caused by lung cancer, breast cancer, or lymphoma. The symptoms and signs reflect the specific location of the nerve injury.[54] Lower plexus involvement (C7, C8, T1 distribution), typically from a superior sulcus lung cancer (known as a Pancoast tumor).[55] causes pain that is often severe, preceding other signs by many months, and located predominantly in the elbow, medial forearm, and fourth and fifth fingers. Horner's syndrome is often present. Severe aching, along with constant or lancinating dysesthesias along the ulnar aspect of the forearm or hand is typical. Weakness and sensory loss occur in the distribution of the lower plexus, starting in the hand and medial arm.

In contrast, the pain accompanying an upper brachial plexopathy (eg, from extension of supraclavicular lymph node metastases) is most severe in the shoulder and upper arm. Pain often precedes by months the development of shoulder weakness and sensory loss across the shoulder and upper arm.

With tumor progression, the presenting pain syndrome may ultimately reflect a panplexopathy, with pain and neurologic abnormalities affecting the entire upper extremity. Early identification of these syndromes encourages obtaining an MRI and starting treatment before neurologic signs develop.[56]

Lumbosacral plexopathy Colorectal, cervical, and breast cancers, sarcoma, and lymphoma are the most common tumors associated with lumbosacral plexopathy. Neuropathic pain symptoms precede the appearance of neurologic signs, and both symptoms and signs point to the site of anatomic involvement.[54] Patients with pelvic sidewall disease typically develop upper plexopathy, with pain in the inguinal region and across the anterior and medial aspects of the thigh, whereas those with more medial or paraspinal lesions develop pain and related phenomena in the distal leg and foot, and posterior thigh. With the development of a panplexopathy, intense neuropathic pain may involve the entire lower extremity.

Deep pelvic tumors that predominantly injure the sacral plexus present with perineal pain and signs of bladder or bowel dysfunction.

Radiculopathies

Any malignant process that compresses, distorts, or inflames nerve roots may cause a painful radiculopathy or polyradiculopathy. A painful radiculopathy may result from leptomeningeal metastases, intradural tumor (such as meningioma, neurofibroma, or ependymoma), or tumor in the epidural space. Radicular pain may be continuous or intermittent, aching or sharp, or dysesthetic (eg, burning or electrical-like) in quality; it may or may not be associated with neurologic signs. When located in the thoracic level and bilateral in distribution, the pain may be experienced as a tight band across the chest or abdomen, a presentation that should signal the possibility of associated epidural disease.

Paraneoplastic painful peripheral neuropathy

Pain is a very common first manifestation of paraneoplastic peripheral neuropathy.[57] The immunologic basis for some of these syndromes is established and there is variation in both etiology and presentation.[58] Most patients have pain consistent with axonopathy, which begins in the feet and ascends, later involving hands and arms as well. Some, however, have asymmetrical pain or regional pain. The diagnosis requires electrophysiologic studies, serologic screening for antibodies associated with paraneoplastic neuropathy, and evaluation of alternative treatable causes, such thyroid disease.

Radiation Therapy-Induced Chronic Pain Syndromes

Neurologic syndromes

Radiation therapy can lead to chronic pain syndromes associated with injury to the viscera, soft tissues, or neural tissue. Radiation-induced cervical, brachial, or lumbosacral plexopathies are best described and may develop many months to years after treatment.[59,60] Pain is usually much less prominent than cancer-related plexopathy; weakness and sensory changes occur earlier with associated lymphedema and focal skin changes. The clinical distinction between radiation-induced plexopathy and malignant plexopathy related to recurrent disease or a second primary can be challenging, requiring repeated imaging and, in some cases, repeated biopsies.

Chronic radiation myelopathy includes sensory symptoms, including pain, that typically precede the development of progressive motor and autonomic dysfunction. The pain is a burning dysesthesia, localized to the area of spinal cord damage or below. The neurologic findings may be consistent with a transverse myelopathy, sometimes in a Brown-Sequard pattern.

Lymphedema

Lymphedema may result from radiation to the breast or shoulder, or to the pelvis. Approximately one-third of patients with cancer with lymphedema experience pain.[61] The pathophysiology is usually musculoskeletal, but some patients experience neuropathic pain from stretch injury of the adjacent plexus or nerve entrapment. However, new onset of severe or progressive pain in a lymphedematous limb suggests tumor recurrence or infection and requires reevaluation.

SUMMARY

Numerous pain syndromes related directly to a neoplasm or to its treatment have been described. Syndrome recognition can guide both evaluation and treatment of pain and should be considered an important objective of pain assessment.

REFERENCES

1. van den Beuken-van Everdingen MH, Hochstenbach LM, Joosten EA, et al. Update on prevalence of pain in patients with cancer: systematic review and meta-analysis. J Pain Symptom Manage 2016;51(6):1070–90.

2. Bryson DJ, Wicks L, Ashford RU. The investigation and management of suspected malignant pathological fractures: a review for the general orthopaedic surgeon. Injury 2015;46(10):1891–9.

3. Jeurnink SM, Steyerberg EW, van Hooft JE, et al. Surgical gastrojejunostomy or endoscopic stent placement for the palliation of malignant gastric outlet obstruction (SUSTENT study): a multicenter randomized trial. Gastrointest Endosc 2010; 71:490.

4. Recordare A, Bonariol L, Caratozzolo E. Management of spontaneous bleeding due to hepatocellular carcinoma. Minerva Chir 2002;57:347–56.

5. Wilson LD, Detterbeck FC, Yahalom J. Clinical practice. Superior vena cava syndrome with malignant causes. N Engl J Med 2007;356:1862–9.

6. Timp JF, Braekkan SK, Versteeg HH, et al. Epidemiology of cancer-associated venous thrombosis. Blood 2013;122:1712–23.

7. Van Sebille YZ, Stansbourough R, Wardill HR, et al. Management of mucosities during chemotherapy: from pathophysiology to pragmatic therapeutics. Curr Oncol Rep 2015;17(11):50–8.

8. Lalla RV, Bowen J, Barasch A, et al. Mucositis Guidelines Leadership Group of the Multinational Association of Supportive Care in Cancer and International Society of Oral Oncology (MASCC/ISOO). MASCC/ISOO clinical practice guidelines for the management of mucositis secondary to cancer therapy. Cancer 2014; 120(10):1453–61.

9. Staff NP, Grisold A, Grisold W, et al. Chemotherapy-induced peripheral neuropathy: a current review. Ann Neurol 2017;81(6):772–81.

10. McCarthy GM, Skillings JR. Jaw and other orofacial pain in patients receiving vincristine for the treatment of cancer. Oral Surg Oral Med Oral Pathol 1992;74: 299–304.

11. Muggia FM, Vafai D, Natale R, et al. Paclitaxel 3-hour infusion given alone and combined with carboplatin: preliminary results of dose-escalation trials. Semin Oncol 1995;22(4 Suppl 9):63–6.

12. Miller KK, Gorcey L, McLellan BN. Chemotherapy-induced hand-foot syndrome and nail changes: a review of clinical presentation, etiology, pathogenesis, and management. J Am Acad Dermatol 2014;71:787.

13. Farr KP, Safwat A. Palmar-plantar erythrodysesthesia associated with chemotherapy and its treatment. Case Rep Oncol 2011;4:229–35.

14. Chanprapaph K, Vachiramon V, Rattanakaemakorn P. Epidermal growth factor receptor inhibitors: a review of cutaneous adverse events and management. Dermatol Res Pract 2014;2014:734249.

15. Reiser M, Bruns C, Hartmann P. Raynaud's phenomenon and acral necrosis after chemotherapy for AIDS-related Kaposi's sarcoma. Eur J Clin Microbiol Infect Dis 1998;17:58–60.

16. De la Riva P, Andres-Marín N, Gonzalo-Yubero N, et al. Headache and other complications following intrathecal chemotherapy administration. Cephalalgia 2017; 37(11):1109–10.

17. Evans RW, Armon C, Frohman EM, et al. Assessment: prevention of post-lumbar puncture headache. Neurology 2000;55(7):909–14.

18. Stewart T, Pavlakis N, Ward M. Cardiotoxicity with 5-fluorouracil and capecitabine: more than just vasospastic angina. Intern Med J 2010;40(4):303–7.

19. Nuttall FQ, Warrier RS, Gannon MC. Gynecomastia and drugs: a critical evaluation of the literature. Eur J Clin Pharmacol 2015;71(5):569–78.

20. Jaaback K, Johnson N, Lawrie TA. Intraperitoneal chemotherapy for the initial management of primary epithelial ovarian cancer. Cochrane Database Syst Rev 2016;(1):CD005340.
21. Shelley MD, Wilt TJ, Court J, et al. Intravesical bacillus Calmette-Guerin is superior to mitomycin C in reducing tumour recurrence in high-risk superficial bladder cancer: a meta-analysis of randomized trials. BJU Int 2004;93:485–90.
22. Packiam VT, Johnson SC, Steinberg GD. Non-muscle-invasive bladder cancer: intravesical treatments beyond Bacille Calmette-Guérin. Cancer 2017;123(3): 390–400.
23. Cheng X, Sun P, Hu QG, et al. Transarterial (chemo)embolization for curative resection of hepatocellular carcinoma: a systematic review and meta-analyses. J Cancer Res Clin Oncol 2014;140(7):1159–70.
24. Fiorentini G, Aliberti C, Benea G, et al. TACE of liver metastases from colorectal cancer adopting irinotecan-eluting beads: beneficial effect of palliative intra-arterial lidocaine and post-procedure supportive therapy on the control of side effects. Hepatogastroenterology 2008;55(88):2077–82.
25. Yildizeli B, Laçin T, Batirel HF, et al. Complications and management of long-term central venous access catheters and ports. J Vasc Access 2004;5:174–8.
26. Kreidieh FY, Moukadem HA, El Saghir NS. Overview, prevention and management of chemotherapy extravasation. World J Clin Oncol 2016;7(1):87–97.
27. Valencak J, Troch M, Raderer M. Cutaneous recall phenomenon at the site of previous doxorubicin extravasation after second-line chemotherapy. J Natl Cancer Inst 2007;99:177–8.
28. Neff SP, Stapelberg E, Warmington A. Excruciating perineal pain after intravenous dexamethasone. Anaesth Intensive Care 2002;30:370–1.
29. Loblaw DA, Wu JS, Kirkbride P, et al. Pain flare in patients with bone metastases after palliative radiotherapy—a nested randomized control trial. Support Care Cancer 2007;15:451–5.
30. Hird A, Chow E, Zhang L, et al. Determining the incidence of pain flare following palliative radiotherapy for symptomatic bone metastases: results from three Canadian cancer centers. Int J Radiat Oncol Biol Phys 2009;75:193–7.
31. Hird A, Zhang L, Holt T, et al. Dexamethasone for the prophylaxis of radiation-induced pain flare after palliative radiotherapy for symptomatic bone metastases: a phase II study. Clin Oncol (R Coll Radiol) 2009;21:329–35.
32. Grabenbauer GG, Holger G. Management of radiation and chemotherapy related acute toxicity in gastrointestinal cancer. Best Pract Res Clin Gastroenterol 2016; 30(4):655–64.
33. Tunio M, Al Asiri M, Al Hadab A, et al. Comparative efficacy, tolerability, and survival outcomes of various radiopharmaceuticals in castration-resistant prostate cancer with bone metastasis: a meta-analysis of randomized controlled trials. Drug Des Devel Ther 2015;9:5291–9.
34. Salner AL, Botnick LE, Herzog AG, et al. Reversible brachial plexopathy following primary radiation therapy for breast cancer. Cancer Treat Rep 1981;65:797–802.
35. Maria OM, Eliopoulos N, Muanza T. Radiation-induced oral mucositis. Front Oncol 2017;7:89–130.
36. Kommalapati A, Tella SH, Esquivel MA, et al. Evaluation and management of skeletal disease in cancer care. Crit Rev Oncol Hematol 2017;120:217–26.
37. Zaporowska-Stachowiak I, Łuczak J, Hoffmann K, et al. Managing metastatic bone pain: new perspectives, different solutions. Biomed Pharmacother 2017; 93:1277–84.

38. Sutcliffe P, Connock M, Shyangdan D, et al. A systematic review of evidence on malignant spinal metastases: natural history and technologies for identifying patients at high risk of vertebral fracture and spinal cord compression. Health Technol Assess 2013;17(42):1–274.
39. Papagelopoulos PJ, Mavrogenis AF, Soucacos PN. Evaluation and treatment of pelvic metastases. Injury 2007;38:509–20.
40. Nader R, Rhines LD, Mendel E. Metastatic sacral tumors. Neurosurg Clin N Am 2004;15:453–7.
41. Laigle-Donadey F, Taillibert S, Martin-Duverneuil N, et al. Skull-base metastases. J Neurooncol 2005;75:63–9.
42. Harris JN, Robinson P, Lawrance J, et al. Symptoms of colorectal liver metastases: correlation with CT findings. Clin Oncol (R Coll Radiol) 2003;15:78–82.
43. Dolan EA. Malignant bowel obstruction: a review of current treatment strategies. Am J Hosp Palliat Care 2011;28(8):576–82.
44. Deraco M, Laterza B, Kusamura S. Updated treatment of peritoneal carcinomas: a review. Minerva Chir 2007;62:459–76.
45. Laval G, Marcelin-Benazech B, Guirimand F, et al, French Society for Palliative Care, French Society for Digestive Surgery; French Society for Gastroenterology, French Association for Supportive Care in Oncology, French Society for Digestive Cancer. Recommendations for bowel obstruction with peritoneal carcinomatosis. J Pain Symptom Manage 2014;48(1):75–91.
46. Lam KY, Lo CY. Metastatic tumours of the adrenal glands: a 30-year experience in a teaching hospital. Clin Endocrinol (Oxf) 2002;56:95–101.
47. Liberman D, McCormack M. Renal and urologic problems: management of ureteric obstruction. Curr Opin Support Palliat Care 2012;6(3):316–21.
48. Taillibert S, Laigle-Donadey F, Chodkiewicz C, et al. Leptomeningeal metastases from solid malignancy: a review. J Neurooncol 2005;75:85–99.
49. Nolan CP, Abrey LE. Leptomeningeal metastases from leukemias and lymphomas. Cancer Treat Res 2005;125:53–69.
50. Drappatz J, Batchelor TT. Leptomeningeal neoplasms. Curr Treat Options Neurol 2007;9:283–93.
51. Mack F, Baumert BG, Schäfer N, et al. Therapy of leptomeningeal metastasis in solid tumors. Cancer Treat Rev 2016;43:83–91.
52. Reis-Pina P, Acharya A, Lawlor PG. Cancer pain with a neuropathic component: a cross-sectional study of its clinical characteristics, associated psychological distress, treatments and predictors at referral to a cancer pain clinic. J Pain Symptom Manage 2018;55(2):297–306.
53. Ribeiro RT, Amorim De Souza N, Carvalho Dde S. Glossopharyngeal neuralgia with syncope as a sign of neck cancer recurrence. Arq Neuropsiquiatr 2007; 65:1233–6.
54. van Alfen N, Malessy MJ. Diagnosis of brachial and lumbosacral plexus lesions. Handb Clin Neurol 2013;115:293–310.
55. Foroulis CN, Zarogoulidis P, Darwiche K, et al. Superior sulcus (Pancoast) tumors: current evidence on diagnosis and radical treatment. J Thorac Dis 2013;5(Suppl 4):S342–58.
56. Van Es HW, Bollen TL, Van Heesewijk HP. MRI of the brachial plexus: a pictorial review. Eur J Radiol 2010;74:391–402.
57. Zis P, Paladini A, Piroli A, et al. Pain as a first manifestation of paraneoplastic neuropathies: a systematic review and meta-analysis. Pain Ther 2017;6(2):143–51.
58. Antoine JC, Camdessanché JP. Paraneoplastic neuropathies. Curr Opin Neurol 2017;30(5):513–20.

59. Delanian S, Lefaix JL, Pradat PF. Radiation-induced neuropathy in cancer survivors. Radiother Oncol 2012;105(3):273–82.
60. Dropcho EJ. Neurotoxicity of radiation therapy. Neurol Clin 2010;28(1):217–34.
61. Paskett ED. Symptoms: lymphedema. Adv Exp Med Biol 2015;862:101–13.

Safe Opioid Use
Management of Opioid-Related Adverse Effects and Aberrant Behaviors

Joseph Arthur, MD[a],*, David Hui, MD, MSc[a,b]

KEYWORDS

- Opioid • Cancer • Aberrant behavior • Adverse effects • Nausea • Constipation
- Tolerance • Sedation

KEY POINTS

- Successful opioid therapy requires the use of opioids in a safe and appropriate way to achieve optimal pain control while minimizing unintended adverse effects and opioid misuse, abuse, or diversion.
- A general approach to the management of opioid-related side effects involves opioid dose reduction, opioid rotation, a change in opioid route of administration, and symptomatic management of the side effects.
- A detailed patient history, risk assessment tools, prescription drug monitoring programs, and urine drug screens are important elements of a comprehensive strategy in the management of aberrant behavior.
- Measures taken to ensure safe opioid use include decreasing the time interval between follow-ups for refills, limiting the opioid quantity and doses at each visit, setting boundaries or limitations, or referring to specialist teams for comanagement.

INTRODUCTION

Opioid analgesics play a central role in the management of cancer pain and other symptoms such as dyspnea and cough; however, the benefits conferred by opioids must be carefully balanced against their potential adverse effects, which could negatively affect symptom management, treatment adherence, psychological wellbeing,

Financial and Competing Interest Disclosure: No relevant conflict of interest. D. Hui is supported in part by National Institutes of Health grants (1R01CA214960-01A1, R21NR016736), an American Cancer Society Mentored Research Scholar grant in Applied and Clinical Research (MRSG-14-1418-01-CCE), and the Andrew Sabin Family Fellowship Award.
[a] Department of Palliative Care, Rehabilitation and Integrative Medicine, The University of Texas MD Anderson Cancer Center, Unit 1414, 1515 Holcombe Boulevard, Houston, TX 77030, USA; [b] Department of General Oncology, The University of Texas MD Anderson Cancer Center, 1515 Holcombe Boulevard, Houston, TX 77030, USA
* Corresponding author.
E-mail address: jaarthur@mdanderson.org

quality of life, and even survival. Many of the adverse effects can be anticipated and mitigated by clinicians with a good working knowledge of the opioid-related adverse effects, and by the provision of skilled patient education, proper monitoring, and timely management. This article provides an up-to-date synopsis on the management of various opioid-related adverse effects. It also discusses the strategies to minimize aberrant opioid use in patients with cancer, which is particularly important during this era of the opioid epidemic.

OPIOID-RELATED ADVERSE EFFECTS

The key determinants of opioid-related adverse effects include both patient-related (genetic variations,[1] age,[2,3] and renal[4,5] and liver dysfunction[6]) and medication-related factors. Medications that alter opioid absorption, metabolism, or clearance may increase their side effects.[7] Moreover, concurrent use of some medications may exacerbate side effects. For example, using opioids and benzodiazepines together could significantly worsen the patient's cognitive function and may precipitate respiratory depression.

Recommendations for management of opioid-related side effects in the literature are mainly based on consensus opinion and clinical experience.[8] There are 4 key strategies to address these adverse effects, including:

1. Opioid dose reduction
2. Opioid rotation
3. Changing the route of opioid administration
4. Symptomatic management of adverse effects.[9]

The prevalence, pathophysiology, and management strategies for several important opioid-related adverse effects, including nausea and vomiting, constipation, sedation, neurotoxicity, pruritus, and respiratory depression, are briefly reviewed (**Table 1**).

Opioid-Induced Nausea and Vomiting

Opioid-induced nausea and vomiting (OINV) occur in approximately 26% of patients treated with opioids.[10] Opioids cause nausea by stimulating receptors in the chemoreceptor trigger zone (CTZ), the gastrointestinal (GI) tract, or the vestibular apparatus to send impulses to the vomiting center located in the medulla oblongata, or by reducing GI motility, resulting in gastroparesis and constipation. Symptomatic management of OINV includes the use of antiemetics (**Table 2**) and treatment of any other coexisting conditions that may contribute to nausea (eg, constipation). See later discussion of the main classes of antiemetics used in the management of OINV.

Antipsychotics are dopamine-2 receptor antagonists that work centrally to block dopamine receptors in the CTZ and the vomiting center. They include butyrophenones (eg, droperidol, and haloperidol) and phenothiazines (eg, prochlorperazine, perphenazine, and promethazine), as well as atypical antipsychotics such as olanzapine, aripiprazole, and risperidone.[9,11] Common adverse effects include sedation, orthostatic hypotension, and extrapyramidal symptoms such as akathisia and dystonic reactions. Olanzapine has a higher affinity for the serotonin receptor than the dopamine receptor and hence has less propensity to cause extrapyramidal symptoms.

Metoclopramide is a unique medication because, apart from being a prokinetic agent by increasing gut motility via acetylcholine release, it can block dopamine receptors both centrally in the CTZ and peripherally in the GI tract. Thus, it is a drug of choice for the management of OINV. At high doses it is capable of blocking both

Table 1
Opioid-related adverse effects

Type of Adverse Effect	Example
Gastrointestinal	Nausea
	Vomiting
	Constipation
	Gastroparesis
Central nervous system	Respiratory depression
	Drowsiness
	Cognitive impairment
	Hallucination
	Allodynia
	Hyperalgesia
	Myoclonus
	Seizure disorder
Cardiovascular	Hypotension
	Bradycardia
	QT prolongation or Torsade des pointes[a]
Autonomic nervous system	Urinary retention
	Xerostomia
Dermatologic	Pruritus
	Sweating
Hormonal or immunologic	Decreased libido
	Sexual dysfunction
	Decreased energy levels
	Osteoporosis
	Amenorrhea or oligomenorrhea
	Depression
	Immunosuppression

[a] In the case of methadone.

dopamine and serotonin receptors.[12] Known side effects include drowsiness, diarrhea, and rarely extrapyramidal symptoms.

Serotonin receptor antagonists act both centrally and peripherally by binding to 5-hydroxytryptamine-3 (5-HT3) receptors in the CTZ and the GI tract. Examples include dolasetron, granisetron, and ondansetron, which are first generation serotonin receptor antagonists; and palonosetron, a second-generation serotonin receptor antagonist. The major side effects of these agents are constipation and headache. Other classes of antiemetics that may be occasionally used include antihistamines, anticholinergics, and corticosteroids (see **Table 2**).

Opioid-Induced Constipation

Opioid-induced constipation (OIC) is the most common opioid-related side effect in cancer pain management, affecting 40% to 80% of patients on opioids. Opioids cause constipation by binding to peripheral receptors in the GI tract; decreasing gastric motility, intestinal water secretion, and blood flow; and increasing anal sphincter tone.[13] OIC is believed to be dose-dependent. Nonpharmacological approaches used in management include increasing hydration, soluble dietary fiber intake, and physical activity.

Due to the paucity of research, there is no established first-line therapy for OIC prevention or treatment. A stimulant is often recommended as part of the initial

Table 2
Common antiemetic medications used in the management of opioid-induced nausea and vomiting

Class	Medication	Common Doses	Comments
Prokinetic agents	Metoclopramide	5–10 mg orally or IV 4/d	Increases peristalsis via acetylcholine release; also blocks both dopamine and serotonin receptors at high doses
	Domperidone (not available in the United States)	10 mg orally every 6 h	Has fewer and less severe extrapyramidal side effects because it crosses the blood–brain barrier to a lesser extent
Antipsychotics	Haloperidol	0.5–2 mg orally 2 to 4/d	—
	Prochlorperazine	5–10 mg orally or IV every 6–8 h or 25 mg rectally every 12 h	Has both antidopaminergic and antihistaminic properties; less sedating than promethazine
	Promethazine	12.5–25 mg orally, IV, or rectally every 4–6 h	Has less dopamine-blocking properties than prochlorperazine; also has antihistaminic properties
	Olanzapine	2.5 to 5 mg orally 2/d	2nd generation antipsychotic; binds to a wide variety of receptors, including dopaminergic, serotonergic, histaminic, and muscarinic receptors
Serotonin antagonists	Ondansetron	4–8 mg orally or IV every 6–8 h	Class is relatively more expensive than other classes of antiemetics and hence considered as second-line agents
	Granisetron	1 mg orally or IV 2/d or 3.1 mg transdermal every 24 h	First-generation agent similar to ondansetron but longer acting
Anticholinergics	Scopolamine	0.3 mg orally every 8 h or 1.5 mg transdermal every 72 h	Can cross the blood–brain barrier and cause central nervous system side effects
Antihistamines	Diphenhydramine	25–50 mg orally or IV every 4–6 h	Very sedating
	Meclizine	12.5–25 mg orally every 6 to 8 h	More effective if nausea is related to motion
Corticosteroids	Dexamethasone	1–4 mg every 6 h	Usually used for short period of time due to the side effects with prolonged use
	Prednisone	5–15 mg every 6–8 h	Similar side effect profile to dexamethasone

Abbreviation: IV, intravenous.

prophylactic bowel regimen.[9] Patients are encouraged to take laxatives on a scheduled basis to ensure regular bowel movements at least every day or every other day.[14] Commonly used laxatives are shown in **Table 3**. Some experts have recommended the use of 2 or more laxatives with different mechanisms of action.[14] Docusate was found in a double-blind randomized control trial to provide limited additional benefit when combined with sennosides.[15] Although some studies have reported that transdermal fentanyl induces less OIC than other opioids, this remains to be confirmed.[16]

Because OIC is mediated predominantly by the peripheral mu-opioid receptors lining the GI tract, selective blockade of these receptors by peripherally acting mu-opioid receptor antagonist (PAMORA), medications such as methylnaltrexone, naloxegol, naldemedine, and alvimopan can relieve constipation without affecting the centrally mediated analgesic effects of opioids or precipitating withdrawal symptoms. A systematic review and meta-analysis on the efficacy of pharmacologic therapies for the treatment of OIC concluded that mu-opioid receptor antagonists are safe and effective for the treatment of OIC.[17]

Methylnaltrexone
In a double-blind, randomized, placebo-controlled trial involving 133 subjects with OIC refractory to other laxatives, 48% of subjects had a bowel movement within 4 hours after the first dose and 52% within 4 hours after 2 or more of the first 4 doses of methylnaltrexone, as compared with 15% and 8% in the placebo group, respectively ($P<.001$). The treatment did not seem to affect central analgesia or cause opioid withdrawal.[18] Methylnaltrexone has been commercially available in subcutaneous formulation at a dosage of 12 mg daily since 2008 and recently received US Food and Drug Administration (FDA) approval for the oral preparation at a dosage of 450 mg daily in 2016.[19] However, clinicians should avoid using this medication in patients with bowel obstruction and GI malignancies because they may develop bowel perforation.

Naloxegol
Naloxegol, a pegylated derivative of naloxone, is approved by the FDA at a dosage of 25 mg daily.[13]

Alvimopan
Alvimopan, the first PAMORA studied for OIC ,was found to potentially cause myocardial infarction with long-term use, resulting in the early termination of a phase III study. It is currently approved only for short-term use in the inpatient setting.[20]

Sedation

Sedation or decreased cognition occurs especially during the initial dosing or at higher doses.[21] The prevalence of opioid-induced cognitive dysfunction is 14% to 77%, depending on the population, opioid doses, and methods and duration of assessment.[22] The effect may be transient in some patients but persistent in others. The first step is to identify and minimize or discontinue any concomitant sedating medications such as antihistamines, anxiolytics, or antidepressants. Opioid dose reduction, opioid rotation, and the use of pharmacologic agents, such as methylphenidate, dextroamphetamine, donepezil, modafinil, and caffeine, have been suggested. Methylphenidate is the most widely studied psychostimulant in randomized clinical trials[23] and is considered the first-line therapy for opioid-induced sedation.[24]

Table 3
Laxatives used for the management of opioid-induced constipation

Class	Medication	Mechanism of Action	Comments
Surfactants	Docusate	Act as detergents to soften fat and increase water penetration to soften stool	Not effective as monotherapy; often used in combination with other laxatives
Emollients	Mineral oil	Act as lubricants to soften stool	May cause lipid pneumonitis if aspiration occurs
Bulk-forming agents	Psyllium Methylcellulose Wheat dextrin (Benefiber)	Absorb water into the intestine, increasing stool bulk, thereby promoting peristalsis	Psyllium and methylcellulose require at least 300–500 mL of water intake, otherwise impaction may occur; not recommended in very sick patients
Stimulants	Bisacodyl Senna	Stimulate peristalsis by irritating the smooth muscle and intramural plexus; increase secretion by inhibiting Na+ and K+ ATPase activity	Activation in colon by bacterial action; side effects include abdominal cramping
Hyperosmolar agents	Lactulose Polyethylene glycol Sorbitol	Increase intestinal fluid retention	Indigestible, unabsorbable compounds; side effects include abdominal bloating, colic, and flatulence; lactulose contraindicated in lactose-deficient patients
Saline laxatives	Magnesium hydroxide Magnesium citrate	Draw fluid into the intestine by osmosis	Avoid in renal or heart failure
Opioid antagonists	Methylnaltrexone Naloxegol	Peripherally acting mu-opioid receptor antagonist	Only works for OIC; contraindicated in bowel obstruction, bowel perforation, pelvic masses; side effects include abdominal pain, nausea, diarrhea
Rectal preparations	Mineral oil enema Sorbitol enema Lactulose enema Saline enema Sodium phosphate enema Glycerin suppository Bisacodyl suppository	In addition to their specific mechanisms of action, they stimulate the anocolonic reflex to induce defecation	Usually used in intractable constipation; contraindicated in thrombocytopenia and neutropenia; repeated saline enemas may cause electrolyte disturbances; glycerin can cause local irritation; sodium phosphate enema is considered the most potent

(continued on next page)

Table 3
(continued)

Class	Medication	Mechanism of Action	Comments
Investigational and new agents	Naldemedine	Peripherally acting mu-opioid receptor antagonist	Currently investigational; side effects include diarrhea and abdominal pain
	Alvimopan	Peripherally acting mu-opioid receptor antagonist	Approved only for short-term use (<16 doses) in a hospital inpatient setting; a phase III trial was terminated early due to potential myocardial infarction with long-term use
	Lubiprostone	Secretagogue; activate chloride receptors on enterocytes to increase intestinal fluid secretion and gut motility	The only secretagogue approved for OIC; not recommended in patients on methadone because its activity is potentially inhibited by methadone; avoid in pregnancy; side effects include nausea, diarrhea, and abdominal pain
	Linaclotide Dolcanatide	Secretagogue; activate guanylate cyclase C receptors on enterocytes to increase intestinal secretion	Currently investigational; side effects include diarrhea

Opioid-Induced Neurotoxicity

Opioid-induced neurotoxicity (OIN) refers to the constellation of neurologic symptoms that may occur due to accumulation of toxic opioid metabolites. Symptoms include confusion, hallucinations, myoclonus, allodynia, or hyperalgesia.[25] Diagnosis of OIN is complicated by concomitant presence of other causes of delirium, such as infection, dehydration, metabolic abnormalities, or advanced cancer.[26] OIN is managed by treating the other precipitating causes of delirium, reducing the dose of opioids, or (most important) switching to a different opioid to prevent further accumulation of toxic metabolites. Some patients with severe or persistent symptoms may require further symptomatic treatment, such as antipsychotics for delirium or benzodiazepines for myoclonic jerks and seizures.[21]

Respiratory Depression

Respiratory depression is the most life-threatening opioid-related side effect. This is due to the effect of opioids on the respiratory centers in the brain stem leading to hypoventilation to the point of apnea. The effect is dose-dependent but tolerance may develop with prolonged opioid use. Hence, it is highly uncommon in patients on chronic opioid therapy with good adherence. Importantly, coadministration with benzodiazepines[27]; alcohol; or the presence of other comorbidities, such as pulmonary embolism, pneumonia, or cardiomyopathy, may precipitate respiratory depression. In addition to decreased respiratory rate (<8 times per minute), pupillary constriction and decreased level of consciousness are often observed. Naloxone, the preferred treatment, should be used only in unresponsive patients breathing less than 8 times per minute because it causes severe opioid withdrawal, even when titrated carefully.[21] It has a relatively short duration of action, so symptomatic patients who were receiving long-acting opioids require careful monitoring to determine the need for repeated naloxone boluses or a naloxone infusion.

Pruritus

Pruritus occurs in less than 10% of patients on oral opioids[9] but in 35% to 90% of those receiving epidural or intrathecal opioids.[28,29] The most compelling pathophysiologic evidence favors the centrally mediated mu-receptor pathway.[30] Others implicated include the histaminic, serotonergic, and the dopaminergic pathways.[31] Opioid-related pruritus is considered an adverse effect rather than an allergic reaction. It is self-limiting and not life-threatening. It is usually managed by reducing the opioid dose, switching to a different opioid, or treating with other medications. In a systematic review, nalbuphine, a mixed opioid agonist-antagonist, was found to be superior to placebo, diphenhydramine, naloxone, or propofol in treating pruritus from neuraxial opioids.[32] Other pharmacologic agents, such as serotonin 5-HT3 receptor antagonists, propofol, nonsteroidal antiinflammatory drugs, and dopamine D2 receptor antagonists, have also been found to be useful.[31]

Physical Dependence and Tolerance

Physical dependence is a physiologic state characterized by the onset of withdrawal symptoms after sudden opioid cessation, dose reduction, or administration of an opioid antagonist. Withdrawal symptoms (eg, piloerection, chills, insomnia, diarrhea, nausea, vomiting, and muscle aches) vary in severity and duration depending on the type, dose, and duration of opioid prescribed.[33] The symptoms are reduced by a gradual taper of opioids.

Tolerance is characterized by the need to use increasing opioid doses to maintain the same effects. It is a form of neuroadaptation to the effects of long-term administration of opioids. Neither physical dependence nor tolerance necessarily indicates addiction.[34] Discontinuing the opioid reverses tolerance and physical dependence within days to weeks, whereas the changes associated with addiction persist for months to years, even after the opioids are stopped. Addicted patients are, therefore, extremely vulnerable to overdosing after a period of abstinence because, although they may still have a persistent desire for opioids, they lose the opioid tolerance which previously protected them from overdosing.[33]

ABERRANT OPIOID-RELATED BEHAVIORS

Aberrant opioid use presents a significant challenge to helping patients with cancer manage their pain. Patients with cancer were previously thought to be less at risk for opioid abuse.[35,36] In 1 study, less than 5% of ambulatory patients with cancer met the criteria for a substance use disorder.[36] The most recent Centers for Disease Control and Prevention guideline for opioid prescriptions exempted patients with cancer pain.[37] However, a more recent study found that chemical coping was diagnosed in 18% of outpatients with cancer.[38] Patients with cancer are also at a risk for aberrant use of prescription drugs if they have a preexisting issue with drug and substance abuse.[39] Clinicians are, therefore, faced with the challenge of helping patients who need to use opioids safely while minimizing opioid misuse and addiction.

Aberrant Behavior: A Spectrum of Conditions

There is a gradation of opioid-related aberrant behaviors from seemingly normal drug-taking behavior to a clear demonstration of addictive behavior (**Fig. 1**). Many patients exhibit different behaviors that fall in between these extremes (**Table 4**). Notably, not all patients who misuse or abuse drugs are addicts. Moreover, some behaviors, such as losing medications, may be relatively less serious than others, such as self-injecting or shooting oral formulations.

Risk Assessment and Monitoring of Aberrant Behaviors

Guidelines that provide specific recommendations for safe opioid prescribing in patients with cancer are limited and, therefore, much of the information is based on the literature about patients who have noncancer pain. **Fig. 2** outlines a recommended approach to patients with cancer on chronic opioid therapy. During the initial visit or before starting opioids, the clinician should carefully screen all patients using a comprehensive clinical history, including psychosocial, substance abuse, and family histories[40]; as well as risk assessment tools (see later discussion). Patients may then be stratified into low risk or high risk for opioid abuse. High-risk patients will require increased monitoring during subsequent clinic visits. Studies have found that patients who are younger, male, have mental health or substance abuse disorders, or have alcohol or tobacco use are at a higher risk of aberrant opioid use.[41]

All patients should give informed consent, detailing the potential risks and benefits of opioid therapy; possible adverse effects; and education on safe opioid use, storage, and disposal strategies.[42] Clinicians should consider using a written opioid management plan, also known as opioid treatment agreement or contract. The plan helps define the goals and expectations of therapy and the responsibilities of both the clinician and patient about how opioids will be prescribed and taken, clinical follow-up, and monitoring.[43] Plans vary, but usually include obtaining opioids from 1 prescriber, filling prescriptions at 1 designated pharmacy, keeping one's scheduled appointments, random urine drug screens (UDS), and the actions that the clinician may take if the patient fails to adhere to the plan.

At every patient visit, monitor for evidence of maladaptive opioid-related behavior, otherwise known as red flags[44,45] (**Box 1**). Also, use prescription monitoring programs,

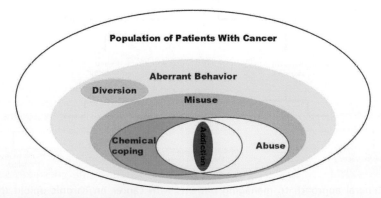

Fig. 1. Spectrum of aberrant opioid-related behavior.

Table 4
Definition of common terms to describe aberrant opioid use

Misuse	The use of a medication for a medical purpose other than as directed or indicated, whether intentionally or unintentionally[63]
Abuse	The intentional self-administration of a medication for a nonmedical purpose, such as altering one's state of consciousness, or the use of any illegal drug[63]
Diversion	The intentional transfer of a controlled substance from legitimate distribution and dispensing channels[63]
Chemical coping	The inappropriate and/or excessive use of opioids to cope with the various stressful events associated with the diagnosis and management of cancer[66,67]
Addiction	A primary chronic neurobiological disease that occurs as result of genetic, psychosocial, and environmental factors It is characterized by 1 or more of the following: • Impaired control during use • Compulsive use • Continued use despite harm • Craving[68]
Pseudoaddiction	The apparent demonstration of a drug-seeking behavior in the setting of undertreated or poorly treated pain[69] It may be erroneously interpreted as addiction but the behavior resolves once adequate pain control is achieved

pain medication diaries, pill counts, and periodic UDS. Routinely conducting and documenting this risk evaluation and monitoring process will allow the clinician to detect when a patient who initially seemed to demonstrate opioid-adherent behavior moves into a pattern of aberrant opioid use.

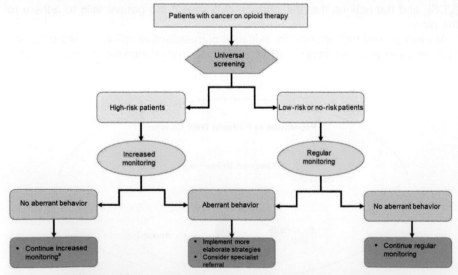

Fig. 2. General approach to managing patients with cancer on chronic opioid therapy.
[a] Consider changing to regular monitoring if adherent pattern observed over a long time.

Box 1
Behaviors suggestive of aberrant opioid use

Frequent unscheduled clinic appointments or telephone calls for early opioid refills

Self-escalation or request for excessive increase in the opioid dosage not consistent with patient's pain syndrome

Reports of lost or stolen opioid prescription or medication

Frequent emergency room visits for opioids

Seeking opioids from multiple providers (doctor shopping)

Requests for a specific opioid

Resistance to changes in the opioid regimen even when clinically indicated

Use of nonprescribed restricted medications or illicit drugs

Requesting opioids for its euphoric effect or for symptoms such as anxiety or insomnia

Reports of impaired functioning in daily activities due to opioid use

Family members expressing concern about patient's use of opioids

Reports of hoarding drugs

Reports of stealing or selling prescription drugs

Obtaining opioids from nonmedical sources

Reports of stealing, tampering, or forging opioid prescriptions

Discrepancy in pill counts without good explanation

Adapted from Arthur JA, Edwards T, Lu Z, et al. Frequency, predictors, and outcomes of urine drug testing among patients with advanced cancer on chronic opioid therapy at an outpatient supportive care clinic. Cancer 2016;122(23):3734; with permission.

Risk assessment tools

Examples of validated risk assessment tools for patient screening include the Cut down, Annoyed, Guilty, and Eye-opener (CAGE) questionnaire; Screener and Opioid Assessment for Patients with Pain (SOAPP) form; the Opioid Risk Tool (ORT); and the Diagnosis, Intractability, Risk, and Efficacy (DIRE) inventory.[46] Although risk assessment and monitoring tools may reveal the possibility of maladaptive behavior, they are based on patient self-reporting, which limits their usefulness.

The CAGE is a clinician-administered 4-item questionnaire that asks about a patient's perceived need to:

1. Cut down on alcohol use
2. Annoyance with questions about alcohol abuse
3. Guilt over drinking habits
4. Use of eye-opener drinks.[47]

Patients score 1 point for every "Yes" answer. A cut-off score of 2 or greater is considered positive and has a sensitivity of 0.93 and a specificity of 0.76 for identifying excessive alcohol use.[48] A positive CAGE may indicate an increased risk of maladaptive opioid use. The CAGE questionnaire was not specifically created for patients with pain; it is also commonly used in other settings. An updated version of the CAGE questionnaire, the CAGE-Adapted to Include Drugs (CAGE-AID) questionnaire, which substitutes "drink" with "drink or drugs," has also been evaluated for the detection of substance use disorder and found to have a sensitivity of 0.88 and a specificity of 0.55 for a score of 2 or greater.[49]

The SOAPP is a patient self-administered screening questionnaire used to help identify patients who may be at risk for aberrant drug-related behavior.[46,50] There are 3 different available versions. The SOAPP-Original, SOAPP-Revised, and SOAPP-Short Form are questionnaires with 14, 24, and 5 items, respectively, and with sensitivity, specificity scores of 0.86, 0.67; 0.81, 0.68; and 0.86, 0.67 for cut-off scores of greater than or equal to 7, greater than or equal to 18, and greater than or equal to 4, respectively.

ORT is a patient self-administered questionnaire that assesses 5 risk factor categories:

1. Family history of substance abuse
2. Personal history of substance abuse
3. Age 16 to 45 years
4. History of preadolescent sexual abuse
5. Psychological disease.[51]

It is a 10-item questionnaire with a possible score ranging from 0 to 26. A score of 0 to 3 is low risk, 4 to 7 is moderate risk, and greater than or equal to 8 is high risk.[52] The ORT has demonstrated excellent discrimination for both the male (c-statistic = 0.82) and the female (c-statistic = 0.85) prognostic models.

The DIRE is a clinician-administered questionnaire that predicts the possibility of patient compliance with long-term opioid therapy and the efficacy of analgesia. It consists of 4 categories of risk factors.[46] Total scores range from 7 to 21, with lower scores indicating greater risk. A cut-off score of 13 has a sensitivity of 0.94 and a specificity of 0.87.

Other tools that are used solely for continued monitoring of patients currently receiving opioid therapy include the Current Opioid Misuse Measure (COMM)[53] and the Addiction Behavior Checklist (ABC).[54]

Prescription drug monitoring programs

Prescription drug monitoring programs (PDMPs) collect data from pharmacies that dispense controlled substances and use it to create secure state-run electronic databases that are made available to authorized users. They provide key information about the patient's prescription history and document when and where patients received opioid prescriptions and who prescribed them.[55] PDMPs are particularly useful in providing objective data on patients who seek opioids from multiple prescribers (doctor shopping) and fill multiple prescriptions at different pharmacies (pharmacy shopping). As of August 24, 2017, every state in the United States had an extensive operational PDMP, except for Missouri, where the PDMP program is not statewide.[56] PDMPs are effective in reducing aberrant opioid use by facilitating clinical decision-making and improving opioid prescribing practices.[57]

Urine drug screens

Two main types of UDS are used in clinical practice. The immunoassays use antibodies to detect the presence of a particular drug or its metabolite. They are more economical and have a quick turnaround time but are unable to distinguish between different drugs in the same class or detect synthetic opioids. The confirmatory or laboratory-based specific drug identification tests use gas or liquid chromatography or mass spectrometry. They can detect specific drugs but are more expensive and have a slower turnaround time.[58] The 3 types of abnormal UDS results are:

1. Absence of prescribed opioids (suggestive of diversion)
2. Presence of unprescribed opioids (suggestive of multiple prescriber involvement or obtaining opioids from unapproved sources)
3. Presence of illicit drugs.

Even these laboratory tests have pitfalls because of the complexity of opioid metabolic pathways. A normal UDS result does not necessarily rule out aberrant behavior. For example, patients who are using opioids for chemical coping may have a normal UDS but may still be using opioids in an excessive or maladaptive manner.

Best practice in the use of UDS in patients with cancer, who have unique symptom burdens and expectations, is not yet defined. UDS seems to be underutilized in patients with cancer as compared with noncancer patients with chronic pain. At the authors' facility, for example, UDS was conducted in only 6% of patients with cancer seen at the palliative care clinic and 54% of these were abnormal.[44]

Management of Detected Aberrant Behavior

When patients demonstrate aberrant behavior, the clinical team needs to have open and nonjudgmental discussions with them, communicating their concerns about patient safety. Measures that should be implemented to ensure that they adhere to safe opioid use include decreasing the time interval between follow-ups for refills, limiting the opioid quantity and dose of refills, setting boundaries or limitations, weaning off the opioids when possible, or referring to a pain or palliative medicine or drug addiction specialist for comanagement. Specific education regarding safe opioid use, storage, and disposal should be provided frequently to the patients and their caregivers.[59] In some patients, complete behavioral change is achievable but not in others. Goals for these patients can, therefore, focus on minimizing harm.

Use nonopioids and adjuvant analgesics

The World Health Organization ladder for management of cancer pain recommends starting pain management with nonopioid and adjuvant analgesics, especially in patients with mild pain. Clinicians should only consider opioids for patients with moderate to severe cancer pain or pain that is unresponsive to nonopioid therapies because these are the populations shown to benefit from opioids in randomized trials.[60] Consider switching patients who demonstrate aberrant behaviors from opioids to nonopioid analgesics or use interventional techniques when possible.

Treat underlying comorbid psychiatric conditions

The prevalence of common psychiatric conditions, such as personality disorder, depression, and anxiety disorders, is extremely high in patients with a history of substance abuse.[61] During the initial, as well as subsequent, patient screenings, evaluate and treat any underlying comorbid psychiatric conditions. Psychological interventions, such as cognitive behavioral therapy, relaxation techniques, biofeedback, distraction techniques, problem-solving techniques, and other coping strategies, in appropriate patients are useful adjunctive therapies.[62] Treatment facilitates recovery from drug addiction and helps minimize the likelihood of relapse.

Adopt an interdisciplinary approach

Management of patients with aberrant opioid-related behavior requires a sound understanding of multiple domains, including biomedical, psychosocial, financial, and legal factors. An interprofessional team is better able to address these multidimensional care needs comprehensively while supporting each other to minimize burnout.[63]

The authors' supportive oncology team recently developed and implemented a specialized interdisciplinary team intervention to standardize care for patients with cancer with aberrant behavior. Using a quasi-experimental design, the intervention resulted in a significant reduction in the frequency of aberrant behaviors from a median of 3 per month before the intervention to 0.4 postintervention ($P<.0001$). There was also a significant reduction in opioid utilization from a median morphine equivalent dose of 165 mg daily at the first intervention visit to 112 mg daily at the last clinic follow-up (P = .02), despite that pain intensity did not change (P = .98).[64]

Consider prescribing intranasal naloxone

Coprescribing naloxone, a short-acting opioid antagonist, to patients on chronic opioids may help reduce opioid-related adverse effects without causing an increase in the dose of prescribed opioids.[65] Patients with a history of drug overdose, a history of a substance use disorder, requiring large opioid doses, or concurrently receiving benzodiazepines may particularly benefit from prescribed intranasal naloxone with instructions for administration by relatives and caregivers.[37]

SUMMARY

Successful opioid therapy requires that opioids be used in a safe and appropriate way to achieve optimal pain control while minimizing unintended adverse effects and aberrant use. A general approach to the management of opioid-related side effects involves opioid dose reduction, opioid rotation, a change in opioid route of administration, and symptomatic management of the side effects. Successful prevention of aberrant opioid use, early identification, and effective management are invaluable practices in managing patients with cancer pain, especially during this era of the opioid epidemic.

REFERENCES

1. Poulsen L, Brosen K, Arendt-Nielsen L, et al. Codeine and morphine in extensive and poor metabolizers of sparteine: pharmacokinetics, analgesic effect and side effects. Eur J Clin Pharmacol 1996;51:289–95.
2. Macintyre PE, Jarvis DA. Age is the best predictor of postoperative morphine requirements. Pain 1996;64:357–64.
3. Vigano A, Bruera E, Suarez-Almazor ME. Age, pain intensity, and opioid dose in patients with advanced cancer. Cancer 1998;83:1244–50.
4. Hagen NA, Foley KM, Cerbone DJ, et al. Chronic nausea and morphine-6-glucuronide. J Pain Symptom Manage 1991;6:125–8.
5. Osborne R, Joel S, Grebenik K, et al. The pharmacokinetics of morphine and morphine glucuronides in kidney failure. Clin Pharmacol Ther 1993;54:158–67.
6. Hasselstrom J, Eriksson S, Persson A, et al. The metabolism and bioavailability of morphine in patients with severe liver cirrhosis. Br J Clin Pharmacol 1990;29: 289–97.
7. Bernard SA, Bruera E. Drug interactions in palliative care. J Clin Oncol 2000;18: 1780–99.
8. Swegle JM, Logemann C. Management of common opioid-induced adverse effects. Am Fam Physician 2006;74:1347–54.
9. Cherny N, Ripamonti C, Pereira J, et al. Strategies to manage the adverse effects of oral morphine: an evidence-based report. J Clin Oncol 2001;19:2542–54.
10. Cepeda MS, Farrar JT, Baumgarten M, et al. Side effects of opioids during short-term administration: effect of age, gender, and race. Clin Pharmacol Ther 2003; 74:102–12.
11. Smith HS, Cox LR, Smith BR. Dopamine receptor antagonists. Ann Palliat Med 2012;1:137–42.
12. Smith HS, Laufer A. Opioid induced nausea and vomiting. Eur J Pharmacol 2014; 722:67–78.

13. Brenner DM, Stern E, Cash BD. Opioid-related constipation in patients with non-cancer pain syndromes: a review of evidence-based therapies and justification for a change in nomenclature. Curr Gastroenterol Rep 2017;19:12.

14. Pappagallo M. Incidence, prevalence, and management of opioid bowel dysfunction. Am J Surg 2001;182:11S–8S.

15. Tarumi Y, Wilson MP, Szafran O, et al. Randomized, double-blind, placebo-controlled trial of oral docusate in the management of constipation in hospice patients. J Pain Symptom Manage 2013;45:2–13.

16. Allan L, Hays H, Jensen NH, et al. Randomised crossover trial of transdermal fentanyl and sustained release oral morphine for treating chronic non-cancer pain. BMJ 2001;322:1154–8.

17. Ford AC, Brenner DM, Schoenfeld PS. Efficacy of pharmacological therapies for the treatment of opioid-induced constipation: systematic review and meta-analysis. Am J Gastroenterol 2013;108:1566–74 [quiz: 1575].

18. Thomas J, Karver S, Cooney GA, et al. Methylnaltrexone for opioid-induced constipation in advanced illness. N Engl J Med 2008;358:2332–43.

19. FDA approves methylnaltrexone bromide for oral use, 2016. Available at: https://www.accessdata.fda.gov/drugsatfda_docs/label/2016/208271s000lbl.pdf. Accessed February 27, 2018.

20. NDA 21-775 ENTEREG (alvimopan) REMS October 6, 2008. Risk Evaluation and Mitigation Strategy (REMS). Available at https://www.accessdata.fda.gov/drugsatfda_docs/label/2009/021775s001REMS.pdf. Accessed February 27, 2018.

21. McNicol E, Horowicz-Mehler N, Fisk RA, et al. Management of opioid side effects in cancer-related and chronic noncancer pain: a systematic review. J Pain 2003; 4:231–56.

22. Lawlor PG. The panorama of opioid-related cognitive dysfunction in patients with cancer: a critical literature appraisal. Cancer 2002;94:1836–53.

23. Bruera E, Miller MJ, Macmillan K, et al. Neuropsychological effects of methylphenidate in patients receiving a continuous infusion of narcotics for cancer pain. Pain 1992;48:163–6.

24. Reissig JE, Rybarczyk AM. Pharmacologic treatment of opioid-induced sedation in chronic pain. Ann Pharmacother 2005;39:727–31.

25. Mercadante S, Portenoy RK. Opioid poorly-responsive cancer pain. Part 1: clinical considerations. J Pain Symptom Manage 2001;21:144–50.

26. Cherny NI. The management of cancer pain. CA Cancer J Clin 2000;50:70–116 [quiz: 117–20].

27. O'Mahony S, Coyle N, Payne R. Current management of opioid-related side effects. Oncology (Williston Park) 2001;15:61–73 [77; discussion 77–8, 80–2].

28. Chaney MA. Side effects of intrathecal and epidural opioids. Can J Anaesth 1995; 42:891–903.

29. Bonnet MP, Mignon A, Mazoit JX, et al. Analgesic efficacy and adverse effects of epidural morphine compared to parenteral opioids after elective caesarean section: a systematic review. Eur J Pain 2010;14:894.e1-9.

30. Liu XY, Liu ZC, Sun YG, et al. Unidirectional cross-activation of GRPR by MOR1D uncouples itch and analgesia induced by opioids. Cell 2011;147:447–58.

31. Ganesh A, Maxwell LG. Pathophysiology and management of opioid-induced pruritus. Drugs 2007;67:2323–33.

32. Jannuzzi RG. Nalbuphine for treatment of opioid-induced pruritus: a systematic review of literature. Clin J Pain 2016;32:87–93.

33. Volkow ND, McLellan AT. Opioid abuse in chronic pain–misconceptions and mitigation strategies. N Engl J Med 2016;374:1253–63.

34. Passik SD, Weinreb HJ. Managing chronic nonmalignant pain: overcoming obstacles to the use of opioids. Adv Ther 2000;17:70–83.

35. World Health Organization. Cancer pain relief with a guide to opioid availability. 2nd edition. Geneva (Switzerland): World Health Organization; 1996. p. 19.

36. Derogatis LR, Morrow GR, Fetting J, et al. The prevalence of psychiatric disorders among cancer patients. JAMA 1983;249:751–7.

37. Dowell D, Haegerich TM, Chou R. CDC guideline for prescribing opioids for chronic pain-United States, 2016. JAMA 2016;315(15):1624–45.

38. Kwon JH, Tanco K, Park JC, et al. Frequency, predictors, and medical record documentation of chemical coping among advanced cancer patients. Oncologist 2015;20:692–7.

39. Starr TD, Rogak LJ, Passik SD. Substance abuse in cancer pain. Curr Pain Headache Rep 2010;14:268–75.

40. Wasan AD, Butler SF, Budman SH, et al. Psychiatric history and psychologic adjustment as risk factors for aberrant drug-related behavior among patients with chronic pain. Clin J Pain 2007;23:307–15.

41. Edlund MJ, Martin BC, Fan MY, et al. Risks for opioid abuse and dependence among recipients of chronic opioid therapy: results from the TROUP study. Drug Alcohol Depend 2010;112:90–8.

42. de la Cruz M, Reddy A, Balankari V, et al. The impact of an educational program on patient practices for safe use, storage, and disposal of opioids at a comprehensive cancer center. Oncologist 2017;22:115–21.

43. Chou R. 2009 clinical guidelines from the American Pain Society and the American Academy of Pain Medicine on the use of chronic opioid therapy in chronic noncancer pain: what are the key messages for clinical practice? Pol Arch Med Wewn 2009;119:469–77.

44. Arthur JA, Edwards T, Lu Z, et al. Frequency, predictors, and outcomes of urine drug testing among patients with advanced cancer on chronic opioid therapy at an outpatient supportive care clinic. Cancer 2016;122:3732–9.

45. Anghelescu DL, Ehrentraut JH, Faughnan LG. Opioid misuse and abuse: risk assessment and management in patients with cancer pain. J Natl Compr Canc Netw 2013;11:1023–31.

46. Moore TM, Jones T, Browder JH, et al. A comparison of common screening methods for predicting aberrant drug-related behavior among patients receiving opioids for chronic pain management. Pain Med 2009;10:1426–33.

47. Williams N. The CAGE questionnaire. Occup Med (Lond) 2014;64:473–4.

48. Bernadt MW, Mumford J, Taylor C, et al. Comparison of questionnaire and laboratory tests in the detection of excessive drinking and alcoholism. Lancet 1982;1:325–8.

49. Dyson V, Appleby L, Altman E, et al. Efficiency and validity of commonly used substance abuse screening instruments in public psychiatric patients. J Addict Dis 1998;17:57–76.

50. Butler SF, Budman SH, Fernandez K, et al. Validation of a screener and opioid assessment measure for patients with chronic pain. Pain 2004;112:65–75.

51. Webster LR, Webster RM. Predicting aberrant behaviors in opioid-treated patients: preliminary validation of the Opioid Risk Tool. Pain Med 2005;6:432–42.

52. Barclay JS, Owens JE, Blackhall LJ. Screening for substance abuse risk in cancer patients using the Opioid Risk Tool and urine drug screen. Support Care Cancer 2014;22:1883–8.

53. Butler SF, Budman SH, Fanciullo GJ, et al. Cross validation of the current opioid misuse measure to monitor chronic pain patients on opioid therapy. Clin J Pain 2010;26:770–6.
54. Wu SM, Compton P, Bolus R, et al. The addiction behaviors checklist: validation of a new clinician-based measure of inappropriate opioid use in chronic pain. J Pain Symptom Manage 2006;32:342–51.
55. Wang J, Christo PJ. The influence of prescription monitoring programs on chronic pain management. Pain Physician 2009;12:507–15.
56. Prescription drug monitoring program training and technical assistance center. Available at: http://www.pdmpassist.org/content/state-pdmp-websites. Accessed February 27, 2018.
57. Feldman L, Skeel Williams K, Knox M, et al. Influencing controlled substance prescribing: attending and resident physician use of a state prescription monitoring program. Pain Med 2012;13:908–14.
58. Magnani B, Kwong T. Urine drug testing for pain management. Clin Lab Med 2012;32:379–90.
59. Lock it up: medicine safety in your home. US Food and Drug Administration Web site. Available at: www.fda.gov/forconsumers/consumerupdates/ucm272905.htm. Accessed February 27, 2018.
60. Kalso E, Edwards JE, Moore RA, et al. Opioids in chronic non-cancer pain: systematic review of efficacy and safety. Pain 2004;112:372–80.
61. Khantzian EJ, Treece C. DSM-III psychiatric diagnosis of narcotic addicts. Recent findings. Arch Gen Psychiatry 1985;42:1067–71.
62. Jamison RN, Ross EL, Michna E, et al. Substance misuse treatment for high-risk chronic pain patients on opioid therapy: a randomized trial. Pain 2010;150:390–400.
63. Passik SD, Portenoy RK, Ricketts PL. Substance abuse issues in cancer patients. Part 1: Prevalence and diagnosis. Oncology (Williston Park) 1998;12:517–21, 524.
64. Arthur J, Edwards T, Reddy S, et al. Outcomes of a specialized interdisciplinary approach for patients with cancer with aberrant opioid-related behavior. Oncologist 2018;23(2):263–70.
65. Coffin PO, Behar E, Rowe C, et al. NOnrandomized intervention study of naloxone coprescription for primary care patients receiving long-term opioid therapy for pain. Ann Intern Med 2016;165:245–52.
66. Kwon JH, Hui D, Bruera E. A pilot study to define chemical coping in cancer patients using the Delphi method. J Palliat Med 2015;18:703–6.
67. Del Fabbro E. Assessment and management of chemical coping in patients with cancer. J Clin Oncol 2014;32:1734–8.
68. Rinaldi RC, Steindler EM, Wilford BB, et al. Clarification and standardization of substance abuse terminology. JAMA 1988;259:555–7.
69. Weissman DE, Haddox JD. Opioid pseudoaddiction–an iatrogenic syndrome. Pain 1989;36:363–6.

Methadone
Maximizing Safety and Efficacy for Pain Control in Patients with Cancer

Mary Lynn McPherson, PharmD, MA, MDE, BCPS, CPE[a],*,
Ryan C. Costantino, PharmD, BCPS, BCGP[b],
Alexandra L. McPherson, PharmD, MPH[b]

KEYWORDS

• Methadone • Analgesics • Pain management • Cancer pain • Opioid

KEY POINTS

• Methadone is an important opioid option in the management of cancer pain. The pharmacodynamics and pharmacokinetics are dissimilar from other opioids.

• Not all patients are appropriate candidates for methadone; providers should perform a risk assessment before initiating methadone therapy.

• Opioid-naïve patients, or patients receiving up to 40 to 60 mg oral morphine equivalents a day should begin methadone at no higher than 7.5 mg a day.

• Opioid-tolerant patients should convert to methadone using a 10:1 or 20:1 (oral morphine/oral methadone) equivalent regimen.

• Providers and informal caregivers must carefully monitor the patient's response to methadone, both therapeutic and potential toxicity.

INTRODUCTION

Methadone is an important therapeutic option in the management of patients who have cancer with pain. Compared with other opioids, methadone offers advantages such as low cost, long half-life (allowing 2 or 3 times daily dosing), lack of active metabolites (advantageous in patients with renal impairment), availability as a high-concentrate oral solution (useful in patients with dysphagia), and benefit in more

None of the authors have any relationship with a commercial company that has a direct financial interest in subject matter or materials discussed in article or with a company making a competing product.
[a] Advanced Post-Graduate Education in Palliative Care, Online Master of Science and Graduate Certificates in Palliative Care, University of Maryland School of Pharmacy, 20 North Pine Street, S405, Baltimore, MD 21201, USA; [b] Pain Management/Palliative Care, University of Maryland School of Pharmacy, 20 North Pine Street, Baltimore, MD 21201, USA
* Corresponding author.
E-mail address: mmcphers@rx.umaryland.edu

Hematol Oncol Clin N Am 32 (2018) 405–415
https://doi.org/10.1016/j.hoc.2018.01.004
0889-8588/18/© 2018 Elsevier Inc. All rights reserved.

complex pain situations.[1] Methadone demands close attention to dosing, both in opioid-naïve and opioid-tolerant patients. Failure to respect best practices in methadone dosing and monitoring may result in serious toxicity or fatality. In recent years, methadone has been reported to cause a growing and disproportionately higher rate of opioid-induced deaths.[2] It is unclear what percentage of these deaths are due to inappropriate prescribing and monitoring of methadone, versus individual misuse or abuse.

PHARMACODYNAMICS AND PHARMACOKINETICS

Methadone is an opioid agonist, binding to the mu-, kappa-, and delta-opioid receptors.[3] Methadone also acts as an N-methyl-D-aspartate (NMDA) antagonist; the NMDA receptor is thought to be associated with opioid tolerance and central hypersensitivity, and to decreased clinical effectiveness of opioids for pain.[4] Methadone is a racemic mixture of 2 enantiomers (R-methadone and S-methadone). A basic and lipophilic opioid, methadone has high oral bioavailability (67%–95%). Onset of action after oral administration is about 30 minutes, with a peak effect at 2.5 hours. Methadone has a long and variable half-life (8–90 hours) but is approximated at 24 hours. Due to its lipophilicity, methadone is widely distributed throughout the body. It exhibits a high degree of protein binding. Methadone is extensively metabolized by the liver (cytochrome P [CYP]2B6, CYP2C19, CYP3A4, and CYP2D6) to pharmacologically inactive metabolites, which are then excreted by the kidneys.[3,5] The extensive hepatic metabolism of methadone predisposes to the numerous drug interactions involving methadone (see later discussion).

EFFICACY OF METHADONE IN CANCER PAIN

Mercadante and colleagues[6] evaluated the effectiveness of oral long-acting morphine, transdermal fentanyl, and oral methadone in cancer pain not responsive to codeine or tramadol. Subjects had mixed nociceptive-neuropathic cancer pain, and the 3 opioids were similarly effective in controlling pain (>30% reduction in pain).

Porta-Sales and colleagues[7] evaluated the efficacy and safety of methadone as a second-line opioid for patients in an outpatient cancer clinic. One hundred forty-five patients were switched to methadone because of poor pain control (77.9% of cases), opioid side effects (2.1%), or both (20%). The outcome measure was worst pain on day 28, and methadone was shown to be statistically superior ($P<.0001$). The median worst pain score decreased from 9 to 6 and no increase in opioid toxicity was noted.

Rhondali and colleagues[4] switched 19 subjects with cancer in an inpatient palliative care unit with refractory pain to methadone. The visual analog scale severity rating decreased by 4 points by day 7 after rotating to methadone, with almost 90% of patients reporting moderate to greater than moderate pain relief.

Reddy and colleagues[8] evaluated overall survival in patients with cancer after rotation to methadone. They compared 76 subjects switched to methadone with 88 subjects switched to other opioids on a follow-up clinic visit. In contrast to the Centers for Disease Control and Prevention report,[2] there were no significant differences between the 2 groups in subject characteristics, performance status, morphine-equivalent daily dose, pain scores, or median overall survival.

RISK ASSESSMENT AND APPROPRIATENESS OF METHADONE THERAPY

In 2014, the American Pain Society (APS) and College on Problems of Drug Dependence, in collaboration with the Heart Rhythm Society, published methadone safety guidelines to provide practitioners with guidance on safer prescribing of methadone for treatment of opioid addiction and chronic pain.[9] The guidelines recommend a comprehensive analysis of the benefit-to-harm ratio for all patients before starting methadone therapy, whether for pain management or treatment of addiction. They further acknowledge that opioid therapy is considered the mainstay of moderate to severe pain in patients with cancer, particularly those with advanced disease. However, the use of methadone warrants careful consideration because of its long and variable terminal elimination half-life, many associated drug–drug interactions, and effects on the electrocardiographic QTc interval and respiratory depression.

Methadone prolongs the QT interval (depolarization and repolarization time of the cardiac ventricles), referred to as the QTc (rate-corrected QT).[10] Prolongation of the QTc can lead to torsades de pointes, a potentially fatal ventricular arrhythmia. Risk factors for acquired QTc prolongation include medications (in addition to methadone), electrolyte disturbances (hypokalemia, hypomagnesemia, and hypocalcemia), structural heart disease, bradycardia, female sex, advanced age, history of QTc prolongation, and genetic polymorphisms.[11]

Despite the acknowledged causal relationship between methadone and QTc prolongation, the clinical significance in unclear. Bart and colleagues[10] recently conducted a retrospective cohort study of 749 subjects on methadone maintenance therapy for opioid use disorder. The mean QTc interval while taking methadone was significantly greater than while subjects were off methadone (436 ms vs 423 ms, respectively). However, the investigators concluded that methadone increased the QTc in a nonclinically significant dose-related manner. They suggested cardiac risk assessment recommendations be modified because their results showed cardiac events were rare and the sudden cardiac death rate was less than that of the general population.[10]

Reddy and colleagues[12] evaluated the effect of oral methadone on the QTc interval in subjects with advanced cancer. One hundred cancer pain subjects taking methadone seen in a palliative care setting were enrolled. Results showed that 28% of subjects had QTc prolongation at baseline (before starting methadone therapy; defined as QTc >430 ms in male patients and >450 ms in female patients). Electrocardiographic follow-up was performed at 2, 4, and 8 weeks after starting methadone therapy. Clinically significant increase in QTc was seen in 1 of 64 subjects at week 2 (defined as greater than 25% increase in QTc from baseline or QTc ≥500 ms), and in no subjects at weeks 4 and 8. The median dose of methadone at 2 weeks was 23 mg and no subjects received methadone in excess of 100 mg. The investigators' conclusion was that clinically significant QTc prolongation rarely occurs in patients with advanced cancer when receiving methadone doses less than 100 mg/d.[12]

The APS recommends obtaining a baseline electrocardiogram (ECG) before beginning methadone therapy in patients at risk for QTc interval prolongation, any prior ECG demonstrating a QTc greater than 450 ms, or a history suggestive of prior ventricular arrhythmia. An ECG obtained anytime in the previous 3 months with a QTC less than 450 ms and no new risk factors is sufficient. Further, they recommend clinicians consider obtaining an ECG if the patient has had an ECG in the previous year with a QTc less than 450 ms and no new risk factors. The panel recommended not using methadone if the QTc is greater than 500 ms, and to consider alternatives if the QTc is greater than or equal to 450 ms but less than 500 ms.[9] Soon after these guidelines were published, a group of hospice and palliative care (HPC) experts convened to interpret the guidelines specifically for HPC patients. The HPC experts were not quite as prescriptive regarding ECG monitoring; instead the group advised that clinicians should be guided by the patient's clinical situation and prognosis. For example, a patient with cancer admitted to hospice with no obvious risk factors for QTc prolongation probably does not require ECG monitoring.[13]

The HPC group of experts suggested that patients who are appropriate candidates for methadone include patients with moderate to severe pain (particularly if methadone is being considered as a second-line opioid), patients with a true morphine or phenanthrene allergy, and those with a preference and/or need for a long-acting opioid that can be administered as an oral solution. In addition to patients at very high risk of QTc prolongation, other potentially inappropriate candidates include patients who are clinically unstable, patients very close to death, and patients or families unable or unwilling to follow the prescribed plan of care.[13]

METHADONE DOSING IN OPIOID-NAÏVE PATIENTS

The APS guidelines define opioid-naïve patients as those receiving up to 40 to 60 mg/d of oral morphine equivalent, and recommend starting methadone at 2.5 mg 3 times daily in these patients. They further recommend increasing the total daily methadone dose by no more than 5 mg per day, and no more frequently than every 5 to 7 days.[9] The HPC expert group was a bit more prescriptive in this recommendation. They too considered patients receiving up to 40 to 60 mg oral morphine or equivalent per day as opioid-naïve, recommending a starting dose of 2 to 7.5 mg oral methadone per day. This more explicitly allows for selecting a starting dose such as 1 mg methadone by mouth twice daily (using the oral solution) as a starting dose. The HPC group agreed with the APS guidelines that the dose should be maintained for 5 to 7 days and increasing the total daily dose by no more than 5 mg per day.[13]

METHADONE DOSING IN OPIOID-TOLERANT PATIENTS

There are many suggested methods used to switch a patient from a different opioid to methadone. McLean and Twomey[14] completed a systematic review of the available evidence on methods to switch to methadone. They summarize the 5 primary methods used to rotate to methadone, which included various models of how and/or when to discontinue the original opioid and how and/or when to start methadone, different mathematical ratios of morphine to methadone, whether or not a higher initial methadone dose should be used, and different dosing intervals. Their conclusion was that there was no clear preferred method and the methodology in many of the studies reviewed was of low quality. Weschules and Bain[15] performed a similar systematic review in 2008 and concluded that "One important distinction that needs to be made is between methadone rotations as a *care process* as opposed to a *dose calculation*. It may be less important to determine an exact opioid ratio when performing a methadone conversion than it is to assure that the patient is an appropriate candidate for methadone rotation, the switch is carried out over a time period consistent with the therapeutic goals, and that the patient is monitored closely by medical staff throughout the process."

When switching opioid-tolerant patients to methadone, the APS guidelines recommend that "clinicians start methadone therapy at a dose 75% to 90% less than the calculated equianalgesic dose and at no higher than 30 to 40 mg/d, with an initial dose increase of no more than 10 mg/d every 5 to 7 days."[9] In other words, the APS guidelines advise that practitioners choose their preferred method but reduce the calculation by 75% to 90%. In an effort to give practitioners a bit more guidance, the HPC expert group recommended the following for converting to methadone[13]:

- For patients receiving less than 60 mg/d oral morphine or equivalent, refer to opioid-naïve dosing (eg, 2–7.5 mg oral methadone per day)
- For patients receiving 60 to 199 mg/d oral morphine equivalent and patients younger than 65 years of age, use a 10:1 conversion (10 mg oral morphine ≈ 1 mg oral methadone)
- For patients receiving greater than or equal to 200 mg/d oral morphine equivalent and/or patients aged 65 years or older, use a 20:1 conversion (20 mg oral morphine ≈ 1 mg oral methadone)
- Convert to no greater than 30 to 40 mg oral methadone per day regardless of the previous opioid regimen
- Dose should not be increased by more than 5 mg/d; when the total daily dose of methadone reaches 30 to 40 mg, it may increase by no more than 10 mg/d. In either case, do not increase dose more frequently than every 5 to 7 days.

METHADONE DOSING AS AN ADJUVANT MEDICATION

An emerging body of literature has demonstrated the benefit of using methadone as an adjuvant analgesic; in other words, adding a small dose of methadone to the patient's current regimen instead of rotating entirely to methadone. Wallace and colleagues[16] assessed the addition of low-dose methadone to the opioid regimen of patients with cancer pain, and showed that 75% of patients had a greater than or equal to 2 point reduction in their pain rating. The mean methadone dose was 4.4 mg at initiation and 15.5 mg at 1 month, and methadone was tolerated well by almost all patients. Salpeter and colleagues[17,18] demonstrated the benefit of adding very low dose methadone (median dose 5 mg) with excellent results. Courtemanche and colleagues[19] evaluated the addition of methadone (median dose 3 mg) to the opioid regimen of 146 subjects with cancer. Approximately half of the subjects were considered significant responders (≥30% reduction in pain intensity). They also concluded that the median time to significant response was 1 week (consistent with achieving steady state).

MONITORING RESPONSE TO METHADONE THERAPY

Patients receiving methadone should be monitored both for therapeutic effectiveness and potential toxicity. Due to its unique pharmacologic properties, including a high volume of distribution; high plasma protein binding; high lipophilicity; and a long, variable half-life and slow elimination phase, caution must be taken when initiating or titrating methadone.

When evaluating the methadone regimen for therapeutic effectiveness, the provider should ask about pain severity. (See Regina M. Fink and Jeannine M. Brant's article, "Complex Cancer Pain Assessment," in this issue.) Providers can ask patients to rate their pain severity on a 0 (no pain) to 10 (worst imaginable pain) scale, in addition to their best and worst severity rating on an average day, and the pain severity at rest and with movement. Even more important is an assessment of the patient's functional ability. Asses whether the methadone regimen improved the patient's functional status, including ambulation, ability to work in the home or at a job, sleep, and their affect (eg, better pain control may relieve depression or anxiety).

As with other opioids, the most common adverse effects associated with methadone include nausea, vomiting, constipation, dizziness, and sedation. With prolonged use, patients typically become tolerant to all of these adverse effects, with the exception of constipation. Less common but potentially serious adverse effects include QTc prolongation and respiratory depression (see previous discussion).

An important monitoring observation is that patients will generally exhibit increasing sedation before progressing to respiratory depression. Methadone has an average terminal elimination half-life of 24 hours; consequently, it takes 4 to 5 days for a patient to achieve steady state (and maximum therapeutic and toxic effect). It is imperative that providers monitor the patient's level of sedation early in therapy to avoid methadone accumulation causing respiratory depression. In fact, when switching a patient in pain to methadone from a different opioid regimen, if the pain is magically eradicated after 1 day of methadone, this is cause for serious consideration of decreasing the dose and for closer monitoring. After 1 day, the patient is only 50% of the way to steady state; after 4 to 5 days of methadone therapy, it may accumulate to a potentially toxic serum level. Therefore, close monitoring is critically important.

When starting methadone in a patient in the community, it is essential to educate both the patient and a reliable family member or caregiver on methadone monitoring. For the first 4 to 5 days after starting methadone, increasing the dose, or starting or stopping a medication that interacts with methadone, a caregiver should closely observe the patient every 2 to 3 hours while awake (eg, 4–5 times per day). To determine whether symptoms of overdose are present, the caregiver should assess the patient using following questions and take the following actions:

- Is the patient asleep? Is she or he easily awakened?
  - If this is a change and the patient is becoming more and more sleepy and harder to wake up, contact the prescriber.
- Is the patient snoring?
  - If the patient's snoring is new or worsening, contact the prescriber.
- Are other symptoms of overdose present?
  - Pinpoint pupils.
  - Slowed or difficult breathing; contact the prescriber.

METHADONE AND DRUG INTERACTIONS

There are numerous potential drug interactions with methadone, both pharmacodynamic and pharmacokinetic in nature. Pharmacodynamics refers to the pharmacologic effect of a medication (ie, what the drug does to the body). In a pharmacodynamic drug interaction, a drug heightens or diminishes the therapeutic effectiveness or toxicity of another drug. For example, a patient taking methadone for persistent pain may also have an order for oral morphine (also a mu-opioid agonist) for breakthrough pain. This is a purposeful drug interaction. It is an additive pharmacologic effect in which the morphine analgesia builds on the analgesia provided by the methadone.

Pharmacodynamic drug interactions are generally thought of as heightening drug toxicity. Methadone (like all opioids) is a central nervous system depressant, potentially causing sedation, sleep-disordered breathing, and respiratory depression. If the patient is taking an additional central nervous system depressant (eg, benzodiazepines, sedative-hypnotics, barbiturates), this increases the risk of sedation and respiratory depression. The US Food and Drug Administration has issued a safety advisory about the concurrent use of benzodiazepines and opioids, and the increased risk of toxicity and death.[20]

As previously discussed, methadone can prolong the QTc interval. If methadone is taken concurrently with other medications that have their own propensity to prolong the QTc interval, this effect will be cumulative, increasing the risk of torsades de pointes and sudden cardiac death. Examples of medications that prolong the QTc include antipsychotics and many antiarrhythmic agents. A useful Web site to determine medications that prolong the QTc is www.crediblemeds.org.[21] Medications that inhibit the metabolism of methadone, resulting in an increased methadone serum concentration, may increase the risk of sedation, respiratory depression, and QTc prolongation. It is crucial that practitioners consider the interactions with methadone when starting new medications or discontinuing medications. **Table 1** provides examples of how interacting medications affect methadone serum concentrations, as well as proposed actions.

PATIENT EDUCATION ABOUT METHADONE

In addition to providing guidance to patients and families about monitoring the patient's response to methadone, the following questions can serve as a guide for facilitating patient and caregiver education on methadone:

What Is This Medication Used for?

Methadone is an opioid analgesic (painkiller) used to treat moderate-to-severe persistent pain. It is also used to treat opioid addiction, which is not why you are receiving it.

Table 1
Methadone metabolism and management with selected enzyme inhibitors and inducers

Clinical Scenario	Drugs	Event	Implications	Actions
Patient taking a drug that is an enzyme-inhibitor	• Amprenavir • Carbamazepine • Efavirenz • Nelfinavir • Nevirapine • Phenobarbital • Phenytoin • Rifabutin • Rifampicin • Rifampin • Ritonavir • Spironolactone • St. John's Wort	• Decreased metabolism of methadone • Increased methadone serum level	• Methadone overdose • Toxicity	• May need to reduce methadone dose by 25% or more • Encourage use of rescue medication
Patient taking a drug that is an enzyme-inducer	• Amiodarone • Amitriptyline • Ciprofloxacin • Citalopram • Clarithromycin • Desipramine • Erythromycin • Fluconazole • Fluoxetine • Fluvoxamine • Itraconazole • Ketoconazole • Paroxetine • Sertraline • Telithromycin • Troleandomycin	• Increased metabolism of methadone • Decreased methadone serum level	• May decrease analgesia	• Encourage use of rescue medication • Reevaluate daily dose requirement

How Is This Medication Supplied?

Methadone is available as both brand and generic, and is available as an oral tablet, oral solution, or injectable formulation. There are several different brand names, including Dolophine and Methadone Intensol. Methadone tablets come in 5 mg and 10 mg, and the Methadone Intensol liquid solution comes as 10 mg/1 mL.[22]

When Do I Take the Medication and for How Long?

It is best to take methadone at evenly spaced times throughout the day (eg, every 8 hours or every 12 hours). Follow the dosage schedule prescribed by your prescriber.

How Should I Take This Medication?

You must take this medication exactly as your prescriber tells you to. Do not increase or decrease your dose, or stop taking this medication unless instructed to do so by your prescriber. Keep in mind, your prescriber may need to change your dose several times to find what works best for you (but do not do this on your own). This medication may be taken with or without food, and the instructions can vary based on the formulation prescribed.[22]

Oral liquid

Measure your dose with the measuring device supplied with the drug (not a household tablespoon). Mix it with 2 tablespoons of liquid (unless your prescriber tells you differently). Drink the medicine right away.

Tablet

Swallow the tablet whole. Do not crush, break, chew, or dissolve it. If you are having difficulty swallowing, speak with your prescriber or pharmacist because there are other formulations available.

What Should I Do if I Forget a Dose?

If you miss a dose, take it as soon as you remember. If it is less than 4 hours before your next dose, skip the missed dose and take your regularly scheduled dose. Never take a double dose to make up for a missed dose.[23]

What Food, Drinks, Dietary Supplements, or Activities Should I Avoid While Taking This Medication?

Do not drink alcohol while taking methadone because that is very dangerous, and you may even die. Methadone may cause dizziness and drowsiness, so you should not drive or operate machinery until you know how your body reacts to the methadone.[22,23]

What Are the Possible Side Effects and What Should I Do if They Occur?

Some of the more common side-effects you may experience include dizziness, drowsiness, nausea, vomiting, constipation, dry mouth, and sweating. Most of these side effects will go away within 2 weeks, when your body gets used to the medication. However, constipation will not go away. Increasing your fluid intake, exercising as tolerated, and taking a laxative regularly can help prevent constipation. If you experience stomach upset, nausea, or vomiting, try taking methadone with food; if still experiencing troublesome symptoms, your prescriber can give you a medicine to prevent them. To prevent dizziness, get up slowly when rising from a sitting or lying position. If you experience dry mouth, it may be helpful to chew sugarless gum or suck on sugar-free hard candy or ice chips. Allergic reactions to methadone are rare, but if you experience rash, hives, swelling, or difficulty breathing seek prompt medical attention. Over time, methadone can lead to physical dependence; therefore, do not stop methadone suddenly; that can lead to symptoms of withdrawal, including body aches, sweating, restlessness, irritability, shakiness, nausea, or vomiting.[24]

When Should I Expect the Medication to Begin to Work and How Will I Know It Is Working?

Methadone starts working with the first dose, but it can take several days for methadone to reach its maximum effect in your body. This is why your prescriber will not increase your dose for approximately 1 week. Your prescriber may also order a shorter-acting medication for breakthrough pain, or pain occurring in between your scheduled methadone doses. Starting methadone is like climbing a mountain. It takes several days to get to the top, so do not be afraid to use the available breakthrough medication.

Will This Medication Interact with the Other Prescription and Nonprescription Medications I Am Taking?

Some medications affect how methadone works. It is important to inform your prescriber of all the medications you are taking before starting methadone, and before starting or stopping other medications. This includes over-the-counter medications, prescription medications, and vitamins or supplements. Tell your prescriber if you are taking any of the medications listed **Box 1**. Also tell your prescriber if you are taking any of the following types of medications[22]:

Box 1
Selected medications that interact with methadone
Carbamazepine (Tegretol)
Desipramine (Norpramin)
Erythromycin
Fluconazole (Diflucan)
Fluvoxamine (Luvox)
Ketoconazole
Mirtazapine (Remeron)
Phenobarbital
Phenytoin (Dilantin)
Rifampin (Rifadin)
Ritonavir
Sertraline (Zoloft)
Stavudine (Zerit)
St. John's wort
Telaprevir (Incivek)
Tramadol (Ultram, Ryzolt)
Trazodone (Desyrel)
Voriconazole (Vfend)
Zidovudine (Retrovir)

- Blood pressure medication
- Diuretic (water pill)
- Depression medication
- Heart rhythm medication
- Triptan medication used to treat migraines.

How Should I Store This Medication at Home?

It is important that you store the methadone in a safe and secure place, away from family, visitors, children, and pets. Methadone should be stored in a closed container at room temperature, away from heat, moisture, and direct light. It is strongly suggested that you store the methadone in a locked box. If there ever comes a time when you are no longer on methadone, do not throw unused drug in the trash. Instead, ask your prescriber or pharmacist about the best way to dispose of unused medication. Some potential options for disposal include flushing your medication down the toilet, mixing it with coffee grounds or kitty litter and throwing it in the trash, or taking your medication to a Drug Enforcement Administration (DEA) Drug Takeback Day.[22,24,25]

REFERENCES

1. Good P, Afsharimani B, Movva R, et al. Therapeutic challenges in cancer pain management: a systematic review of methadone. J Pain Palliat Care Pharmacother 2014;28:197–205.
2. Centers for Disease Control and Prevention. Vital signs: risk for overdose from methadone used for pain relief – United States, 1999-2010. MMWR Morb Mortal Wkly Rep 2012;61:493–7.
3. Neto JOB, Garcia MA, Garcia JBS. Revisiting methadone: pharmacokinetics, pharmacodynamics and clinical indication. Rev Dor. São Paulo 2015;16(1):60–6.
4. Rhondali W, Tremellat F, Ledoux M, et al. Methadone rotation for cancer patients with refractory pain in a palliative care unit: an observational study. J Palliat Med 2013;16(11):1382–7.
5. Gerber JG, Rhodes RJ, Gal J. Stereoselective metabolism of methadone N-demethylation by cytochrome P4502B6 and 2C19. Chirality 2004;16(16):36–44.
6. Mercadante S, Porzio G, Ferrera P, et al. Sustained-release oral morphine versus transdermal fentanyl and oral methadone in cancer pain management. Eur J Pain 2008;12:1040–6.
7. Porta-Sales J, Garzon-Rodriguez C, Villavicencio-Chavez C, et al. Efficacy and safety of methadone as a second-line opioid for cancer pain in an outpatient clinic: a prospective open-label study. Oncologist 2016;21:981–7.
8. Reddy A, Schuler US, de la Cruz M, et al. Overall survival among cancer patients undergoing opioid rotation to methadone compared to other opioids. J Palliat Med 2017;20:656–61.
9. Chou R, Cruciani RA, Fiellin DA, et al. Methadone safety: a clinical practice guideline from the American Pain Society and College of Problems on Drug Dependence, in collaboration with the Heart Rhythm Society. J Pain 2014;15:321–37.
10. Bart G, Wyman Z, Wang Q, et al. Methadone and the QTc interval: paucity of clinically significant factors in a retrospective cohort. J Addict Med 2017;11(6):489–93.
11. Trinkley KE, Page RL, Lien H, et al. QT interval prolongation and the risk of torsades de pointes: essentials for clinicians. Curr Med Res Opin 2013;29(12):1719–26.
12. Reddy S, Hui D, Osta BE, et al. The effect of oral methadone on the QTc interval in advanced cancer patients: a prospective pilot study. J Palliat Med 2010;13(1):33–8.

13. McPherson ML. Methadone safety guidelines for hospice and palliative care. AAHPM Quarterly 2016;17(2):8–9.
14. McLean S, Twomey F. Methods of rotation from another strong opioid to methadone for the management of cancer pain: a systematic review of the available evidence. J Pain Symptom Manage 2015;50(2):248–59.
15. Weschules DJ, Bain KT. A systematic review of opioid conversion ratios used with methadone for the treatment of pain. Pain Med 2008;9(5):595–612.
16. Wallace E, Ridley J, Bryson J, et al. Addition of methadone to another opioid in the management of moderate to severe cancer pain: a case series. J Palliat Med 2013;16(3):305–9.
17. Salpeter SR, Buckley J, Bruera E. The use of very-low-dose methadone for palliative pain control and the prevention of opioid hyperalgesia. J Palliat Med 2013; 16(6):1–7.
18. Salpeter SR, Buckley JS, Buckley NS, et al. The use of very-low-dose methadone and haloperidol for pain control in the hospital setting: a preliminary report. J Palliat Med 2015;18(2):114–9.
19. Courtemanche F, Dao D, Gagne F, et al. Methadone as a coanalgesic for palliative care cancer patients. J Palliat Med 2016;19(9):1–7.
20. U.S. Food & Drug Administration. FDA Drug Safety Communication: FDA warns about serious risks and death when combining opioid pain or cough medicines with benzodiazepines; requires its strongest warning. 2016. Available at: https://www.fda.gov/Drugs/DrugSafety/ucm518473.htm. Accessed October 15, 2017.
21. Credible Meds. Available at: https://crediblemeds.org/. Accessed October 15, 2017.
22. Methadone. Micromedex solutions. Ann Arbor (MI): Truven Health Analytics, Inc. Available at: http://www.micromedexsolutions.com. Accessed October 10, 2017.
23. Nova Scotia Health Authority. Using methadone for chronic pain: patient & family guide. 2017. Available at: https://www.cdha.nshealth.ca/patientinformation/nshealthnet/0686.pdf. Accessed October 8, 2017.
24. VA National Pain Management Program. Available at: https://www.ethics.va.gov/docs/policy/Taking_Opioids_Responsibly_2013528.pdf. Accessed October 10, 2017.
25. Leavitt SB. Methadone safety handout for patients. Glenview (IL): Pain Treatment Topics; 2008. Available at: https://depts.washington.edu/fammed/files/Pt_Ed_Leavitt_Methadone_Handout%20for%20Pt_English_Spanish.pdf. Accessed October 8, 2017.

Cancer-Related Neuropathic Pain: Review and Selective Topics

Mellar P. Davis, MD

KEYWORDS

- Neuropathic • Pain • Neuroinflammation • Neuroplasticity • Analgesics
- Cannabinoids

KEY POINTS

- Neuropathic pain arises from neuroinflammation and neuroplasticity involving the somato-sensory system.
- Guidelines for treating cancer-related neuropathic pain rely on trials involving patients with noncancer neuropathic pain. Few trials are limited to cancer-related neuropathic pain.
- Opioid effectiveness in treating neuropathic pain is poorly defined with few high-quality studies. Combinations of antidepressants, anticonvulsants, and opioids are better than monotherapy and should be considered for patients not responding to single analgesics.
- Cannabinoids are popular, but benefits in managing neuropathic pain are not well defined with few high-quality trials. Many cannabinoids other than THC may have analgesic properties that should be explored.
- Scrambler therapy is a noninvasive modality with low risks as demonstrated in small single-arm studies.

INTRODUCTION

Neuropathic pain is defined by the International Association for the Study of Pain as "pain arising as a direct consequence of a lesion or disease which affects the somato-sensory system."[1] Central neuropathic pain arises largely from spinal cord injury, demyelinating diseases, or transverse myelitis. Peripheral neuropathic pain arises from damage to peripheral nerves and is more common than central neuropathic pain. Peripheral neuropathic pain will likely increase as the elderly population increases, and because of the increased incidence of diabetes mellitus, cancer, and cancer treatment-related neuropathy. Treatable causes of neuropathic pain include nutritional deficiencies (B_{12}, thiamine), cancer-induced nerve compression, spinal

Disclosure Statement: The author has no COI to disclose.
Department of Palliative Care, Geisinger Medical Center, 100 North Academy Avenue, Danville, PA 17822, USA
E-mail address: mdavis2@geisinger.edu

Hematol Oncol Clin N Am 32 (2018) 417–431
https://doi.org/10.1016/j.hoc.2018.01.005
0889-8588/18/© 2018 Elsevier Inc. All rights reserved.

cord compression, and brain metastases. Radiation-induced nerve damage and plex-opathy, diagnostic and therapeutic surgery-induced injury, and paraneoplastic syndromes are not preventable and require palliation.[2]

Physical findings, symptoms, and radiographs define cancer pain syndromes[3] (See Russell K. Portenoy and Ebtesam Ahmed's article, "Cancer Pain Syndromes," in this issue, for a full discussion). Patients should be assessed for depression, insomnia, quality of life, and reduced function, which occur with increasing frequency in patients with neuropathic pain, and complicate management.

Epigenetic changes from nerve injury, neuronal microRNA (miRNA) changes, activation of certain histone deacetylases, and DNA (deoxyribonucleic acid) methylation contribute to neuropathic pain and diminish analgesic responses. These epigenetic changes are biomarkers and potential targets for personalized pain management.

Treatment algorithms for cancer-related neuropathic pain are largely based on noncancer-related neuropathic pain guidelines; there are few studies restricted to patients with cancer-related pain. Recent studies suggest that in patients with noncancer neuropathic pain, therapy can be directed by phenotyping pain using specific questionnaires and quantitative sensory testing. Additional research studies examine the role of functional MRI (fMRI) and magnetic resonance spectroscopy.

EPIDEMIOLOGY OF NEUROPATHIC PAIN IN CANCER

Several studies explore the prevalence and associated morbidities of neuropathic pain in patients with cancer. Of 371 patients surveyed using the neuropathic pain questionnaire, the Douleur Neuropathique en 4, one-third had mixed nociceptive and neuropathic pain. Individuals with neuropathic pain more often had depression and insomnia compared with those who had nociceptive pain. Patients with neuropathic pain had a greater frequency of incident pain (odds ratio [OR], 2.63) and spontaneous breakthrough pain (OR, 3.67), were more likely to have received chemotherapy (OR, 2.93) and/or undergone surgery (OR, 3.6), and were on adjuvant analgesics (OR, 2.93). Pain lasted greater than 3 months (OR, 2.35) more often, and was of greater intensity (OR, 1.47).[4]

In a second survey of more than 1000 patients, one-third of whom had neuropathic pain,[5] the most common descriptor "pins and needles" (65%) was associated with greater pain severity than nociceptive pain and poorer quality of life.

MECHANISMS OF NEUROPATHIC PAIN

Cancer, its treatment, or related infections damage inhibitory interneurons within the superficial lamina of the dorsal horn, and cause alterations in anterior cingulate and amygdala connections to periaqueductal gray and loss of downward inhibition from the periaqueductal gray to the dorsal horn through the dorsal funiculus, in part from neuroplasticity involving receptors and neurotransmitters or microglia activation (neuroinflammation).[6–9]

Dorsal horn A-beta low-threshold afferents change from mechanical to sensory sensors, causing allodynia. Neuromas form and spontaneously discharge causing lightning-like pain. Upregulation of surviving neuron sodium and voltage-gated calcium channels cause continuous dysesthesia, spontaneous breakthrough pain, and allodynia. Loss of repolarizing potassium channels leads to spontaneous pain. Central sensitization causes more widespread pain outside of the injured dermatome.

The periaqueductal gray facilitates transmission of pain signals when the balance between inhibition and facilitation ("off" and "on" cells, respectively) is lost. With chronic pain, increased wide dynamic range neuron activity within the spinal cord causes temporal summation of pain. Brain default networks are altered causing increased insular cortex connectivity with other parts of the brain, promoting central sensitization. The subnucleus reticularis dorsalis responsible for conditioned pain modulation becomes impaired. In addition, "offset analgesia," governed by an unknown modulatory pathway through the brainstem, is impaired.[10]

Neuropathic pain is accompanied by neuroinflammation. Injured neuron central endings within the dorsal horn secrete chemokines (CX3CL1, CCL2, CCL21) that activate microglia. ATP from injured neurons activates microglia purinergic receptors. In return, microglia secrete brain-derived neurotrophic factor, which stimulates surviving neuron receptors, upregulates N-methyl-D-aspartate receptor (NMDA) receptors, and downregulates potassium repolarizing channels and γ-aminobutyric acid (GABA) receptors. Inhibitory signals through GABA receptors therefore diminish.[11]

Pain from peripheral nerve injury versus central sensitization can be clinically differentiated. Peripheral nerve injury produces positive or negative symptoms and signs (see later for symptoms) within a dermatome. Central sensitization is often widespread; pain extends to uninjured areas. It produces disproportionate pain to the degree of injury and correlates poorly with imaging studies. Central sensitization causes pain to multiple stimuli, including changes in weather.[12]

EPIGENETICS AND NEUROPATHIC PAIN

miRNAs regulate gene expression by preventing gene translation.[13] Neuropathic injury changes neuronal miRNA. It reduces expression of Beta-site Amyloid Precursor Protein Clearing enzyme-1, which increases miRNA-15b in animal models. Alternatively, miRNAs may be downregulated causing increased expression of trophic factors, such as brain-derived neurotrophic factor.[14] Dysregulation also influences expression of ion channels, glutamate receptors, and opioid receptors and modulates microglia activity.[15] Circulating miRNAs are promising diagnostic biomarkers of pain and potential targets for analgesics.[16]

Neuropathic injury upregulates histone deacetylases that downregulates opioid receptors, glutamate transporters, and potassium channels.[17] Histone deacetylase inhibitors improve opioid receptor expression and morphine analgesia in animal models. Valproic acid, a histone deacetylase inhibitor, restores glutamate transporters function in neuropathic-injured animals and reduces pain behaviors.[18] The Nicotinamide Adenine Dinucleotide dependent acetylase SIRT-1, critical for maintaining axon function, is downregulated with chronic constrictive injury. Resveratrol upregulates SIRT-1 and reduces neuropathic pain behaviors in animals.

DNA methylation enzymes act on promoter site CpG islands and 5″ untranslated sites of the mu gene receptor site resulting in downregulation of receptor expressions diminishing opioid responses.[19] Methylation of voltage-gated potassium channel genes impairs expression of these repolarization channels.[20]

Epigenetic changes alter morphine distribution in neuropathy. Neuropathic injured animals have reduced morphine brain levels compared with uninjured animals, from upregulation of the conjugase family UGT 2B and P-glycoprotein.[21] Epigenetic changes in opioid receptors and altered drug distribution contribute to poor opioid responses in patients with neuropathic pain.

CLINICAL AND RESEARCH EVALUATION OF PATIENTS WITH NEUROPATHIC PAIN

Diagnosis is based on the history and physical examination. Patients present with dysesthesias/paresthesias[22] (so-called positive symptoms) or negative symptoms (numbness) within a dermatome or "stocking and glove" distribution. Other positive symptoms are tingling, pins and needles sensations, prickling, burning, electric shock, or squeezing. In response to heat cold or touch, patients experience allodynia or hyperpathia. Negative symptoms are numbness, loss of sensation, loss of reflexes, and motor weakness in painful areas. Neuropathic screening questionnaires include Douleur Neuropathique en 4, the Neuropathic Pain Inventory, Pain DETECT, Leeds Assessment of Neuropathic Pain Symptoms, Neuropathic Pain Questionnaire, and the Short Form of the McGill Pain Questionnaire.[23]

On examination, patients have hypoesthesia to tactile stimulus, cold or warmth, or paradoxic hypoalgesia to painful stimuli. Hyperalgesia to pinprick, blunt pressure, and cold or heat allodynia to pin prick or soft brush across the dermatome also helps confirm neuropathic pain.[24]

Quantitative sensory testing assists in defining three clusters of pain phenotypes that are not disease specific, but can guide further therapy: (1) cluster 1, patients with pronounced deficits in temperature and mechanical sensation; (2) cluster 2, patients with normal thermal thresholds and a gain in sensory pain, particularly thermal pain; and (3) cluster 3, patients with pronounced deficits in thermal sensation and gain in mechanical pain.[25]

Patients with preserved sensory function and gain in sensory pain (subtype Cluster 2) are more likely to respond to sodium channel blockers, such as oxcarbazepine, than those with profound sensory loss (number needed to treat [NNT], 3.9 vs 13).[26] Individuals with postherpetic neuralgia and high heat pain thresholds are more likely to respond to tricyclic antidepressants than those with normal heat pain thresholds.[27] Patients with diabetes with increased spontaneous pain from capsaicin are more likely to respond to topical clonidine.[28] Patients with diabetes with impaired conditioned pain modulators are more likely to respond to duloxetine.[29] Unfortunately, these personalized approaches have not been tested in patients with cancer with neuropathic pain.

Research tools can identify neuropathic pain before clinical symptoms develop. Pseudomotor function, tested by iontophoretic-stimulated sweat output, is impaired early in neuropathic pain. Changes reflect small fiber neuropathy common with diabetes and chemotherapy-induced peripheral neuropathy (CIPN).[30] Punch skin biopsies detect small fiber neuropathy early, showing small nerve fiber swelling, reduced fiber length, reduced fiber density, and diminished sweat gland innervation. Intradermal nerve fiber density has better utility and sensitivity than quantitative sensory testing in detecting CIPN.[31]

Used as research tools, fMRI and magnetic resonance spectroscopy provide additional insights. fMRI demonstrates a complex relationship between pain intensity, symptoms, and brain structure through altered connectivity among brain areas involved in pain processing.[32] Chronic pain reduces gray matter, changes white matter, and alters connectivity among brain default networks.[33] Chronic pain increases glutamate in insula cortex, which is associated with increased connectivity between insular cortex and other brain areas within the "pain matrix." Pregabalin, interestingly, reduces insula glutamate levels and connectivity between insula and other brain areas.[34]

THE MANAGEMENT OF CANCER-RELATED NEUROPATHIC PAIN: SELECTIVE TOPICS
Gaps in Guidelines for Neuropathic Pain

A systematic review of nine guidelines for cancer-related neuropathic pain found more than 70% of the references for recommendations involved treatment of patients with noncancer neuropathic pain; only 11% involved treatment of cancer-related neuropathy and only 18% of references were shared between two guidelines.[35]

A systematic review of 30 studies involving drug management of neuropathic pain in patients with cancer included 16 prospective studies and 14 randomized controlled trials. Outcome was the absolute risk benefits; that is, the total number of responders (those experiencing a 30%–50% reduction in pain intensity) divided by the total number of patients treated. Because more than half of trials were nonrandomized, the risk of bias was significant. The absolute risk benefits for antidepressants was 0.55 (95% confidence interval [CI], 0.4–0.69), anticonvulsants 0.57 (95% CI, 0.44–0.7), opioids 0.95 (95% CI 0.93–0.96) and other adjuvants 0.45 (95% CI, 0.33–0.57). Patients with mixed neuropathic and nociceptive pain benefitted to the same degree as patients with neuropathic pain only. Pain intensity differences compared with baseline were 25% for antidepressants, 48% for anticonvulsants, 82% for opioids, and 68% for other adjuvant analgesics. Dropout rates for all classes of medications was less than 15%.[36]

Antidepressants

Tricyclic antidepressants

Tricyclic antidepressants are the oldest class of analgesics for neuropathic pain. Doses needed for neuropathic pain are lower than those for depression; analgesia occurs sooner than antidepressant effects.[37] Amitriptyline, imipramine, desipramine, and nortriptyline have been used with the latter two preferred because of fewer anticholinergic side effects. Tricyclic antidepressants block NMDA receptors and sodium channels, block uptake of spinal noradrenaline (which facilitates brainstem downward inhibition) and adenosine (which binds to adenosine receptors), and blunt neuroinflammation.[38] Tricyclic antidepressants are helpful for those with pain and insomnia.[39] The NNT for tricyclic antidepressants in several trials ranged between 1.9 and 4.5 for desipramine, 1.7 and 3.2 for imipramine, and 2.5 and 4.2 for amitriptyline.[40] These benefits might be an overestimate because of the small number of patients in each trial and the trial designs.[41]

Cytochrome CYP2D6 is important to amitriptyline and imipramine clearance. The Food and Drug Administration recommends monitoring tricyclic antidepressant levels when coadministered with drugs known to block CYP2D6.[42] Initial doses are 10 to 25 mg at night with slow titration to 150 mg if needed.[43] Tricyclic antidepressants can cause dizziness, sedation, orthostatic hypotension, dry mouth, and other anticholinergic side effects. Avoid tricyclic antidepressants in patients with cardiac arrhythmias and heart failure.

Selective norepinephrine reuptake inhibitors

Selective norepinephrine reuptake inhibitors (SNRIs), but not selective serotonin reuptake inhibitors, have demonstrated efficacy in patients with neuropathic pain. All selective serotonin reuptake inhibitors and SNRI antidepressants can cause a serotonin syndrome when combined with tramadol or certain potent opioids.[44] This drug interaction is common.

Venlafaxine

Venlafaxine is an SNRI at doses greater than 150 mg/d. It is O-demethylated by CYP2D6 to desvenlafaxine that is more potent than the parent drug. Venlafaxine is 40% bioavailable; steady state concentrations are reached at 3 days. Starting doses are 37.5 mg daily and are doubled weekly. Analgesia for neuropathic pain (excluding acute pain with taxanes and oxaliplatin) requires doses of 150 mg to 225 mg for noradrenaline reuptake inhibition.[45]

Six trials, involving 460 patients, were included in a systematic review of randomized trials.[46] Most patients had diabetic neuropathy. There were no trials of venlafaxine for cancer-related neuropathic pain. Four of six trials were positive. In the largest trial the NNT was 4.5 compared with placebo.[47]

A narrative review of venlafaxine for neuropathic pain found 13 studies of which 11 were randomized controlled trials. Two trials involved patients with oxaliplatin or taxane acute neuropathy.[48] In this review, venlafaxine was inferior to pregabalin, equivalent to imipramine, and superior or equivalent to carbamazepine, although studies were small and involved heterogeneous populations. Doses of 37.5 mg to 50 mg per day up to 75 mg daily reduced acute neuropathic pain from taxanes and oxaliplatin, although these studies were small and one was a case control study.

Venlafaxine can cause hypertension and prolong the QTc interval. Use caution when adding venlafaxine to other QTc-prolonging medications, such as haloperidol or methadone. Venlafaxine produces a severe withdrawal syndrome if abruptly stopped.

Duloxetine

Duloxetine has oral bioavailability of 50% and elimination half-life of 10 to 12 hours. It is metabolized through CYP1A2 and CYO2D6. Inhibitors of CYP2D6 increase plasma levels. Unlike venlafaxine, duloxetine metabolites are not active. Duloxetine should be avoided in advanced liver disease and renal failure.[49]

Duloxetine is licensed to treat diabetic neuropathy. Doses of 60 mg daily improve pain with an NNT of five. Duloxetine improves fibromyalgia, painful physical symptoms arising from depression, chronic osteoarthritis pain, and low back pain but not central neuropathic pain.[50] There are no trials in cancer-related neuropathic pain.

Initial doses are 20 mg to 30 mg daily, increasing to 60 mg daily 1 week later. There are no benefits to doses of 120 mg daily. Side effects include nausea, dizziness, headache, irritability, dry mouth, constipation and hyperhidrosis.[51] Nausea and other side effects diminish over time.[52] Duloxetine lacks cardiovascular adverse effects, unlike venlafaxine and tricyclic antidepressants.[53] Duloxetine has the best evidence for treating CIPN.[54]

Other antidepressants

Paroxetine and citalopram improve diabetic neuropathic pain in small randomized trials. No studies are reported for treating cancer-related neuropathic pain.[55]

Mirtazapine increases pain tolerance in healthy individuals but has weak evidence for reducing pain in patients with cancer.[56] Mirtazapine, 7.5 mg every 12 hours, was compared with pregabalin, 150 mg every 8 hours, in patients with metastatic bone pain; mirtazapine was superior, particularly in relieving paroxysmal pain.[57] Mirtazapine facilitates serotonin neurotransmission through 5HT1a receptors while blocking postsynaptic 5HT2 and 5HT3 receptors and enhances noradrenaline levels in the spinal cord as a second mechanism.[58] Mirtazapine improves sleep, reversing the lowered pain threshold from the decrease in nonrapid eye movement sleep caused by neuropathic pain.[59] Side effects include drowsiness, daytime sedation, increased appetite, and weight gain.

Anticonvulsants

Gabapentinoids

Gabapentin blocks voltage gated calcium channel expression by binding to alpha-2 delta subunits, increases central nervous system GABA levels, improves cholinergic neurotransmission, and prevents neuroactive transmitter release (glutamate) indirectly blocking NMDA receptors. Gabapentin enhances inhibitory neurotransmission through the periaqueductal gray, and blunts neuroinflammatory responses to neuropathic injury and neuroplastic synaptogenesis.[60] Increased central nervous system GABA levels lead to improved sleep, reduced anxiety, mood stabilization, and antiseizure activity.[61] Gabapentin stabilizes sleep disorders in medical illnesses, which can be particularly helpful in patients with neuropathic pain and insomnia.[62]

Gabapentin is absorbed through a small bowel transporter, causing a dose-dependent reduction in bioavailability from transporter saturation. Bioavailability is reduced from 60% to 33% as doses are increased from 900 mg to 3600 mg daily.[63] Gabapentin is not metabolized by hepatic enzymes nor inhibits cytochromes or conjugases. Dose reductions are needed in renal failure. Elimination half-life is 5 to 9 hours so that dosing should be three times daily.[64] Initial doses are 100 mg three times a day or 100 mg twice a day and 300 mg at nighttime. Doses can be increased by 300 mg daily.[65]

In a randomized trial involving 121 patients with cancer, gabapentin was opioid sparing and reduced pain with toxicities similar to placebo. The NNT was 7.3 for a 33% reduction in pain intensity; doses ranged in this study from 600 to 1800 mg daily.[66] In a systematic review, 9 of 14 randomized gabapentin trials were positive. Four of six randomized trials involving extended-release gabapentin or gabapentin enacarbil were positive. The NNT was 6.3 (95% CI, 5–8.3) with a number needed to harm (NNH) for withdrawal from trial of 25.6 (95% CI, 15.3–78.6). Doses ranged from 900 to 3600 mg daily.[43] An updated Cochrane Database Review found 37 gabapentin studies involving 5914 patients. The NNT was 6.7 (95% CI, 5.4–8.7) for a 50% reduction in pain and 4.8 (95% CI, 4.1–6.0) for a 30% reduction in pain. The NNH was 30 (95% CI, 20–65).[67] Side effects were dizziness (19%), somnolence (14%), peripheral edema (7%), and gait disturbances (14%). The average dose was 1200 mg daily.

Gabapentin has been used to treat CIPN. Although a small nonrandomized trial was positive,[68] gabapentin failed to improve CIPN in the randomized trial.[69]

Pregabalin

The mechanisms by which pregabalin reduces pain are similar to gabapentin.[70] However, pregabalin reduces pain in patients who have not responded to gabapentin.[71]

Oral bioavailability is 90% with peak concentrations occurring earlier than gabapentin (0.7–1.3 hours vs 2–4 hours). Food delays pregabalin absorption and reduces maximum concentration but not overall bioavailability. Pregabalin is not metabolized by the liver, does not interact with hepatic enzymes, and is highly dependent on renal clearance.[63] It is 2.5 times more potent than gabapentin. Starting doses are 50 to 75 mg twice daily, which is doubled every 1 to 2 days to a maximum of 600 mg daily. Side effects are like gabapentin. Both gabapentinoids can be abused.[72]

Pregabalin reduces dysesthesia, lancinating pain, and opioid doses more than amitriptyline or gabapentin.[73] Seventy-three percent of pregabalin-treated patients had a 30% reduction in pain intensity compared with 37% of fentanyl-treated patients (P<.001).[74] Maximum doses were 600 mg daily and transdermal fentanyl 150 μg/h.

A systematic review of pregabalin found 18 of 25 randomized trials positive. Pregabalin doses ranged from 150 to 600 mg daily. Patients receiving 600 mg daily had better responses than those on 300 mg daily. The NNT was 7.7 (95% CI, 6.5–9.4) and NNH 13.9 (95% CI, 11.6–17.4).[43] Pregabalin is effective regardless of the duration of neuropathic pain before treatment.[75]

Other anticonvulsants

There is weak evidence and poor safety profile for carbamazepine (except for trigeminal neuralgia), oxcarbazepine, valproic acid, topiramate, and zonisamide in patients with cancer with neuropathic pain. The NNH is 6.3 (95% CI, 5.1–8) indicating a narrow therapeutic index. Levetiracetam trials are negative.[43]

Opioids

The quality of evidence supporting the use of buprenorphine,[76] fentanyl,[77] morphine,[78] oxycodone, or hydromorphone[79] alone for neuropathic pain is low. Methadone is reviewed extensively by Mary Lynn McPherson and colleagues' article, "Methadone: Maximizing Safety and Efficacy for Pain Control in Patients with Cancer," in this issue. Tramadol, a nonopioid that binds opiate receptors, showed improved efficacy compared with placebo.[80]

A Cochrane database systematic review of 31 randomized trials and 10 different opioids found the NNT to reduce pain severity by 33% was 4.0 and by 50% was 5.9. Toxicities were significant. The NNH for constipation was 4.0, drowsiness 7.1, nausea 6.3, dizziness 7.1, and withdrawal because of toxicity 12.5.[80] This systematic review demonstrated weak evidence for opioids and a narrow therapeutic index. When treating cancer-related neuropathic pain, consider starting with gabapentinoids, tricyclic antidepressants, and SNRIs, even if their neuropathic pain is a mixed neuropathic and nociceptive pain.[74]

Analgesic Combinations

Randomized trials demonstrate that adding either a tricyclic antidepressant (nortriptyline or amitriptyline) or gabapentinoid (gabapentin or pregabalin) to opioids (morphine or oxycodone) or tramadol improves dysesthesias, pain, and vitality and social functioning in patients with cancer and noncancer-related neuropathic pain.[81–83] That a lower dose of gabapentin is needed in the combination may be related to delayed renal clearance caused by morphine or morphine metabolites.[81] There have been no trials comparing opioids and SNRIs in combination.

Combinations of antidepressants (mirtazapine, duloxetine, nortriptyline, or imipramine) with anticonvulsants (gabapentin or pregabalin) are more effective than either agent alone in reducing cancer-related pain.[83] For patients not responding to gabapentin (at doses >900 mg per day), a switch to pregabalin or duloxetine or the addition of duloxetine to gabapentin were successful in improving pain control.[82]

A systematic review using a Delphi-guided guideline and a Cochrane database systematic review recommended the combination of an opioid and either a tricyclic antidepressant or gabapentinoid or the combination of a gabapentinoid plus tricyclic antidepressant or duloxetine as evidence-based combinations for patients not responding to monotherapy.[83] Tricyclic antidepressants should not be combined with SNRIs. SNRIs and tricyclic antidepressants should not be combined with tramadol because of drug interactions and the risk of developing a serotonin syndrome.[84]

Cannabinoids

There is a significant public interest in the use of medical cannabis to treat pain.[85] It is estimated that 17% to 18% of patients in pain try medical cannabis in some form. Smoked cannabis has been associated with pulmonary aspergillus, so the cannabis should be radiated or smoking should be discouraged in those undergoing active cancer treatment.[86]

Opioid use and deaths diminish in states that have decriminalized medical cannabis, and some advocates suggest that cannabis is a safe substitution for opioids.[87] Although many animal studies suggest that cannabis has antitumor activity, patients should be cautioned that cannabis has also been shown to stimulate tumor growth.[88] Plant cannabis does not cause respiratory depression because cannabis receptors (CB1 and CB2) are absent in brainstem respiratory centers. However, synthetic cannabinoids, which are sometimes mixed with plant cannabis, can cause respiratory depression.[89]

Patients with advanced cancer and pain are attracted to cannabis because it is reported to stimulate appetite, reduce nausea, and have anticancer activity. There is little randomized trial evidence that substantiates these claims. Cannabis stimulates appetites in patients with human immunodeficiency virus but not cancer. Cannabis antiemetic activity is through 5HT3 receptors, which are blocked more effectively by 5HT3 antagonists.[90,91]

The evidence for cannabis as an analgesic for neuropathic pain is far from robust.[92] In the meta-analysis pain was reduced relative to placebo; 37% versus 31%, respectively (OR, 1.41; 95% CI, 0.99–2.00) in eight trials. The average reduction in numerical rating scale pain assessment (on a 0–10-point scale; weighted mean difference), was −0.46 (95% CI, −0.80 to −0.11) in six trials.[92] Three additional systematic reviews had mixed enthusiasm.[93] There are also negative trials and a lack of evidence for comparative effectiveness with nonopioid active analgesics.[94] Some guidelines place cannabis as third-line therapy for neuropathic pain, whereas others exclude cannabinoids because of the weak evidence and side effects.[43] The Canadian Agency for Drugs and Technologies in Health in a Rapid Response Report stated that the evidence for oromucosal THC/CBD (which has had nine trials) is insufficient to make well-founded conclusions about the benefits in neuropathic pain.[94]

Noninvasive Neuromodulation (Scrambler Therapy)

Scrambler therapy (MC5-A Calmare, Competitive Technologies Inc, Fairfield, CT) is Food and Drug Administration–approved. It is based on the premise that nerve stimulation across an area of neuropathic pain reduces ectopic pulses from surviving sensory nerves, enhancing inhibitory gating of pain in the dorsal horn and/or reducing wind up.[95] Although no randomized trials are reported, there are several small studies involving patients with cancer and neuropathic pain.[96,97] The procedure requires placement of surface silver gel electrodes proximal and distal to the painful site. Electrical stimulus is increased up to maximum tolerated levels using a frequency of 43 to 52 Hz. If pain is not relieved, the stimulus is turned off and the electrode pair is repositioned. One to five sets of electrodes may be placed. Sessions last approximately 30 to 40 minutes daily, 5 days a week for 2 weeks.[98] Responses are reported to last for months. Scrambler therapy can be repeated if pain relapses.

SUMMARY AND FUTURE DIRECTION

Neuropathic pain arises from neuroinflammation and neuroplasticity. Further studies using quantitative sensory testing and fMRI are needed to better phenotype and classify neuropathic pain, with the hope that more effective analgesics can be selected. Guidelines for treating cancer-related neuropathic pain are largely dependent on trials involving patients with noncancer neuropathic pain. Specific trials in cancer-related neuropathic pain would provide a better basis for treatment. CIPN is resistant to standard analgesics. Future investigations should also focus on mechanisms of CIPN and preventive therapies. Few high-quality studies provide guidance on the use of opioids alone. It is clear, however, that combinations of antidepressants, gabapentinoids, and opioids are better than monotherapy. Additional trials are needed to define the optimal combinations. The benefits of cannabinoids are ill-defined with few high-quality trials. Scrambler therapy is a noninvasive modality with low risks and should be tested in randomized trials.

REFERENCES

1. Merskey H. Clarifying definition of neuropathic pain. Pain 2002;96(3):408–9.
2. Vadalouca A, Raptis E, Moka E, et al. Pharmacological treatment of neuropathic cancer pain: a comprehensive review of the current literature. Pain Pract 2012; 12(3):219–51.
3. Kocoglu H, Pirbudak L, Pence S, et al. Cancer pain, pathophysiology, characteristics and syndromes. Eur J Gynaecol Oncol 2002;23(6):527–32.
4. Bouhassira D, Luporsi E, Krakowski I. Prevalence and incidence of chronic pain with or without neuropathic characteristics in patients with cancer. Pain 2017; 158(6):1118–25.
5. Lu F, Song L, Xie T, et al. Current status of malignant neuropathic pain in Chinese patients with cancer: report of a hospital-based investigation of prevalence, etiology, assessment, and treatment. Pain Pract 2017;17(1):88–98.
6. Zhao H, Alam A, Chen Q, et al. The role of microglia in the pathobiology of neuropathic pain development: what do we know? Br J Anaesth 2017;118(4):504–16.
7. Samineni VK, Premkumar LS, Faingold CL. Neuropathic pain-induced enhancement of spontaneous and pain-evoked neuronal activity in the periaqueductal gray that is attenuated by gabapentin. Pain 2017;158(7):1241–53.
8. Tsuda M, Koga K, Chen T, et al. Neuronal and microglial mechanisms for neuropathic pain in the spinal dorsal horn and anterior cingulate cortex. J Neurochem 2017;141(4):486–98.
9. Khangura RK, Bali A, Jaggi AS, et al. Histone acetylation and histone deacetylation in neuropathic pain: an unresolved puzzle? Eur J Pharmacol 2017;795:36–42.
10. Colloca L, Ludman T, Bouhassira D, et al. Neuropathic pain. Nat Rev Dis Primers 2017;3:17002.
11. Tsuda M. Microglia in the spinal cord and neuropathic pain. J Diabetes Investig 2016;7(1):17–26.
12. Nijs J, Goubert D, Ickmans K. Recognition and treatment of central sensitization in chronic pain patients: not limited to specialized care. J Orthop Sports Phys Ther 2016;46(12):1024–8.
13. Lopez-Gonzalez MJ, Landry M, Favereaux A. MicroRNA and chronic pain: from mechanisms to therapeutic potential. Pharmacol Ther 2017;180:1–15.
14. Bali KK, Hackenberg M, Lubin A, et al. Sources of individual variability: miRNAs that predispose to neuropathic pain identified using genome-wide sequencing. Mol Pain 2014;10:22.
15. Zhao X, Tang Z, Zhang H, et al. A long noncoding RNA contributes to neuropathic pain by silencing Kcna2 in primary afferent neurons. Nat Neurosci 2013;16(8): 1024–31.
16. Cogswell JP, Ward J, Taylor IA, et al. Identification of miRNA changes in Alzheimer's disease brain and CSF yields putative biomarkers and insights into disease pathways. J Alzheimers Dis 2008;14(1):27–41.
17. Uchida H, Sasaki K, Ma L, et al. Neuron-restrictive silencer factor causes epigenetic silencing of Kv4.3 gene after peripheral nerve injury. Neuroscience 2010; 166(1):1–4.
18. Hobo S, Eisenach JC, Hayashida K. Up-regulation of spinal glutamate transporters contributes to anti-hypersensitive effects of valproate in rats after peripheral nerve injury. Neurosci Lett 2011;502(1):52–5.
19. Sun L, Zhao JY, Gu X, et al. Nerve injury-induced epigenetic silencing of opioid receptors controlled by DNMT3a in primary afferent neurons. Pain 2017;158(6): 1153–65.

20. Zhao JY, Liang L, Gu X, et al. DNA methyltransferase DNMT3a contributes to neuropathic pain by repressing Kcna2 in primary afferent neurons. Nat Commun 2017;8:14712.

21. Ochiai W, Kaneta M, Nagae M, et al. Mice with neuropathic pain exhibit morphine tolerance due to a decrease in the morphine concentration in the brain. Eur J Pharm Sci 2016;92:298–304.

22. Gilron I, Watson CP, Cahill CM, et al. Neuropathic pain: a practical guide for the clinician. CMAJ 2006;175(3):265–75.

23. Dworkin RH, Turk DC, Revicki DA, et al. Development and initial validation of an expanded and revised version of the short-form McGill Pain Questionnaire (SF-MPQ-2). Pain 2009;144(1–2):35–42.

24. Hansson P, Backonja M, Bouhassira D. Usefulness and limitations of quantitative sensory testing: clinical and research application in neuropathic pain states. Pain 2007;129(3):256–9.

25. Baron R, Maier C, Attal N, et al. Peripheral neuropathic pain: a mechanism-related organizing principle based on sensory profiles. Pain 2017;158(2):261–72.

26. Demant DT, Lund K, Vollert J, et al. The effect of oxcarbazepine in peripheral neuropathic pain depends on pain phenotype: a randomised, double-blind, placebo-controlled phenotype-stratified study. Pain 2014;155(11):2263–73.

27. Edwards RR, Haythornthwaite JA, Tella P, et al. Basal heat pain thresholds predict opioid analgesia in patients with postherpetic neuralgia. Anesthesiology 2006; 104(6):1243–8.

28. Campbell CM, Kipnes MS, Stouch BC, et al. Randomized control trial of topical clonidine for treatment of painful diabetic neuropathy. Pain 2012;153(9):1815–23.

29. Yarnitsky D, Granot M, Nahman-Averbuch H, et al. Conditioned pain modulation predicts duloxetine efficacy in painful diabetic neuropathy. Pain 2012;153(6): 1193–8.

30. Thaisetthawatkul P, Fernandes Filho JA, Herrmann DN. Contribution of QSART to the diagnosis of small fiber neuropathy. Muscle Nerve 2013;48(6):883–8.

31. Devigili G, Tugnoli V, Penza P, et al. The diagnostic criteria for small fibre neuropathy: from symptoms to neuropathology. Brain 2008;131(Pt 7):1912–25.

32. Brodersen KH, Wiech K, Lomakina EI, et al. Decoding the perception of pain from fMRI using multivariate pattern analysis. Neuroimage 2012;63(3):1162–70.

33. Baliki MN, Schnitzer TJ, Bauer WR, et al. Brain morphological signatures for chronic pain. PLoS One 2011;6(10):e26010.

34. Harris RE, Napadow V, Huggins JP, et al. Pregabalin rectifies aberrant brain chemistry, connectivity, and functional response in chronic pain patients. Anesthesiology 2013;119(6):1453–64.

35. Piano V, Verhagen S, Schalkwijk A, et al. Diagnosing neuropathic pain in patients with cancer: comparative analysis of recommendations in national guidelines from European countries. Pain Pract 2013;13(6):433–9.

36. Jongen JL, Huijsman ML, Jessurun J, et al. The evidence for pharmacologic treatment of neuropathic cancer pain: beneficial and adverse effects. J Pain Symptom Manage 2013;46(4):581–90.e1.

37. Mika J, Zychowska M, Makuch W, et al. Neuronal and immunological basis of action of antidepressants in chronic pain: clinical and experimental studies. Pharmacol Rep 2013;65(6):1611–21.

38. Wolff M, Czorlich P, Nagaraj C, et al. Amitriptyline and carbamazepine utilize voltage-gated ion channel suppression to impair excitability of sensory dorsal horn neurons in thin tissue slice: an in vitro study. Neurosci Res 2016;109:16–27.

39. Gilron I, Baron R, Jensen T. Neuropathic pain: principles of diagnosis and treatment. Mayo Clin Proc 2015;90(4):532–45.
40. Saarto T, Wiffen PJ. Antidepressants for neuropathic pain. Cochrane Database Syst Rev 2007;(4):CD005454.
41. Moore RA, Derry S, Aldington D, et al. Amitriptyline for neuropathic pain in adults. Cochrane Database Syst Rev 2015;(7):CD008242.
42. Dean L. Amitriptyline therapy and CYP2D6 and CYP2C19 genotype. In: Pratt V, McLeod H, Dean L, et al, editors. Medical genetics summaries. Bethesda (MD): National Center for Biotechnology Information (US); 2012. p. 1–21.
43. Finnerup NB, Attal N, Haroutounian S, et al. Pharmacotherapy for neuropathic pain in adults: a systematic review and meta-analysis. Lancet Neurol 2015; 14(2):162–73.
44. Rastogi R, Swarm RA, Patel TA. Case scenario: opioid association with serotonin syndrome: implications to the practitioners. Anesthesiology 2011;115(6):1291–8.
45. Laird B, Colvin L, Fallon M. Management of cancer pain: basic principles and neuropathic cancer pain. Eur J Cancer 2008;44(8):1078–82.
46. Gallagher HC, Gallagher RM, Butler M, et al. Venlafaxine for neuropathic pain in adults. Cochrane Database Syst Rev 2015;(8):CD011091.
47. Rowbotham MC, Goli V, Kunz NR, et al. Venlafaxine extended release in the treatment of painful diabetic neuropathy: a double-blind, placebo-controlled study. Pain 2004;110(3):697–706.
48. Trouvin AP, Perrot S, Lloret-Linares C. Efficacy of venlafaxine in neuropathic pain: a narrative review of optimized treatment. Clin Ther 2017;39(6):1104–22.
49. Lobo ED, Heathman M, Kuan HY, et al. Effects of varying degrees of renal impairment on the pharmacokinetics of duloxetine: analysis of a single-dose phase I study and pooled steady-state data from phase II/III trials. Clin Pharmacokinet 2010;49(5):311–21.
50. Pergolizzi JV Jr, Raffa RB, Taylor R Jr, et al. A review of duloxetine 60 mg once-daily dosing for the management of diabetic peripheral neuropathic pain, fibromyalgia, and chronic musculoskeletal pain due to chronic osteoarthritis pain and low back pain. Pain Pract 2013;13(3):239–52.
51. Hauser W, Petzke F, Sommer C. Comparative efficacy and harms of duloxetine, milnacipran, and pregabalin in fibromyalgia syndrome. J Pain 2010;11(6): 505–21.
52. Norman TR, Olver JS. Continuation treatment of major depressive disorder: is there a case for duloxetine? Drug Des Devel Ther 2010;4:19–31.
53. Hunziker ME, Suehs BT, Bettinger TL, et al. Duloxetine hydrochloride: a new dual-acting medication for the treatment of major depressive disorder. Clin Ther 2005; 27(8):1126–43.
54. Duloxetine reduces chemotherapy induced peripheral neuropathy. BMJ 2013; 346:f2199.
55. Lee YC, Chen PP. A review of SSRIs and SNRIs in neuropathic pain. Expert Opin Pharmacother 2010;11(17):2813–25.
56. Arnold P, Vuadens P, Kuntzer T, et al. Mirtazapine decreases the pain feeling in healthy participants. Clin J Pain 2008;24(2):116–9.
57. Nishihara M, Arai YC, Yamamoto Y, et al. Combinations of low-dose antidepressants and low-dose pregabalin as useful adjuvants to opioids for intractable, painful bone metastases. Pain Physician 2013;16(5):E547–52.
58. de Boer T. The effects of mirtazapine on central noradrenergic and serotonergic neurotransmission. Int Clin Psychopharmacol 1995;10(Suppl 4):19–23.

59. Enomoto T, Yamashita A, Torigoe K, et al. Effects of mirtazapine on sleep distur-bance under neuropathic pain-like state. Synapse 2012;66(6):483–8.
60. Hayashida K, Parker R, Eisenach JC. Oral gabapentin activates spinal cholin-ergic circuits to reduce hypersensitivity after peripheral nerve injury and interacts synergistically with oral donepezil. Anesthesiology 2007;106(6):1213–9.
61. Cai K, Nanga RP, Lamprou L, et al. The impact of gabapentin administration on brain GABA and glutamate concentrations: a 7T (1)H-MRS study. Neuropsycho-pharmacology 2012;37(13):2764–71.
62. Liu GJ, Karim MR, Xu LL, et al. Efficacy and tolerability of gabapentin in adults with sleep disturbance in medical illness: a systematic review and meta-analysis. Front Neurol 2017;8:316.
63. Bockbrader HN, Wesche D, Miller R, et al. A comparison of the pharmacokinetics and pharmacodynamics of pregabalin and gabapentin. Clin Pharmacokinet 2010;49(10):661–9.
64. McLean MJ. Clinical pharmacokinetics of gabapentin. Neurology 1994;44(6 Suppl 5):S17–22 [discussion: S31–2].
65. Backonja M, Glanzman RL. Gabapentin dosing for neuropathic pain: evidence from randomized, placebo-controlled clinical trials. Clin Ther 2003;25(1):81–104.
66. Caraceni A, Zecca E, Bonezzi C, et al. Gabapentin for neuropathic cancer pain: a randomized controlled trial from the Gabapentin Cancer Pain Study Group. J Clin Oncol 2004;22(14):2909–17.
67. Wiffen PJ, Derry S, Bell RF, et al. Gabapentin for chronic neuropathic pain in adults. Cochrane Database Syst Rev 2017;(6):CD007938.
68. Tsavaris N, Kopterides P, Kosmas C, et al. Gabapentin monotherapy for the treat-ment of chemotherapy-induced neuropathic pain: a pilot study. Pain Med 2008; 9(8):1209–16.
69. Rao RD, Michalak JC, Sloan JA, et al. Efficacy of gabapentin in the management of chemotherapy-induced peripheral neuropathy: a phase 3 randomized, double-blind, placebo-controlled, crossover trial (N00C3). Cancer 2007;110(9):2110–8.
70. Horga de la Parte JF, Horga A. Pregabalin: new therapeutic contributions of cal-cium channel alpha2delta protein ligands on epilepsy and neuropathic pain. Rev Neurol 2006;42(4):223–37 [in Spanish].
71. Chiechio S, Zammataro M, Caraci F, et al. Pregabalin in the treatment of chronic pain: an overview. Clin Drug Investig 2009;29(3):203–13.
72. Schifano F, D'Offizi S, Piccione M, et al. Is there a recreational misuse potential for pregabalin? Analysis of anecdotal online reports in comparison with related ga-bapentin and clonazepam data. Psychother Psychosom 2011;80(2):118–22.
73. Mishra S, Bhatnagar S, Goyal GN, et al. A comparative efficacy of amitriptyline, gabapentin, and pregabalin in neuropathic cancer pain: a prospective random-ized double-blind placebo-controlled study. Am J Hosp Palliat Care 2012;29(3): 177–82.
74. Raptis E, Vadalouca A, Stavropoulou E, et al. Pregabalin vs. opioids for the treat-ment of neuropathic cancer pain: a prospective, head-to-head, randomized, open-label study. Pain Pract 2014;14(1):32–42.
75. Perez C, Latymer M, Almas M, et al. Does duration of neuropathic pain impact the effectiveness of pregabalin? Pain Pract 2017;17(4):470–9.
76. Simpson RW, Wlodarczyk JH. Transdermal buprenorphine relieves neuropathic pain: a randomized, double-blind, parallel-group, placebo-controlled trial in dia-betic peripheral neuropathic pain. Diabetes Care 2016;39(9):1493–500.
77. Derry S, Stannard C, Cole P, et al. Fentanyl for neuropathic pain in adults. Cochrane Database Syst Rev 2016;(10):CD011605.

78. Cooper TE, Chen J, Wiffen PJ, et al. Morphine for chronic neuropathic pain in adults. Cochrane Database Syst Rev 2017;(5):CD011669.
79. Stannard C, Gaskell H, Derry S, et al. Hydromorphone for neuropathic pain in adults. Cochrane Database Syst Rev 2016;(5):CD011604.
80. McNicol ED, Midbari A, Eisenberg E. Opioids for neuropathic pain. Cochrane Database Syst Rev 2013;(8):CD006146.
81. Eckhardt K, Ammon S, Hofmann U, et al. Gabapentin enhances the analgesic effect of morphine in healthy volunteers. Anesth Analg 2000;91(1):185–91.
82. Irving G, Tanenberg RJ, Raskin J, et al. Comparative safety and tolerability of duloxetine vs. pregabalin vs. duloxetine plus gabapentin in patients with diabetic peripheral neuropathic pain. Int J Clin Pract 2014;68(9):1130–40.
83. Holbech JV, Jung A, Jonsson T, et al. Combination treatment of neuropathic pain: Danish expert recommendations based on a Delphi process. J Pain Res 2017;10: 1467–75.
84. Feng XQ, Zhu LL, Zhou Q. Opioid analgesics-related pharmacokinetic drug interactions: from the perspectives of evidence based on randomized controlled trials and clinical risk management. J Pain Res 2017;10:1225–39.
85. Park JY, Wu LT. Prevalence, reasons, perceived effects, and correlates of medical marijuana use: a review. Drug Alcohol Depend 2017;177:1–13.
86. Nugent SM, Morasco BJ, O'Neil ME, et al. The effects of cannabis among adults with chronic pain and an overview of general harms: a systematic review. Ann Intern Med 2017;167(5):319–31.
87. Olfson M, Wall MM, Liu SM, et al. Cannabis use and risk of prescription opioid use disorder in the United States. Am J Psychiatry 2017;175(1):47–53.
88. Takeda S, Yamamoto I, Watanabe K. Modulation of Delta9-tetrahydrocannabinol-induced MCF-7 breast cancer cell growth by cyclooxygenase and aromatase. Toxicology 2009;259(1–2):25–32.
89. Alon MH, Saint-Fleur MO. Synthetic cannabinoid induced acute respiratory depression: case series and literature review. Respir Med Case Rep 2017;22: 137–41.
90. Davis MP. Cannabinoids for symptom management and cancer therapy: the evidence. J Natl Compr Canc Netw 2016;14(7):915–22.
91. Cannabis In Cachexia Study Group, Strasser F, Luftner D, Possinger K, et al. Comparison of orally administered cannabis extract and delta-9-tetrahydrocannabinol in treating patients with cancer-related anorexia-cachexia syndrome: a multicenter, phase III, randomized, double-blind, placebo-controlled clinical trial from the Cannabis-In-Cachexia-Study-Group. J Clin Oncol 2006;24(21):3394–400.
92. Whiting PF, Wolff RF, Deshpande S, et al. Cannabinoids for medical use: a systematic review and meta-analysis. JAMA 2015;313(24):2456–73.
93. Boychuk DG, Goddard G, Mauro G, et al. The effectiveness of cannabinoids in the management of chronic nonmalignant neuropathic pain: a systematic review. J Oral Facial Pain Headache 2015;29(1):7–14.
94. Cannabinoid buccal spray for chronic non-cancer or neuropathic pain: a review of clinical effectiveness, safety, and guidelines. Ottawa (ON): Canadian Agency for Drugs and Technologies in Health; 2016.
95. Lee SC, Park KS, Moon JY, et al. An exploratory study on the effectiveness of "Calmare therapy" in patients with cancer-related neuropathic pain: a pilot study. Eur J Oncol Nurs 2016;21:1–7.
96. Starkweather AR, Coyne P, Lyon DE, et al. Decreased low back pain intensity and differential gene expression following Calmare(R): results from a double-blinded randomized sham-controlled study. Res Nurs Health 2015;38(1):29–38.

97. Smith TJ, Auwaerter P, Knowlton A, et al. Treatment of human immunodeficiency virus-related peripheral neuropathy with scrambler therapy: a case report. Int J STD AIDS 2017;28(2):202–4.
98. Majithia N, Smith TJ, Coyne PJ, et al. Scrambler therapy for the management of chronic pain. Support Care Cancer 2016;24(6):2807–14.

Interventional Anesthetic Methods for Pain in Hematology/Oncology Patients

Holly Careskey, MD, MPH, Sanjeet Narang, MD*

KEYWORDS

• Anesthetic techniques • Regional • Cancer pain • Intrathecal drug delivery

KEY POINTS

• Approximately 20% of patients with cancer do not receive adequate pain control despite following the WHO pain stepladder; for these patients interventional measures may provide relief.

• There are several single-injection interventions to treat pain that is in an anatomic location clearly supplied by one or more neural pathways, including peripheral or central nerve blocks, plexus injections, and sympathetic nerve neurolysis.

• Continuous infusion therapy through epidural, intrathecal, and perineural infusions can relieve pain with logarithmic medication dose reduction compared with oral route of administration and with significant decreases in side effects.

INTRODUCTION

When cancer pain cannot be adequately treated with traditional medication administration routes, there are numerous interventional procedures that can aid in the management of intractable pain. It has been estimated that cancer pain is well managed for 75% to 90% of patients with cancer by following the World Health Organization (WHO) stepladder for medication escalation.[1,2] However, for the remaining 10% to 25% of patients who have failed conventional treatment, poor pain control is associated with decreased quality of life for patients and their families.[3,4] Additionally, some patients experience intolerable systemic side effects from traditional pain management approaches that necessitate consideration of alternative approaches and routes of administration to achieve relief.[5,6] For these patients, interventional anesthetic procedures are critical in improving daily functioning and quality of life, and reducing medication side effects.

Disclosure Statement: S. Narang: Consultant for Medtronic, Inc. H. Careskey: No disclosures.
Department of Anesthesiology, Perioperative and Pain Medicine, Brigham and Women's Hospital, Harvard Medical School, 75 Francis Street, Boston, MA 02115, USA
* Corresponding author.
E-mail address: snarang@bwh.harvard.edu

Hematol Oncol Clin N Am 32 (2018) 433–445
https://doi.org/10.1016/j.hoc.2018.01.007
0889-8588/18/© 2018 Elsevier Inc. All rights reserved.

hemonc.theclinics.com

This article introduces and reviews the wide variety of interventional techniques available in the treatment of simple and complex cancer-related pain. Reviewed are the epidemiology, assessment of pain, specific causes, and progression of pain as they pertain to interventional approaches to cancer-related pain (a discussion of general assessment of the patient in pain is found in Regina M. Fink and Jeannine M. Brants' article, "Complex Cancer Pain Assessment," in this issue). Also reviewed are the indications for and efficacy of various interventional procedures for targeted pain control in the patient suffering from cancer. The goal is to provide an understanding of when to consider interventional pain management for patients with cancer-related pain and to define the role of the pain physician as part of the oncology team.

EPIDEMIOLOGY OF CANCER PAIN

Estimates of prevalence of cancer pain vary widely because of lack of standardization in definition and reporting variability. The highest rates of pain reported are for head and neck cancer, prostate, uterine, other genitourinary, breast, and pancreatic cancers.[7,8] The prevalence of pain in patients in active treatment is estimated to be between 24% and 73%.[9] Those patients with advanced or terminal disease are estimated to have a pain prevalence between 58% and 69%. Surprisingly, patients in remission from their disease report a pain prevalence between 21% and 46%.[8] Of all patients with cancer pain, more than one-third grade their pain as moderate or severe. Cancer pain is multifactorial in origin and thus there does not exist a one size fits all treatment protocol.[10,11] Cancer pain negatively affects sleep,[12] social life,[13] and compromises enjoyment of life.[14]

Reviews of the WHO ladder of cancer pain management estimate that this management strategy provides adequate pain relief for 75% to 90% of patients.[1,15,16] This ladder begins with nonopioid analgesics with gradual escalation to mild opioids with the addition of more potent opioids as the last step. At every level, the option of additional adjuvant medication is present. Although opioid medication is introduced early on the WHO cancer pain relief ladder, globally opioid use and availability vary widely.[17] With opioid availability limited in many parts of the world, consideration of alternate therapies and interventions is crucial. Furthermore, it has been traditionally considered that patients should first be given conventional therapies, reserving interventional cancer pain procedures for patients who do not respond. However, this strategy may lead to delayed referrals and uncontrolled pain. Moreover, patients who are referred late in the course of their disease may not be candidates for interventional procedures because they are too debilitated from the advanced disease and from side effects of treatment. A more inclusive, efficient, and humane approach may be to consider multimodal interventions, including interventional therapies, as part of the same toolbox, all concurrent modalities to be applied throughout the course of the disease process.

GENERAL CONSIDERATIONS FOR INTERVENTIONAL PROCEDURES

The application of regional anesthetic techniques through the use of nerve blocks, neurolysis, or continuous peripheral and neuraxial catheter infusions often provides a high quality of pain control with decreased need for systemic opioids. Patients typically are relieved of one or more components of their pain more profoundly than with opioid therapy alone. The use of interventional procedures in patients suffering from cancer is not without added risks. These patients are by definition immunocompromised and are therefore at a higher baseline risk to acquire infection. Additionally, the hypercoagulable state of many cancer states necessitates anticoagulation therapy for either prophylaxis or treatment of thromboembolic disease. For many interventional procedures, these medications need to be withheld during the periprocedural period, thereby exposing the patient to potential thrombosis. The procedures themselves may be uncomfortable, distressing, and have the potential for minor and significant complications. The decision to proceed must be made after a careful risk and benefit assessment by the care team and patient.

The incidence, severity, and type of pain syndrome vary by location and type of cancer (see Russell K. Portenoy and Ebtesam Ahmeds' article, "Cancer Pain Syndromes," in this issue). The feasibility of an intervention also depends on the region of the body affected. Finally, the rate of progress of disease influences choice and timing of procedures. Hence, with lung cancer, where pain is a major symptom, and 5-year survival postdiagnosis is low, there may be an accelerated urgency to offer advanced procedures earlier than, for example, a patient with breast cancer, where even with lung or bone metastases median survival is 18 to 29 months and a more, stepwise approach might be permitted.[18,19] This is by no means a rule, because the course of either disease could be indolent or rapidly progressive or markedly improved by targeted therapies or immunotherapies.

The most common pain conditions that are amenable to anesthetic interventions are related to the abdomen and pelvis, with solid organ tumors of the pancreas, kidney, ovarian, and cervical cancer. Infusion therapy through indwelling catheters in the periphery and neuraxis is feasible for pain of the torso and extremities, and depending on the skill and comfort level of the practitioner, less so for cancers of the head and neck.

Characteristics of Cancer Pain

The dominant characteristic of cancer-related pain is that it can (and usually does) change over time. It is also often a mixed pattern, with components of acute and chronic pain, and nociceptive and neuropathic in nature. Additionally, pain may arise from several origins, involve multiple sites, and different processes may affect the patient at the same time, and some of these may arise outside the area covered by an intervention. Patients therefore often need to receive multiple modalities. For example, even in a patient with an intrathecal pump for severe pelvic pain, draining ascetic fluid, bracing a foot drop, or irradiating a clavicular metastasis can all contribute to the overall comfort of the patient, as would a sleep aid and increased pain medication at night if pain is worse at that time. As with any other modality, an increase in pain may indicate cancer progression and should prompt investigation.

Interventional Considerations in Patient Assessment and Diagnosis

Each patient requires a thorough evaluation and timeline of previous symptoms and treatment. A list of all the pains and related symptoms, such as constipation, sedation/insomnia, and mood, should be made. It is important to determine exactly how patients are taking their pain medication and what is its effect. Often asking the patient to describe a typical day and the exacerbating and relieving factors in detail is useful. The examination must be gentle, but complete. Previous scars, any deformities or areas of skin breakdown, and obvious items, such as a colostomy or a G tube, must be noted. Images from recent scans should be examined with special regard to the area of pain, and laboratory results should be checked, especially platelet counts, coagulation assays, and liver function tests. The purpose of the assessment is to postulate the anatomic structures affected (soft tissue, nerve, bone, hollow viscus, or solid organ) and create a mental picture of the pain as it projects on the patient's body. One should prioritize the more severe and/or the most bothersome pains for intervention.

Unique Considerations

Patients who have cancer-related pain present with a unique set of considerations when compared with those who have chronic noncancer pain. The cancer pain specialist must work closely with the oncologist and the palliative care teams and obtain their cooperation and collaboration at all times. An assessment of prognosis is necessary, as is classifying whether the patient is in active treatment or in a purely palliative and supportive mode. It is prudent to ask the oncologist in writing if the patient has days to weeks, or weeks to months, or months to years to live. This helps choose the appropriate interventions.

Additional questions about the effects of chemotherapy on healing or cytopenia are important. If the absolute neutrophil count is less than 1000, most interventions are contraindicated. The timing of the chemotherapy and the nadir of the cytopenic effect may dictate scheduling the intervention at a specific time point. If patients are participants in clinical trials certain interventions might be precluded. If a continuous intervention, such as an intrathecal pump, is planned chemotherapy may have to be suspended temporarily until incisions heal. It is important to obtain the consent of the patient and the assent of the oncologist before proceeding.

Cancer affects the patient's metabolism in variable and unpredictable ways; hence, caution in following guidelines for drug pharmacokinetics is needed, especially if there is hepatic dysfunction. Usual wait times for stopping and starting anticoagulation are sometimes much longer. Constitutional factors influence the procedures in various ways; patients might need sedation for procedures that in the chronic noncancer pain population are done with only local anesthesia. This is because they may be opioid tolerant and suffering from severe acute-on-chronic nociceptive pain and unable to assume the position required for the injection. The physiologic trespass of a minor operation in this population may have prolonged recovery time, and could require a longer inpatient hospitalization. Even the presence of infection sometimes becomes only a relative contraindication, because some patients have conditions that may never heal or are related to their tumor. The risk of patients having infection during operations is considered higher than the noncancer population and aggressive antibiosis is advised periprocedurally. This is because the consequences of an infected implant are more problematic in the patient who already has unmanageable pain, a limited life span, and requires further chemotherapy.

When to Refer

For patients with chronic noncancer pain, pain providers have the option of exhausting conservative measures before pursuing interventional techniques. However, when it comes to patients with cancer pain, the luxury of time is not always available. Because every patient has a different progression and presentation of pain, there is not always a singular "action moment" for referral for interventional pain procedures. We propose the time points listed next as action moments for consideration of interventional pain procedures for the patient with cancer pain:

- Pain that is distributed in a regional or localized body area
- Pain that is distributed along a known nerve distribution
- When pain control requires rapid escalation in opioid doses
- Patients with daily opioid requirements more than 300 morphine equivalents
- When pain is progressing rapidly in the face of poor prognosis
- When the thought occurs to a member of the oncologic care team

Even if pain seems controlled an early referral is wise in patients where an intervention is anticipated to begin a relationship with the interventional pain physician. There is a school of thought that believes in prophylactic placement of an intrathecal device before initiating chemotherapy with the belief that cancer treatment may continue longer if pain is controlled.

TYPES OF INTERVENTIONS

It is convenient to consider interventional pain management to be of two main types (with overlap). There are single interventions that provide benefit at one treatment session (nerve blocks, neurolytic procedures, or cordotomy), and those that need a more continuous or ongoing treatment (usually infusion therapy) requiring an external or internalized pump.[20] Sometimes in the cancer-related pain population, combinations of single procedures and/or continuous infusions are pursued. For example, a patient may get a nerve block and a trial or placement of an indwelling device at the same time; or multiple blocks may be done at one time.

SINGLE INTERVENTIONS

A single injection or series of injections of local anesthetic with or without corticosteroids is helpful for diagnosing and treating cancer-related pain. Often the duration of pain relief extends beyond the expected duration (from pharmacokinetic data) of the local anesthetic blockade, especially when an adjuvant, such as a corticosteroid, has also been injected.[20]

The use of regional anesthetic procedures can lead to increased comfort despite dose reduction of oral and intravenous medication, therefore reducing side effects, such as impaired cognition, fatigue, respiratory compromise, and constipation. Alternatively, the injections may allow for increased medication efficacy of a systemic opioid dose that was previously ineffective and thereby facilitate outpatient pain control.

Single injections are as simple as trigger point injections for myofascial pain related to cutaneous or bony metastases, the more complex temporary nerve blocks, or the even more complicated and longer-lasting neurolytic procedures. Limited only by operator skill and imaging modality availability, a wide array of cranial or spinal nerves and peripheral nerves or neural plexuses can be "blocked." Blocks can typically be performed in awake or sedated patients using surface anatomy, ultrasound guidance, and fluoroscopic or tomographic imaging, to anesthetize a nerve plexus or specific peripheral nerve. Virtually any nerve can be "blocked" with a combination of local anesthetic and corticosteroid with the expectation of relief on the order of weeks. Although nerve blocks with local anesthetic with or without adjuvant medications are a well-described and frequent tool in the anesthesiologist's armamentarium, standardization of practice and clearly defined therapeutic mechanism for the duration of action and degree of pain control are not well established.[21,22] The expectation is for the pain relief to last from 2 to 6 weeks similar to injections for chronic pain and injections can be repeated, eventually with diminishing results.[23,24]

Mixed spinal or cranial nerves and autonomic plexuses can also be targeted for a similar temporary nerve block, and, if that is effective, for neurolysis, which may offer relief for some months. Neurolysis involves a physical (thermal radiofrequency lesioning [RFL] or cryoablation) or chemical (alcohol or phenol) treatment to a peripheral nerve to temporarily inhibit transmission of signals to the central nervous system and prolong the duration of pain relief for a few months. For bony metastases, intralesional injections with corticosteroids[25,26] are helpful, whereas kyphoplasty or vertebroplasty procedures can be performed for patients with intractable bone pain from vertebral fractures. Kyphoplasty and vertebroplasty are discussed in Nicholas Figura and colleagues' article, "Mechanisms of and Adjuvants for Bone Pain," in this issue.

Peripheral Nerve Blocks

When a patient has pain along the territory of a peripheral nerve or plexus, a peripheral nerve block is used to anesthetize along its distribution to provide short term relief. The nerves of interest are located using surface anatomy projection or under ultrasound visualization with care to identify surrounding vascular structures. A needle is advanced to the neural sheath and local anesthetic is injected in a targeted manner with subsequent analgesia in the distribution of the neurosensory pathway. Numerous adjuvant medications can be injected including epinephrine, corticosteroids, opioids, and α_2-agonists to enhance and prolong the block.[25–27]

Peripheral nerve blocks are used as a diagnostic tool to determine a source of pain or for periprocedural anesthesia, such as before tumor biopsy or fracture fixation. Nearly every region of the upper and lower extremities and most areas of the head, neck and trunk can be anesthetized by peripheral nerve blocks.[28–30] Blockade of the thorax, abdomen, and trunk is also possible through peripheral blocks, although for neoplastic radiculopathy in the extremities, more commonly neuraxial injections in the epidural space are used.[31]

When longer term relief is desired, a catheter is placed in the region with a continuous infusion of local anesthetic and other adjuvants. These catheters are tunneled or port-a-cath placement is pursued along the nerve trajectory to allow long-term infusion and decrease the risk of infection associated with nontunneled devices. The contraindications to nerve blocks include patient refusal, true allergy to local anesthetic, significant coagulopathy, or systemic or overlying infection. In patients with end-stage disease, a risk-benefit assessment may be performed by the clinicians, patient, and family regarding risk of significant bleeding and infection spread versus establishing comfort at the end of life. Technically, these blocks and catheters may be difficult to perform because of distorted anatomy from surgery, radiation, or effects of tumor or edema.[32] In the hands of an experienced practitioner, complications are generally rare and minor. They include block failure, catheter misplacement or migration, neural injury, and damage to surrounding structures.[33–35] Individual blocks have specific risks associated with their anatomic location. Overall, complication rates drop when ultrasound guidance is used to perform the injection.[36]

Neurolysis with Chemical or Physical Agents

Autonomic plexus neurolysis procedures have been shown to provide significant pain relief that can last on the order of months. These blocks can target visceral pain in the head, trunk, abdomen, pelvis, and extremities. **Table 1** lists common sympathetic plexus blocks and their indications. The injections are typically performed under fluoroscopic, computed tomography, or ultrasound guidance. Typically, chemical neurolysis is performed using high-concentration alcohol (97.5%) or 6% phenol.

Neurolytic injections for cancer pain result in improvement in pain score, decreased opioid intake, and decreased side effects related to opioid intake.[37] Management of visceral abdominal pain, such as from metastatic pancreatic cancer, with celiac plexus neurolysis has been shown in a meta-analysis to have 90% pain relief for at least 3 months following the intervention.[37,38] Superior hypogastric plexus neurolysis is a performed for visceral pain related to pelvic cancers (including gynecologic, genitourinary, and colorectal disease). Studies suggest between a 53% and 72% success

Table 1
Common neurolytic blocks for cancer pain

Neurolytic Block	Indication	Anatomic Location	Complications
Stellate ganglion block	Upper extremity and facial pain	Anterior to transverse process of C7	Vascular injury Pneumothorax Brachial plexus and vagus nerve injury Hematoma
Celiac plexus block	Visceral abdominal pain including pain from pancreatic, gastric, biliary, and esophageal malignancies	Anterior to the L1 vertebral body	Orthostatic hypotension Diarrhea Hemorrhage (rare) Paraplegia (rare)
Lumbar sympathetic block	Sympathetically mediated pain of the lower extremities	Anterior to the L3 vertebral body	Intravascular injection Vascular injury Renal or ureteral injury
Superior hypogastric plexus block	Visceral pelvic pain	Anterior to the L5 vertebral body	Intravascular injection Vascular injury
Ganglion impar block	Rectal and coccygeal pain	Anterior to the sacrococcygeal junction	Rectal perforation Fistula formation

rate (>50% improvement of visual analogue scale [VAS] for at least 1 month) of this injection in patients with cancer-related pelvic pain.[37,38] Ganglion impar neurolysis is especially effective for lower pelvic visceral pain and the procedure itself is fairly low risk.[39,40] This is often combined with bilateral S3 nerve root block to target additional somatic components of pelvic pain associated with cancer.[41–43] A small study of 15 patients with cancer-related pelvic pain demonstrated at least a short-term benefit (decreased pain score and decrease morphine consumption) of pelvic pain following combination ganglion impar injection and superior hypogastric plexus injection.[44] Historically, intrathecal phenol was used widely to treat cancer-related pelvic pain. However, with the advent of effective neuraxial infusions, and the necessity for the phenol to be compounded often at an extramural pharmacy, phenol injection has become less common. Nevertheless, it is useful in the patient too ill for other procedures, especially when patients may have already compromised bowel and bladder function.[39]

Peripheral neurotomy through RFL is also a well-described practice for chronic, noncancer pain.[45] RFL has been used to target and kill metastatic cells in a manner similar to RFL for neuroablation.[46] This technique involves directing alternating current at a high frequency through a needle to heat surrounding tissue. This creates scar and cell necrosis, which when involving affected nerves can provide significant relief. Intralesional RFL has also been described for bony metastases[47] and soft tissue lesions.[48] One major benefit of all of these procedures is their relative degree of minimal invasiveness and the ability to repeat the procedures should pain progress or return. A similar process with the use of extreme cold, cryoanalgesia and cryosurgery, also has application. This procedure uses a freezing and thawing technique to induce cellular apoptosis and regional ischemia to cause cellular death of desired tumor lesions by forming an "iceball."[49,50] It is performed as part of cancer treatment or for symptom management alone.[49,51]

Neurosurgical Intervention and Spinal Cord Stimulation

A brief mention of neurosurgical interventions for intractable cancer pain is warranted, although the details are outside the scope of this review. Surgical cordotomy is a procedure that involves severing of the spinothalamic tracts to arrest pain signal transmission to the thalamus.[46,52–54] Surgical destruction of the ventrolateral portion of the dorsal rootlet entry zone, known as DREZotomy, has also been reported to improve neuropathic pain in a variety of conditions including cancer pain.[55] Dorsal root ganglion stimulation and spinal cord stimulation through implantable stimulators is a growing treatment of complex regional pain syndrome and other neuropathic pain syndromes.[56] These technologies have not been well studied in cancer-related pain and pose some potential areas of challenge with regards to the patient with cancer. Typically for noncancer pain, these devices necessitate a stable pain syndrome (not one that is expected to progress significantly over time), which is unusual in cancer. Moreover, previous technology was not MRI-compatible, which limited its use in the patient with cancer who might need frequent imaging. However, with the availability of MRI-compatible electrodes and battery packs these devices present an avenue for future application.[57]

CONTINUOUS NEURAXIAL INTERVENTIONS

Neuraxial medication delivery through epidural and intrathecal catheters is a growing field in the management of cancer and chronic noncancer pain. This therapy takes advantage of the logarithmic dose reduction of opioid analgesics in the cerebrospinal fluid compared with oral and intravenous doses required to achieve equivalent analgesia. This dose reduction leads to a decrease in unpalatable side effects including cognitive slowing, gastrointestinal upset, constipation, and respiratory depression; however, pruritus and peripheral edema are more common with intrathecal administration. Patients who have (or are expected to develop) escalating opioid requirements, difficult-to-control pain, or intolerance to medication regimen should be considered for continuous neuraxial therapy.[58] Typically, patients undergo a trial of epidural or intrathecal therapy before proceeding with a semipermanent or permanent implant. A trial requires first establishing clear goals of care and expectations with the patient, their family, and care team. The primary purpose of pursuing continuous neuraxial infusion is to decrease pain with secondary benefits of improving quality of life, allowing tolerance of treatment and rehabilitation programs. Formal psychological assessment before a trial (a standard of care for intrathecal modalities for nonmalignant pain), maybe considered but is not essential in many cases. However, patients who are unable to report symptoms reliably, or who have difficulty complying with follow up visits, may not be suitable candidates for continuous interventions.

Once the patient and care team have decided to proceed, a trial of epidural or intrathecal medication is given through a percutaneously placed catheter or a single injection.[59] Adherence to the American Society of Regional Anesthesia and Pain Medicine guidelines with regards to anticoagulation is essential to prevent the devastating consequence of epidural hematoma formation with subsequent spinal cord compression.[60] Additional considerations include anatomic evaluation of the spine to ensure there is no involvement of the epidural space, dura, or thecal sac especially at or near the thoracolumbar spine, although this is a relative contraindication.

Occasionally, in the patient who finds positioning for radiation therapy or lying still for any length of time impossible because of intolerable pain, epidural analgesia is immensely beneficial; the insertion of an epidural catheter for the duration of treatment, typically 7 to 10 days, and infusing analgesic solution during the periods of therapy can safely accomplish the desired goals, albeit at the expense of a longer inpatient stay.

A trial may last anywhere from 1 to 7 days. During this time, frequent assessment of pain control, along with vital signs and neurologic examination, is necessary. For this reason, trial periods nearly always occur in the inpatient setting. The goal of a trial is to establish efficacy and additionally conduct a dose-ranging study of medications at which a noticeable improvement in symptoms occurs. There are currently three medications that are approved by the Food and Drug Administration for the intrathecal route: (1) morphine, (2) ziconotide, and (3) baclofen. However, there are a plethora of other medications that are now widely used via intrathecal delivery in routine clinical practice. Commonly used neuraxial medications include opioids (morphine, hydromorphone, fentanyl, sufentanil), local anesthetics (bupivacaine), and adjuvant medications (clonidine). Occasionally, the trial period is bypassed in the patient with cancer with end-stage disease, severe immunodepression, or concern that trial will significantly prolong the patient's suffering.[59]

A trial is typically considered successful if a VAS reduction by 50% is obtained. Clinical practice varies widely, however, and ultimately the definition of a successful trial must be tailored to each patient.[50] Once a patient has been deemed a candidate for continuous neuraxial infusion, there are several options for medication delivery. Depending on prognosis and anatomy, the patient may have an external system (either tunneled or via a port-a-cath) or an implantable system placed to aid in long-term pain control. Placement of an implanted drug delivery system is minor surgery. In a fragile and complicated patient with limited reserve, and an unknown velocity of tumor progression, it still cannot be undertaken lightly.

Frail patients and patients with a predicted life expectancy less than 3 months are often better candidates for externalized epidural infusion systems. Because of the open connection with the skin, externalized systems are at increased risk of infection compared with indwelling devices. Tunneling the catheter under the skin can reduce the risk of infection and prevent catheter migration.[59]

Before placement of an internal or external infusion device, it is critical to determine insurance coverage for home care of external infusion devices, and to coordinate with hospital and/or hospice staff and the patients' informal caregivers regarding their ability to manage postprocedure wound care and the infusion. It is common for dosing and medication regimens to change over time and thus close follow-up of these patients by the pain service is crucial to ensure that the patient's symptoms are optimally controlled. If patients experience waxing and waning pain symptoms, the ability to add a patient-controlled bolus dose allows for rapid treatment of pain without increasing the basal infusion. This is incorporated easily into a patient-controlled epidural pump using a button similar to a Patient Controlled Analgesia. For surgically implanted intrathecal pumps, an external remote control communicates wirelessly with the pump to deliver an on-demand dose for patient-controlled intrathecal analgesia.[61]

CHOICE OF INTERVENTION

When the pain syndrome is easily identified, the appropriate single intervention (eg, a celiac plexus block) is offered in a straightforward manner. More commonly, if the patient's pain is complex and multifactorial, more than one procedure may be needed to treat the spectrum of the patient's symptoms. If a patient's pain spans more than four to six dermatomal levels, it is unlikely to completely respond to injections and an epidural or intrathecal infusion should be offered. Often after the dominant pain has been successfully treated, other subsidiary pains emerge and acquire importance and urgency. Infusions, nerve blocks, and neurolysis can reduce the need for systemic opioids but not eliminate them. Systemic opioids and adjuvants are often still needed, albeit usually at lower doses.

An estimate of prognosis is a vital consideration; when it is clear a patient will live months to years a completely implantable pump is appropriate. If it seems a patient is days or weeks away from the end of life, an external infusion is probably the path to be adopted. It is when the patient is likely to live weeks to months that the decision is more nuanced. Secondary factors, such as psychosocial situation, home environment, distance from the hospital, language or communication barriers, insurance coverage, and the availability of domiciliary services, all need to be considered as part of the final decision.

SUMMARY

Within the interdisciplinary cancer care team, the interventional pain physician is often the last resort to manage patients with cancer pain syndromes that have failed to respond to oral medication. By involving a pain care physician early in the process patients may receive superior quality pain relief before side effects from progressively increasing doses of opioids cause general malaise, fatigue, constipation, and cognitive decline. This may permit tolerating chemotherapy for longer periods and eventually increase survival times. A continual reassessment of a patient's pain location, quality, nature, and evolution is imperative to proactively address the changing nature of cancer pain that a patient is likely to experience. An attempt should be made to stay "a step ahead" of a patient's pain and predict what pain problems may occur next. Adopting an aggressive pain management strategy can help patients with devastating disease states live the best possible quality of life during the course of the disease. Although the complete eradication of cancer pain is a lofty goal that may not be possible with every patient, certainly it is an aspiration all team members can support. Finally, caregiver stress in pain management professionals who are unused to end-of-life situations demands co-training in palliative care to avoid compassion fatigue and physician burnout.

REFERENCES

1. Zech DF, Grond S, Lynch J, et al. Validation of World Health Organization guidelines for cancer pain relief: a 10-year prospective study. Pain 1995; 63(1):65–76.
2. Jain PN, Pai K, Chatterjee AS. The prevalence of severe pain, its etiopathological characteristics and treatment profile of patients referred to a tertiary cancer care pain clinic. Indian J Palliat Care 2015;21(2):148–51.
3. Deandrea S, Montanari M, Moja L, et al. Prevalence of undertreatment in cancer pain. A review of published literature. Ann Oncol 2008;19(12):1985–91.
4. Vayne-Bossert P, Afsharimani B, Good P, et al. Interventional options for the management of refractory cancer pain: what is the evidence? Support Care Cancer 2016;24(3):1429–38.
5. Meuser T, Pietruck C, Radbruch L, et al. Symptoms during cancer pain treatment following WHO-guidelines: a longitudinal follow-up study of symptom prevalence, severity and etiology. Pain 2001;93(3):247–57.
6. Bhatnagar S, Gupta M. Evidence-based clinical practice guidelines for interventional pain management in cancer pain. Indian J Palliat Care 2015;21(2):137–47.
7. Vainio A, Auvinen A. Prevalence of symptoms among patients with advanced cancer: an international collaborative study. Symptom prevalence group. J Pain Symptom Manage 1996;12(1):3–10.

8. van den Beuken-van Everdingen MH, de Rijke JM, Kessels AG, et al. Prevalence of pain in patients with cancer: a systematic review of the past 40 years. Ann Oncol 2007;18(9):1437–49.
9. van den Beuken-van Everdingen MH, Hochstenbach LM, Joosten EA, et al. Update on prevalence of pain in patients with cancer: systematic review and meta-analysis. J Pain Symptom Manage 2016;51(6):1070–90.
10. Caraceni A, Weinstein SM. Classification of cancer pain syndromes. Oncology Dec 2001;15(12):1627–40.
11. Paice JA, Mulvey M, Bennett M, et al. AAPT diagnostic criteria for chronic cancer pain conditions. J Pain 2017;18(3):233–46.
12. Hu DS, Silberfarb PM. Management of sleep problems in cancer patients. Oncology 1991;5(9):23–7.
13. Strang P. Emotional and social aspects of cancer pain. Acta Oncol 1992;31(3): 323–6.
14. Daut RL, Cleeland CS. Prevalence and severity of pain in cancer. Cancer 1982; 50(9):1912–8.
15. Hanks GW, Justins DM. Cancer pain: management. Lancet 1992;339(8800): 1031–6.
16. Jacox A, Carr DB, Payne R. Management of cancer pain. AHCPR clinical practice guideline No. 9. Agency for Health Care Policy and Research. N Engl J Med 1994;330:651–5.
17. Pain & Policy Studies Group. Global opioid consumption. 2015. Available at: http://painpolicy.wisc.edu/global. Accessed November 17, 2017.
18. Swenerton KD, Legha SS, Smith T, et al. Prognostic factors in metastatic breast cancer treated with combination chemotherapy. Cancer Res 1979;39(5): 1552–62.
19. Smalley RV, Lefante J, Bartolucci A, et al. A comparison of cyclophosphamide, adriamycin, and 5-fluorouracil (CAF) and cyclophosphamide, methotrexate, 5-fluorouracil, vincristine, and prednisone (CMFVP) in patients with advanced breast cancer. Breast Cancer Res Treat 1983;3(2):209–20.
20. Fitzgibbon D. Interventional procedures for cancer pain management: selecting the right procedure at the right time. J Support Oncol 2010;8(2):60–1.
21. Vlassakov KV, Narang S, Kissin I. Local anesthetic blockade of peripheral nerves for treatment of neuralgias: systematic analysis. Anesth Analg 2011;112(6): 1487–93.
22. Carr DB. Local anesthetic blockade for neuralgias: "why is the sky blue, daddy?". Anesth Analg 2011;112(6):1283–5.
23. Roberts ST, Wilick SE, Rho ME, et al. Efficacy of lumbosacral transforaminal epidural steroid injections: a systematic review. PM R 2009;1(7):657–68.
24. Eckel TS, Bartynski WS. Epidural steroid injections and selective nerve root blocks. Tech Vasc Interv Radiol 2009;12(1):11–21.
25. Rowell NP. Intralesional methylprednisolone for rib metastases: an alternative to radiotherapy? Palliat Med 1988;2(2):153–5.
26. Rousseff RT, Simeonov S. Intralesional treatment in painful rib metastases. Palliat Med 2004;18:259.
27. Cummings KC III, Napierkowski DE, Parra-Sanchez I, et al. Effect of dexamethasone on the duration of interscalene nerve blocks with ropivacaine or bupivacaine. Br J Anaesth 2011;107(3):446–53.
28. Khor KE, Ditton JN. Femoral nerve blockade in the multidisciplinary management of intractable localized pain due to metastatic tumor: a case report. J Pain Symptom Manage 1996;11(1):57–60.

29. Smith BE, Fischer HB, Scott PV. Continuous sciatic nerve block. Anaesthesia 1984;39(2):155–7.
30. Neill RS. Ablation of the brachial plexus: control of intractable pain, due to a pathological fracture of the humerus. Anaesthesia 1979;34(10):1024–7.
31. Manchikanti L, Buenaventura RM, Manchikanti KN, et al. Effectiveness of therapeutic lumbar transforaminal epidural steroid injections in managing lumbar spinal pain. Pain 2012;15(3):E199–245.
32. Chambers WA. Nerve blocks in palliative care. Br J Anaesth 2008;101(1):95–100.
33. Ilfeld BM. Continuous peripheral nerve blocks: an update of the published evidence and comparison with novel, alternative analgesic modalities. Anesth Analg 2017;124(1):308–55.
34. Knight JB, Schott NJ, Kentor ML, et al. Neurotoxicity of common peripheral nerve block adjuvants. Curr Opin Anaesthesiol 2015;28(5):598–604.
35. Kirksey MA, Haskins SC, Cheng J, et al. Local anesthetic peripheral nerve block adjuvants for prolongation of analgesia: a systematic qualitative review. PLoS One 2015;10(9):e0137312.
36. Lewis SR, Price A, Walker KJ, et al. Ultrasound guidance for upper and lower limb blocks. Cochrane Database Syst Rev 2015;(9):CD006459.
37. de Oliveira R, dos Reis MP, Prado WA. The effects of early or late neurolytic sympathetic plexus block on the management of abdominal or pelvic cancer pain. Pain 2004;110(1–2):400–8.
38. Eisenberg E, Carr DB, Chalmers TC. Neurolytic celiac plexus block for treatment of cancer pain: a meta-analysis. Anesth Analg 1995;80(2):290–5.
39. Raphael J, Hester J, Ahmedzai S, et al. Cancer pain: part 2: physical, interventional and complimentary therapies; management in the community; acute, treatment-related and complex cancer pain: a perspective from the British Pain Society endorsed by the UK Association of Palliative Medicine and the Royal College of General Practitioners. Pain Med 2010;11(6):872–96.
40. Scott-Warren JT, Hill V, Rajasekaran A. Ganglion impar blockade: a review. Curr Pain Headache Rep 2013;17:306.
41. Plancarte R, Amescua C, Patt RB, et al. Presacral blockade of the ganglion of Walther (ganglion impar). Anesthesiology 1990;73:A751.
42. Kroll CE, Schartz B, Gonzalez-Fernandez M, et al. Factors associated with outcome after superior hypogastric plexus neurolysis in cancer patients. Clin J Pain 2014;30(1):55–62.
43. Plancarte R, de Leon-Casasola OA, El-Helaly M, et al. Neurolytic superior hypogastric plexus block for chronic pelvic pain associated with cancer. Reg Anesth 1997;22(6):562–8.
44. Ahmed DG, Mohamed MF, Mohamed SA. Superior hypogastric plexus combined with ganglion impar neurolytic blocks for pelvic and/or perineal cancer pain relief. Pain Physician 2015;18(1):E49–56.
45. Lord SM, Bogduk N. Radiofrequency procedures in chronic pain. Best Pract Res Clin Anaesthesiol 2002;16(4):597–617.
46. Munk PL, Rashid F, Heran MK, et al. Combined cementoplasty and radiofrequency ablation in the treatment of painful neoplastic lesions of bone. J Vasc Interv Radiol 2009;20(7):903–11.
47. Goetz MP, Callstrom MR, Charboneau JW, et al. Percutaneous image-guided radiofrequency ablation of painful metastases involving bone: a multicenter study. J Clin Oncol 2004;22(2):300–6.
48. Patti JW, Neeman Z, Wood BJ. Radiofrequency ablation for cancer-associated pain. J Pain 2002;3(6):471–3.

49. Niu L-Z, Li J-L, Xu K-C. Percutaneous cryoablation for liver cancer. J Clin Transl Hepatol 2014;2(3):182–8.

50. Niu L, Wang Y, Yao F, et al. Alleviating visceral cancer pain in patients with pancreatic cancer using cryoablation and celiac plexus block. Cryobiology 2013;66(2):105–11.

51. Zugaro L, Di Staso M, Gravina GL, et al. Treatment of osteolytic solitary painful osseous metastases with radiofrequency ablation or cryoablation: a retrospective study by propensity analysis. Oncol Lett 2016;11(3):1948–54.

52. Lahuerta J, Bowsher D, Lipton S, et al. Percutaneous cervical cordotomy: a review of 181 operations on 146 patients with a study on the location of "pain fibers" in the C-2 spinal cord segment of 29 cases. J Neurosurg 1994;80(6):975–85.

53. Spiller WG, Martin E. The treatment of persistent pain of organic origin in the lower part of the body by division of the anterolateral column of the spinal cord. JAMA 1912;58(20):1489–90.

54. Raslan AM, Cetas JS, McCartney S, et al. Destructive procedures for control of cancer pain: the case for cordotomy. J Neurosurg 2011;114(1):155–70.

55. Gadgil N, Viswanathan A. DREZotomy in the treatment of cancer pain: a review. Stereotact Funct Neurosurg 2012;90(6):356–60.

56. Pope JE, Deer TR, Kramer J. A systematic review: current and future directions of dorsal root ganglion therapeutics to treat chronic pain. Pain Med 2013;14(10): 1477–96.

57. Belberud S, Mogilner A, Schulder M. Intrathecal pumps. Neurotherapeutics 2008; 5(1):114–22.

58. Horlocker TT, Wedel DJ, Rowlingson JC, et al. Regional anesthesia in the patient receiving antithrombotic or thrombolytic therapy: American Society of Regional Anesthesia and Pain Medicine evidence-based guidelines (third edition). Reg Anesth Pain Med 2010;35(1):64–101.

59. Narang S, Weisheipl A, Ross EL, editors. Surgical pain management. New York: Oxford University Press; 2016.

60. Deer TR, Hayek SM, Pope JE, et al. The Polyanalgesic Consensus Conference (PACC): recommendations for trialing of intrathecal drug delivery infusion therapy. Neuromodulation 2017;20(2):133–54.

61. Maeyaert J, Busher E, Van Buyten JP, et al. Patient-controlled analgesia in intrathecal therapy for chronic pain: safety and effective operative of the Model 8831 Personal Therapy Manager with a pre-implanted SynchroMed infusion system. Neuromodulation 2003;6(3):133–41.

Mechanisms of, and Adjuvants for, Bone Pain

Nicholas Figura, MD[a],*, Joshua Smith, MD[b], Hsiang-Hsuan Michael Yu, MD, ScM[a]

KEYWORDS

- Metastatic • Bone • Pain • NGF • Bisphosphonate • RANKL inhibitor • Kyphoplasty
- Vertebroplasty

KEY POINTS

- Bone metastasis is a heterogeneous compilation of diseases that require a multidisciplinary approach to personalize treatment to the patient's individual needs.
- Metastatic bone pain is caused by several mechanisms, including osteoclast activation within the tumor microenvironment, inflammatory factors at the tumor-nociceptor interface, mechanical nerve damage, and neuroplastic changes.
- Several adjuvant therapies are available to alleviate metastatic bone pain, including nonsteroidal analgesics, bisphosphonates, RANKL inhibitors, surgery, kyphoplasty, vertebroplasty, and radiofrequency ablation.

INTRODUCTION

Each year, approximately 400,000 people in the United States are diagnosed with metastatic bone cancer.[1] Bone is the third most common site of metastases, after the lung and the liver.[2] As cancer screening and treatments improve and patients experience longer life expectancies, they are at increasing odds of developing bone metastases, which may lead to chronic pain, pathologic fractures, and spinal cord compression.

Approximately 30% to 50% of all patients who have cancer will experience moderate to severe pain; of those with advanced or metastatic disease, as many as 75% to 95% of patients will report severe pain.[3-5] Complications from bone metastasis appear an average of 7 months after the patient first reports bone pain.[6] Chronic cancer-induced bone pain (CIBP) negatively affects a patient's quality of life, increases

---

Disclosure Statement: None of the authors have any relationship with a commercial company that has a direct financial interest in the subject matter or materials discussed in this article or with a company making a competing product.
[a] Department of Radiation Oncology, Moffitt Cancer Center, 12902 Magnolia Drive, Tampa, FL 33612, USA; [b] Department of Supportive Care Medicine, Moffitt Cancer Center, 12902 Magnolia Drive, Tampa, FL 33612, USA
* Corresponding author.
E-mail address: nicholas.figura@moffitt.org

Hematol Oncol Clin N Am 32 (2018) 447–458
https://doi.org/10.1016/j.hoc.2018.01.006
hemonc.theclinics.com

patient morbidity, and decreases overall functional status. The current paradigm in managing metastatic bone disease focuses on preventing CIBP, pathologic fractures, and spinal cord compression, which are collectively known as skeletal-related events (SREs).

Bone metastasis is actually a heterogeneous collection of diseases made up of various primary cancers occurring in various sites of metastases and with baseline functional statuses. Accordingly, metastatic bone pain requires a multidisciplinary approach to personalize treatment to the patient's individual needs and performance status.

This article discusses the mechanisms of metastatic bone pain and the many adjuvant treatment options available to alleviate it.

BONE METASTASES

Cancers of the lung, breast, and prostate cause approximately 80% of all bone metastases. As many as 70% of all patients who have breast or prostate cancer develop skeletal metastases as compared with only 20% to 30% of patients with gastrointestinal cancers.[7]

Cancer commonly metastasizes to bone because of the high blood flow and concentration of immobilized cellular growth factors residing in the red marrow. Metastatic disease most commonly deposits in the axial skeleton, such as the vertebral column and pelvis, or in the medullary portions of the appendicular skeleton, such as the proximal femur.[8,9]

Bone metastases are frequently asymptomatic and incidentally found on initial staging evaluation. For symptomatic patients, pain is the most common and earliest manifestation of bone metastases. (See Regina M. Fink and Jeannine M. Brants' article, "Complex Cancer Pain Assessment," in this issue.)

Metastatic bone pain has a gradual onset that worsens over time and typically increases in intensity at night. The pain may be described as somatic (musculoskeletal) or neuropathic but commonly presents with mixed aspects of each. The intensity or nature of the pain cannot be predicted by tumor size, location, or histology, and the pain is often disproportionate to the degree of bone involvement.[3]

As the disease progresses, patients may begin to experience breakthrough pain. Breakthrough pain is an acute and unpredictable flare of pain not controlled with long-acting pain medications. It may occur spontaneously or be reproducible with nonnoxious movements and/or mechanical weightbearing of the involved bone. Breakthrough pain is often difficult to manage owing to its rapid, striking onset and it frequently results in the decline of a patient's functional status.[10,11]

MECHANISMS OF PAIN PERCEPTION

Pain is the cognitive perception of potentially harmful environmental stimuli. It requires the synchronization of complex processes, including the (1) detection of an environmental stimuli that is (2) converted to an electrochemical signal and (3) transmitted along the nervous system, where it is (4) cognitively perceived as an unpleasant sensation.

Primary afferent sensory neurons are the pathways on which sensory information is received and transmitted. These sensory neurons provide innervation throughout every organ of the body, except for the brain. The cell bodies of the primary afferent sensory neurons that innervate the body and the face reside in the dorsal root and the trigeminal ganglia, respectively. The nerve fibers of these sensory neurons are divided into 2 main categories: myelinated A fibers and unmyelinated C fibers, each with their own respective subgroups. The small-diameter unmyelinated C-fibers and A-delta fibers are called nociceptors, which specialize in detecting pain.

Nociceptors are specialized peripheral receptors that respond to environmental stimuli and transmit the electrochemical signals perceived as pain. Compared with other primary sensory receptors that respond to only 1 type of input, nociceptors are unique in the range and variability of possible input signals. For example, the vanilloid receptors (VRs) are able to respond to heat, acidity (via proton concentration), and specific lipid metabolites.[12–14] Other nociceptors are able to respond to thermal, mechanical, and/or inflammatory factors, such as tumor necrosis factor (TNF)-alpha, interleukins, bradykinin, chemokines, prostaglandins, nerve growth factor (NGF), and endothelins.[15,16] Because these stimuli each contribute to the sensation of pain, each may prove to be potential targets in the treatment of metastatic bone pain.

The tenets of generalized pain management have changed little in the last several decades. In 1982, the World Health Organization (WHO) developed the WHO analgesic ladder that promoted a 3-step approach:

(Step 1) Nonopioids, such as nonsteroidal antiinflammatory drugs (NSAIDs) for mild pain
(Step 2) Weak opioids for moderate pain
(Step 3) Strong opioids for severe pain.

However, as many as 45% of patients who have cancer continue to report insufficient or ineffective pain control,[17,18] so new therapies are needed.

CANCER BONE PAIN MECHANISMS

Understanding the intricate mechanisms that cause metastatic bone pain may allow for the development of novel targeted therapies. In 1999, the first mouse model was developed by infusing sarcoma cells into the intramedullary portion of a mouse femur,[19] creating the first reproducible model to study isolated bone metastases without an associated systemic burden.

Metastatic bone pain is caused by several distinct mechanisms, all of which contribute to the sensation of bone pain. This article discusses the effects of sustained osteoclast activation within the tumor microenvironment; the role of inflammatory factors at the tumor-nociceptor interface; the development of structural instability, causing mechanical nerve damage; and, ultimately, the plasticity of the central and peripheral nervous system in the setting of sustained nerve stimulation.

OSTEOCLASTS

Osteoclasts play an important role in the development and perpetuation of CIBP. Osteoclasts are multinucleated, differentiated cells derived from the monocyte lineage that regulate bone resorption in physiologic bone remodeling.

Healthy bone has a highly regulated process of constant bone turnover, consisting of simultaneous osteoblastic and osteolytic activity. Metastatic bone disease disrupts this well-balanced system, leading to bone destruction and its subsequent complications. Traditionally, bone metastases have been characterized as osteolytic, osteoblastic, or mixed. However, rather than strictly resorbing or forming bone, metastatic cancer seems to stimulate both osteoblastic and osteolytic activity. The overstimulation of both processes leads to functional unit disorganization with a relative predominance of either excess bone formation or resorption.

As cancer deposits and proliferates in the bone, the tumor and associated stromal cells express the receptor-activator of nuclear factor κ-β (RANK) ligand (RANKL), which binds to and activates the RANK receptor on osteoclast precursors,[20] causing maturation and proliferation of osteoclasts. Osteoclasts resorb healthy bone by forming highly acidic, inflammatory microenvironments that lower the activation threshold of nociceptors. Prolonged and disorganized bone turnover eventually may compromise the structural integrity of the bone, causing pathologic fractures and mechanical nerve entrapment. Bisphosphonates, which cause the death of osteoclasts, and RANKL antagonists that prevent osteoclast activation are, therefore, used to treat CIBP.

Bisphosphonates were originally developed to prevent SREs in patients with osteopenia or osteoporosis. They are pyrophosphate analogues that are endocytosed by osteoclasts and, once internalized, disrupt adenosine triphosphate (ATP) metabolism (nonnitrogenous bisphosphonates) or cholesterol metabolism (nitrogenous bisphosphonates), leading to cell death.[21] By inhibiting osteoclastic activity in patients who have cancer, they each prevent the development of SREs and they decrease CIBP by reducing the tumor burden and decreasing its associated inflammatory response.[22,23]

Newer generations of bisphosphonates, such as zoledronate, are more potent, allowing for decreased dosing and potentially fewer adverse effects.[24] One recent meta-analysis evaluating 12 studies and more than 1700 subjects with lung cancer concluded that zoledronate plus chemotherapy significantly decreased rates of developing SREs (relative risk [RR] 0.81, 95% CI 0.67–0.97) and improved pain control when added either to chemotherapy or radiation therapy (RT; RR 1.18, 95% CI 1.0–1.4).[25] A Cochrane review analyzing 30 randomized trials agreed that bisphosphates provide some pain relief for bone metastases but did not find enough evidence to recommend bisphosphonates as first-line therapy for immediate pain control.[26]

RANKL-inhibitors prevent the activation of osteoclasts and treat CIBP by inhibiting the RANK–RANKL interaction. Osteoprotegerin (OPG), also known as osteoclastogenesis inhibitory factor, is a naturally occurring soluble receptor that binds to RANKL, preventing osteoclast activation. Denosumab is a human immunoglobulin monoclonal antibody that mimics OPG by selectively binding to and sequestering RANKL, consequently preventing CIBP and SREs caused by osteoclast overstimulation.

A phase III trial evaluating 2046 subjects who have metastatic breast cancer demonstrated that, compared with zoledronate, denosumab caused a significant delay in the development to first SRE (median time 32.4 vs 26.4 months; hazard ratio 0.82, 95% CI 0.71–0.95, P<.001) and a significant decrease in reported bone pain.[27] Ongoing studies are evaluating the role of denosumab in both delaying SREs and relieving CIBP in other primary cancers.

ROLE OF TUMOR CELLS AND INFLAMMATION

CIBP is also caused by local inflammation within a tumor microenvironment at the nociceptor–tumor interface. Metastatic lesions are predominantly composed of stroma and inflammatory cells, such as macrophages, neutrophils, mast cells, and T-lymphocytes[28]; cancer cells are only a fraction of the cells in the lesion. Both tumor and inflammatory cells secrete inflammatory factors, such as protons, prostaglandins, bradykinin, endothelin, TNF-alpha, and cytokines, which sensitize or excite primary afferent neurons by lowering their excitation-threshold.[28–30]

Nociceptors sensitized or stimulated by inflammatory or tumor-induced acidosis are an important cause of CIBP. A tumor's microenvironment is relatively acidic compared with nearby healthy tissue owing to several mechanisms.[31] First, its hypermetabolic activity leads to the production of acidic metabolites. Second, because tumors reside in relatively hypoxic conditions, they preferentially use the anaerobic cellular metabolic pathway, creating significant acidic byproducts. The high turnover rate and cell death within a tumor then releases those intracellular acidic products into the microenvironment, further lowering the local pH. Infiltrating inflammatory cells also release protons and cytotoxic factors that propagate additional tissue destruction and local acidosis.

The increased concentration of protons directly activates and sensitizes nearby nociceptors. Large proportions of nerves express acid-sensing ion channel 3 (ASIC3) and VR1, both of which are stimulated by increased proton concentration.[32,33] Inhibition of the receptor may produce pain control. Mouse studies found that the acute and chronic administration of VR1 antagonists demonstrated significant attenuation of pain-behaviors. The efficacy was maintained in settings of acute, moderate, and late tumor burden.[34]

Along with decreasing the local pH, both cancer and inflammatory cells release prostaglandins that directly act on prostanoid receptors of nociceptors to produce pain.[30] Prostaglandins are lipid metabolites of the cyclooxygenase (COX) enzyme. Whereas COX1 isoform is constitutionally active in tissues, COX2 is primarily active in the setting of inflammation and tissue injury. COX2 has been found to be associated with angiogenesis, tumor proliferation, and inhibition of apoptosis.[35,36] NSAIDs, such as aspirin and ibuprofen, nonselectively inhibit both COX1 and COX2 enzymes to reduce prostaglandin levels and attenuate pain. Doses of nonselective NSAIDs, however, are limited by their side-effect profile, which includes gastric ulcers and/or bleeding and nephrotoxicity.

Selective COX2 inhibitors, such as celecoxib, were developed to minimize systemic side effects while preferentially acting at sites of inflammation. COX2 inhibitors assist in inflammatory-mediated pain control and provide a synergistic effect with opioids.[37] In mouse models, selective COX2 inhibitors decreased cancer pain–related behaviors while also decreasing the expression of c-Fos and dynorphin in the dorsal roots of the spinal cord.[38]

NERVE GROWTH FACTOR

Early research is evaluating the role of NGF in CIBP. NGF is a neurotrophic factor responsible for the maintenance and survival of neurons. It was also found to be associated with the signaling and transmission of pain after elevated NGF levels were correlated with increased pain-associated behaviors in early mouse models.[39,40] Further studies in humans found that the administration of NGF led to increased reports of hyperalgesia and allodynia.[41,42]

NGF can directly stimulate nociceptors by binding to TrkA and p75, which alters the synthesis and expression of pain-inducing neurotransmitters, such as substance P and calcitonin gene-related peptide.[43] It may also sensitize afferent neurons by increasing the expression of $Na_V1.8$ sodium channels and lowering their activation threshold. Because many primary cancers overexpress or are stimulated by NGF,[44–48] anti-NGF therapies may be particularly effective in metastatic bone pain.

Tanezumab is a humanized monoclonal antibody that selectively binds to NGF, preventing its normal function. Clinical studies have demonstrated significant improvement in pain and functional status with the use of tanezumab for subjects with osteoarthritis and chronic low back pain.[49] Current research is evaluating the role of anti-NGF in the setting of CIBP. Early mouse studies found anti-NGF agents were able to reduce pain-related behaviors more effectively than either 10 or 30 mg/kg of morphine sulfate.[50,51] A recent phase 2 randomized clinical trial demonstrated no increase of adverse events or treatment-related toxicities with the use of tanezumab when compared with a placebo group.[52] Clinical trials evaluating the efficacy of tanezumab in attenuating metastatic bone pain are currently ongoing.

ENDOTHELINS

The role of endothelins in cancer pain is not fully understood but may present another avenue for treating CIBP. Endothelins are peptides secreted by tumors and associated inflammatory cells that act directly on primary afferent neurons.[53,54] Initial studies found a correlation of elevated endothelin levels to nociceptive behavior and that an injection of endothelin led to localized hyperalgesia.[55] Endothelins bind to G-coupled endothelin A receptor (ETAR) and endothelin B receptor (ETBR).

Atrasentan is an oral ETAR antagonist that has been previously studied in preventing prostate cancer progression. Studies for efficacy in CIBP have to date been negative. Subjects in 1 study were randomized to receive either a placebo, low-dose (2.5 mg) or high-dose (10 mg) atrasentan. There was no difference in pain control of 3 arms.[56] A recent phase III study that evaluated 811 men with prostate cancer confirmed no significant pain improvement with the use of a selective ETAR antagonist.[57]

Whereas ETAR are found on peripheral sensory neurons, ETBR is expressed by Schwann cells and dorsal root ganglion satellite cells.[58] Compared with ETAR, ETBR stimulation was shown to have antinociceptive effects in mouse studies.[59] Early studies suggest that ETBR agonists may increase the endogenous release of endorphins to attenuate pain.[60]

Future research is needed to evaluate whether a combination of ETAR antagonists and ETBR agonists is beneficial in treating CIBP.

MECHANICAL STIMULATION

Although tumor cells are rarely innervated, bone and the surrounding periosteum are diffusely innervated with afferent sensory nerves.[61] Rapid tumor growth may cause mechanical distension, leading to nerve entrapment or compression causing pain from continuous nerve stimulation. Nociceptors detect noxious mechanical stimuli through either purinergic receptors that are activated by changes in the concentration of ATP, or mechanically gated ion channels that are activated by physical distension.[62,63] Furthermore, osteoclastic activity can destroy sensory nerve fibers, leading to neuropathic pain.[64]

As bone metastases grow, the reorganized bone loses its structural integrity, increasing the risk for destabilization and fracture. This is of particular concern for spinal disease because of the intricate relationship between the spinal cord and its protective vertebral column. Even minor areas of spinal destabilization may lead to spinal root injury or cord compression.

NERVOUS SYSTEM PLASTICITY

In response to sustained stimulation, the nervous system undergoes plastic changes at the levels of the peripheral and central nervous system, contributing to CIBP.

In a process called peripheral sensitization, primary afferent sensory neurons exposed to chronic stimulation are altered to become more sensitive to excitation. In peripheral sensitization, nociceptors alter the expression of ion-channels and/or receptors, lowering the activation threshold.[65,66] This may lead to the phenomena in which mild stimuli may be perceived as painful (hyperalgesia) or in which nonnoxious stimuli may be perceived as noxious (allodynia).

Similar to the peripheral system, chronic CIBP may lead to changes within the central nervous system in a process called central sensitization.[67] Studies have shown that the spinal cord and its associated segmental neurons will undergo plastic changes when exposed to chronic neuropathic injury.[65,66] In normal tissue, substance P is synthesized by nociceptors and only released onto the spinal cord in response to noxious stimuli. However, in murine models, the spinal segments receiving input from tumor sites had increased levels of c-Fos, dynorphin, and substance-P markers, which indicate increased transmission of pain signals.[68] Along with neurochemical changes, there seems to be a redistribution in the proportion of nerve fibers, potentiating greater transmission of pain signals.[69]

ADJUVANT THERAPEUTIC OPTIONS FOR METASTATIC BONE PAIN

External beam RT, stereotactic body RT, radiopharmaceuticals, surgery, and radiofrequency ablation (RFA) can all alleviate CIBP. (See Ron Shiloh and Monica Krishnan's article, "Radiation for Treatment of Painful Bone Metastases," in this issue.)

SURGERY

Surgical interventions in metastatic bone disease are strictly palliative, relieving pain, restoring mechanical stability, and/or improving a patient's functional status. Surgical intervention is typically reserved for those lesions with unstable or impending pathologic fractures, particularly in the long bones or in the spine, where vertebral instability increases the risk for metastatic spinal cord compression.

Pain is the most common symptom of vertebral or long bone involvement. Up to 29% of patients with metastatic bone disease may develop a pathologic fracture.[70] The most common location of a pathologic fracture is within the femur owing to its weightbearing nature.[71] Formal staging systems provide guidelines to determine whether surgery followed by radiation or radiation alone is needed. One such staging system, Mirels criteria, predicts the risk of an impending fracture through the summation of 4 variables: the site of disease (upper extremity, lower extremity, or peritrochanteric), the intensity of pain (mild, moderate, or functional), the type of lesion (blastic, mixed, or lytic), and lesion size (<one-third, one-third–two-thirds, or >two-third–three-thirds). A score of 8 or greater indicates that surgery followed by radiation may be an appropriate treatment.[72] Algorithms using advanced imaging to determine the structural integrity of long bone and type of therapy recommended are under study.[73]

Surgery is also integral in the treatment of spinal metastases. Scales to determine whether to recommend surgical intervention measure the degree of spinal instability, mechanical pain, performance status, number of extraspinal, bone metastases, number of vertebral metastases, extent of visceral metastases, tumor histology, and neurologic status to determine whether to recommend surgical intervention.[74]

Ten percent of patients with malignant cancer will, at some point, develop spinal metastases and, of those, approximately 10% to 20% of patients will develop cord compression.[75] For spinal cord compression, the Patchell and colleagues[76] study demonstrated that selected subjects with radio-resistant tumors and a single site of spinal cord compression benefit from surgery followed by postoperative RT (PORT). The study was discontinued early because at interim analysis 84% (42/50) of the subjects were able to walk following surgery and PORT compared with only 57% (29/51) treated with RT alone (OR 6.2, $P = .001$). The subjects who underwent surgery and PORT retained the ability to walk for a significantly longer period of time (122 days vs 13 days; $P = .003$).[76] Overall, of patients undergoing spinal surgery for metastatic bone disease, 5% to 10% develop surgical site infections and up to 25% can develop perioperative complications.[77,78]

Patients who are not surgical candidates may be eligible for vertebral augmentation with either kyphoplasty or vertebroplasty, which allow for the injection of a cement formulation, most commonly polymethyl-methacrylate (PMMA), to restore mechanical stability. Vertebral augmentation has been shown to improve pain control in most patients.[79]

RADIOFREQUENCY ABLATION

RFA has only recently been used in treating painful bone metastases. Originally used in benign disease, it has become the standard treatment of osteoid osteomas. RFA generates heat by running an electrical current through image-guided–placed electrodes that ablate nearby tissue.

RFA is currently restricted to those patients who fail previous treatment and who have limited metastatic disease. Two trials have demonstrated effective pain control in patients at up to 3 months. However, given concern for potential damage to nearby tissue, it is essential to ensure proper patient selection to minimize adverse effects.[80,81]

SUMMARY

Metastatic bone pain is a complex, poorly understood process. Although significant progress has been made in understanding the unique mechanisms of CIBP, significant controversies remain. Understanding these mechanisms may allow for the development of novel therapeutic targets. By appreciating bone metastasis as a group of heterogeneous diseases, a multimodality approach can be used to personalize treatment for patients and their particular diseases, improving survival and optimizing quality of life.

REFERENCES

1. Mundy GR. Metastasis to bone: causes, consequences and therapeutic opportunities. Nat Rev Cancer 2002;2(8):584–93.
2. Greenlee RT, Murray T, Bolden S, et al. Cancer statistics, 2000. CA Cancer J Clin 2000;50(1):7–33.
3. Mercadante S. Malignant bone pain: pathophysiology and treatment. Pain 1997; 69(1–2):1–18.
4. Mercadante S, Arcuri E. Breakthrough pain in cancer patients: pathophysiology and treatment. Cancer Treat Rev 1998;24(6):425–32.
5. Portenoy RK, Lesage P. Management of cancer pain. Lancet 1999;353(9165): 1695–700.
6. Gabriel K, Schiff D. Metastatic spinal cord compression by solid tumors. Semin Neurol 2004;24(4):375–83.
7. Coleman RE, Rubens RD. The clinical course of bone metastases from breast cancer. Br J Cancer 1987;55(1):61–6.
8. Krishnamurthy GT, Tubis M, Hiss J, et al. Distribution pattern of metastatic bone disease. A need for total body skeletal image. JAMA 1977;237(23):2504–6.
9. Tubiana-Hulin M. Incidence, prevalence and distribution of bone metastases. Bone 1991;12(Suppl 1):S9–10.
10. Mercadante S, Fulfaro F. Management of painful bone metastases. Curr Opin Oncol 2007;19(4):308–14.

11. Coleman RE. Skeletal complications of malignancy. Cancer 1997;80(8 Suppl): 1588–94.
12. Julius D, Basbaum AI. Molecular mechanisms of nociception. Nature 2001; 413(6852):203–10.
13. Bevan S, Geppetti P. Protons: small stimulants of capsaicin-sensitive sensory nerves. Trends Neurosci 1994;17(12):509–12.
14. Kirschstein T, Greffrath W, Busselberg D, et al. Inhibition of rapid heat responses in nociceptive primary sensory neurons of rats by vanilloid receptor antagonists. J Neurophysiol 1999;82(6):2853–60.
15. McMahon SB. NGF as a mediator of inflammatory pain. Philos Trans R Soc Lond B Biol Sci 1996;351(1338):431–40.
16. Nelson JB, Carducci MA. The role of endothelin-1 and endothelin receptor antagonists in prostate cancer. BJU Int 2000;85(Suppl 2):45–8.
17. Meuser T, Pietruck C, Radbruch L, et al. Symptoms during cancer pain treatment following WHO-guidelines: a longitudinal follow-up study of symptom prevalence, severity and etiology. Pain 2001;93(3):247–57.
18. de Wit R, van Dam F, Loonstra S, et al. The Amsterdam Pain Management Index compared to eight frequently used outcome measures to evaluate the adequacy of pain treatment in cancer patients with chronic pain. Pain 2001;91(3):339–49.
19. Schwei MJ, Honore P, Rogers SD, et al. Neurochemical and cellular reorganization of the spinal cord in a murine model of bone cancer pain. J Neurosci 1999; 19(24):10886–97.
20. Peng X, Guo W, Ren T, et al. Differential expression of the RANKL/RANK/OPG system is associated with bone metastasis in human non-small cell lung cancer. PLoS One 2013;8(3):e58361.
21. Price N. Bisphosphonates to prevent skeletal morbidity in patients with lung cancer with bone metastases. Clin Lung Cancer 2004;5(5):267–9.
22. Ripamonti C, Fulfaro F, Ticozzi C, et al. Role of pamidronate disodium in the treatment of metastatic bone disease. Tumori 1998;84(4):442–55.
23. Conte PF, Latreille J, Mauriac L, et al. Delay in progression of bone metastases in breast cancer patients treated with intravenous pamidronate: results from a multinational randomized controlled trial. The Aredia Multinational Cooperative Group. J Clin Oncol 1996;14(9):2552–9.
24. Gatti D, Adami S. New bisphosphonates in the treatment of bone diseases. Drugs Aging 1999;15(4):285–96.
25. Lopez-Olivo MA, Shah NA, Pratt G, et al. Bisphosphonates in the treatment of patients with lung cancer and metastatic bone disease: a systematic review and meta-analysis. Support Care Cancer 2012;20(11):2985–98.
26. Wong R, Wiffen PJ. Bisphosphonates for the relief of pain secondary to bone metastases. Cochrane Database Syst Rev 2002;(2):CD002068.
27. Stopeck AT, Lipton A, Body JJ, et al. Denosumab compared with zoledronic acid for the treatment of bone metastases in patients with advanced breast cancer: a randomized, double-blind study. J Clin Oncol 2010;28(35):5132–9.
28. Joyce JA, Pollard JW. Microenvironmental regulation of metastasis. Nat Rev Cancer 2009;9(4):239–52.
29. Mantyh PW. Cancer pain and its impact on diagnosis, survival and quality of life. Nat Rev Neurosci 2006;7(10):797–809.
30. Vasko MR. Prostaglandin-induced neuropeptide release from spinal cord. Prog Brain Res 1995;104:367–80.
31. Griffiths JR. Are cancer cells acidic? Br J Cancer 1991;64(3):425–7.

32. Tominaga M, Caterina MJ, Malmberg AB, et al. The cloned capsaicin receptor integrates multiple pain-producing stimuli. Neuron 1998;21(3):531–43.

33. Lingueglia E, de Weille JR, Bassilana F, et al. A modulatory subunit of acid sensing ion channels in brain and dorsal root ganglion cells. J Biol Chem 1997;272(47):29778–83.

34. Ghilardi JR, Rohrich H, Lindsay TH, et al. Selective blockade of the capsaicin receptor TRPV1 attenuates bone cancer pain. J Neurosci 2005;25(12):3126–31.

35. Moore BC, Simmons DL. COX-2 inhibition, apoptosis, and chemoprevention by nonsteroidal anti-inflammatory drugs. Curr Med Chem 2000;7(11):1131–44.

36. Masferrer JL, Leahy KM, Koki AT, et al. Antiangiogenic and antitumor activities of cyclooxygenase-2 inhibitors. Cancer Res 2000;60(5):1306–11.

37. Farooqui M, Li Y, Rogers T, et al. COX-2 inhibitor celecoxib prevents chronic morphine-induced promotion of angiogenesis, tumour growth, metastasis and mortality, without compromising analgesia. Br J Cancer 2007;97(11):1523–31.

38. Sabino MA, Ghilardi JR, Jongen JL, et al. Simultaneous reduction in cancer pain, bone destruction, and tumor growth by selective inhibition of cyclooxygenase-2. Cancer Res 2002;62(24):7343–9.

39. Aloe L, Tuveri MA, Carcassi U, et al. Nerve growth factor in the synovial fluid of patients with chronic arthritis. Arthritis Rheum 1992;35(3):351–5.

40. Hefti FF, Rosenthal A, Walicke PA, et al. Novel class of pain drugs based on antagonism of NGF. Trends Pharmacol Sci 2006;27(2):85–91.

41. Apfel SC, Schwartz S, Adornato BT, et al. Efficacy and safety of recombinant human nerve growth factor in patients with diabetic polyneuropathy: a randomized controlled trial. rhNGF Clinical Investigator Group. JAMA 2000;284(17):2215–21.

42. Dyck PJ, Peroutka S, Rask C, et al. Intradermal recombinant human nerve growth factor induces pressure allodynia and lowered heat-pain threshold in humans. Neurology 1997;48(2):501–5.

43. Mantyh PW, Koltzenburg M, Mendell LM, et al. Antagonism of nerve growth factor-TrkA signaling and the relief of pain. Anesthesiology 2011;115(1):189–204.

44. Dolle L, El Yazidi-Belkoura I, Adriaenssens E, et al. Nerve growth factor overexpression and autocrine loop in breast cancer cells. Oncogene 2003;22(36):5592–601.

45. Davidson B, Reich R, Lazarovici P, et al. Expression and activation of the nerve growth factor receptor TrkA in serous ovarian carcinoma. Clin Cancer Res 2003;9(6):2248–59.

46. Davidson B, Reich R, Lazarovici P, et al. Expression of the nerve growth factor receptors TrkA and p75 in malignant mesothelioma. Lung Cancer 2004;44(2):159–65.

47. Singer HS, Hansen B, Martinie D, et al. Mitogenesis in glioblastoma multiforme cell lines: a role for NGF and its TrkA receptors. J Neurooncol 1999;45(1):1–8.

48. Astolfi A, Nanni P, Landuzzi L, et al. An anti-apoptotic role for NGF receptors in human rhabdomyosarcoma. Eur J Cancer 2001;37(13):1719–25.

49. Katz N, Borenstein DG, Birbara C, et al. Efficacy and safety of tanezumab in the treatment of chronic low back pain. Pain 2011;152(10):2248–58.

50. Halvorson KG, Kubota K, Sevcik MA, et al. A blocking antibody to nerve growth factor attenuates skeletal pain induced by prostate tumor cells growing in bone. Cancer Res 2005;65(20):9426–35.

51. Sevcik MA, Ghilardi JR, Peters CM, et al. Anti-NGF therapy profoundly reduces bone cancer pain and the accompanying increase in markers of peripheral and central sensitization. Pain 2005;115(1–2):128–41.

52. Sopata M, Katz N, Carey W, et al. Efficacy and safety of tanezumab in the treatment of pain from bone metastases. Pain 2015;156(9):1703–13.
53. Gokin AP, Fareed MU, Pan HL, et al. Local injection of endothelin-1 produces pain-like behavior and excitation of nociceptors in rats. J Neurosci 2001;21(14):5358–66.
54. Davar G. Endothelin-1 and metastatic cancer pain. Pain Med 2001;2(1):24–7.
55. Wacnik PW, Eikmeier LJ, Ruggles TR, et al. Functional interactions between tumor and peripheral nerve: morphology, algogen identification, and behavioral characterization of a new murine model of cancer pain. J Neurosci 2001;21(23):9355–66.
56. Carducci MA, Padley RJ, Breul J, et al. Effect of endothelin-A receptor blockade with atrasentan on tumor progression in men with hormone-refractory prostate cancer: a randomized, phase II, placebo-controlled trial. J Clin Oncol 2003;21(4):679–89.
57. Nelson JB, Love W, Chin JL, et al. Phase 3, randomized, controlled trial of atrasentan in patients with nonmetastatic, hormone-refractory prostate cancer. Cancer 2008;113(9):2478–87.
58. Pomonis JD, Rogers SD, Peters CM, et al. Expression and localization of endothelin receptors: implications for the involvement of peripheral glia in nociception. J Neurosci 2001;21(3):999–1006.
59. Khodorova A, Fareed MU, Gokin A, et al. Local injection of a selective endothelin-B receptor agonist inhibits endothelin-1-induced pain-like behavior and excitation of nociceptors in a naloxone-sensitive manner. J Neurosci 2002;22(17):7788–96.
60. Quang PN, Schmidt BL. Peripheral endothelin B receptor agonist-induced antinociception involves endogenous opioids in mice. Pain 2010;149(2):254–62.
61. Seifert P, Spitznas M. Tumours may be innervated. Virchows Arch 2001;438(3):228–31.
62. Price MP, McIlwrath SL, Xie J, et al. The DRASIC cation channel contributes to the detection of cutaneous touch and acid stimuli in mice. Neuron 2001;32(6):1071–83.
63. Krishtal OA, Marchenko SM, Obukhov AG. Cationic channels activated by extracellular ATP in rat sensory neurons. Neuroscience 1988;27(3):995–1000.
64. Sevcik MA, Luger NM, Mach DB, et al. Bone cancer pain: the effects of the bisphosphonate alendronate on pain, skeletal remodeling, tumor growth and tumor necrosis. Pain 2004;111(1–2):169–80.
65. Honore P, Menning PM, Rogers SD, et al. Neurochemical plasticity in persistent inflammatory pain. Prog Brain Res 2000;129:357–63.
66. Honore P, Schwei J, Rogers SD, et al. Cellular and neurochemical remodeling of the spinal cord in bone cancer pain. Prog Brain Res 2000;129:389–97.
67. Gordon-Williams RM, Dickenson AH. Central neuronal mechanisms in cancer-induced bone pain. Curr Opin Support Palliat Care 2007;1(1):6–10.
68. Honore P, Rogers SD, Schwei MJ, et al. Murine models of inflammatory, neuropathic and cancer pain each generates a unique set of neurochemical changes in the spinal cord and sensory neurons. Neuroscience 2000;98(3):585–98.
69. Urch CE, Donovan-Rodriguez T, Dickenson AH. Alterations in dorsal horn neurones in a rat model of cancer-induced bone pain. Pain 2003;106(3):347–56.
70. Aaron AD. Treatment of metastatic adenocarcinoma of the pelvis and the extremities. J Bone Joint Surg Am 1997;79(6):917–32.
71. Weikert DR, Schwartz HS. Intramedullary nailing for impending pathological subtrochanteric fractures. J Bone Joint Surg Br 1991;73(4):668–70.

72. Mirels H. Metastatic disease in long bones. A proposed scoring system for diagnosing impending pathologic fractures. Clin Orthop Relat Res 1989;(249): 256–64.
73. Hong J, Cabe GD, Tedrow JR, et al. Failure of trabecular bone with simulated lytic defects can be predicted non-invasively by structural analysis. J Orthop Res 2004;22(3):479–86.
74. Tokuhashi Y, Matsuzaki H, Oda H, et al. A revised scoring system for preoperative evaluation of metastatic spine tumor prognosis. Spine (Phila Pa 1976) 2005; 30(19):2186–91.
75. Siegal T, Siegal T. Current considerations in the management of neoplastic spinal cord compression. Spine (Phila Pa 1976) 1989;14(2):223–8.
76. Patchell RA, Tibbs PA, Regine WF, et al. Direct decompressive surgical resection in the treatment of spinal cord compression caused by metastatic cancer: a randomised trial. Lancet 2005;366(9486):643–8.
77. Smith JS, Shaffrey CI, Sansur CA, et al. Rates of infection after spine surgery based on 108,419 procedures: a report from the Scoliosis Research Society Morbidity and Mortality Committee. Spine (Phila Pa 1976) 2011;36(7):556–63.
78. Wise JJ, Fischgrund JS, Herkowitz HN, et al. Complication, survival rates, and risk factors of surgery for metastatic disease of the spine. Spine (Phila Pa 1976) 1999;24(18):1943–51.
79. Fourney DR, Schomer DF, Nader R, et al. Percutaneous vertebroplasty and kyphoplasty for painful vertebral body fractures in cancer patients. J Neurosurg 2003;98(1 Suppl):21–30.
80. Goetz MP, Callstrom MR, Charboneau JW, et al. Percutaneous image-guided radiofrequency ablation of painful metastases involving bone: a multicenter study. J Clin Oncol 2004;22(2):300–6.
81. Dupuy DE, Liu D, Hartfeil D, et al. Percutaneous radiofrequency ablation of painful osseous metastases: a multicenter American College of Radiology Imaging Network trial. Cancer 2010;116(4):989–97.

Radiation for Treatment of Painful Bone Metastases

Ron Shiloh, MD*, Monica Krishnan, MD

KEYWORDS

- Bone metastases • External beam radiation therapy
- Stereotactic body radiation therapy • Radiopharmaceuticals • Hypofractionation

KEY POINTS

- External beam radiation therapy (EBRT) effectively relieves symptoms for most individuals with painful bone metastases.
- Hypofractionated EBRT is as effective as a multiple fraction radiotherapy course in most cases, although retreatment rates are higher after a single dose of radiation.
- Stereotactic body radiation is a highly focused form of radiation that may be used in cases of oligometastatic disease, repeat irradiation, and radiation-resistant tumors.
- Radiopharmaceuticals may be used for diffuse bone metastases and have a proven overall survival benefit in patients with castrate-resistant prostate cancer.

INTRODUCTION

Pain related to bone metastases may be effectively treated with radiation therapy. Patients with bone metastases represent a heterogeneous population in terms of prognosis and extent of disease, some with widespread metastases, and others with oligometastatic disease. Various modalities employ radiation to treat pain, including external beam radiation therapy (EBRT), its offshoot stereotactic body radiation therapy (SBRT), and radiopharmaceutical therapy. Several variables may be considered when deciding on the optimal modality of radiation therapy for each patient, including prognosis, tumor histology, location and extent of metastases, and association with cord compression.

EXTERNAL BEAM RADIATION THERAPY

External beam radiation therapy (EBRT) is effective at pain improvement in most patients with bone metastases. Various dose and fractionation schedules have been studied and compared, and the optimal approach for every patient may differ.

Disclosure Statement: Nothing to disclose.
Department of Radiation Oncology, Dana-Faber Cancer Institute, Brigham and Women's Cancer Center, 20 Prospect Street, Boston, MA 01757, USA
* Corresponding author.
E-mail address: ron_shiloh@dfci.harvard.edu

Hematol Oncol Clin N Am 32 (2018) 459–468
https://doi.org/10.1016/j.hoc.2018.01.008
0889-8588/18/© 2018 Elsevier Inc. All rights reserved.

hemonc.theclinics.com

Several major prospective clinical trials have evaluated the efficacy of different radiotherapy approaches, including single fraction versus multiple fraction. Overall, the results of the studies suggest that a single fraction of higher-dose radiation may be as effective as a more protracted course of radiation in many patients.[1–6]

Fractionation

The first large-scale study to investigate different fractionation schedules was an RTOG study that enrolled patients between 1974 and 1980 and randomized patients with solitary and multiple bone metastases to different regimens.[1] Of the 1016 patients enrolled in the trial, 266 had solitary metastases, and 750 had multiple metastases. Patients with solitary metastases were randomly assigned to treatment with 40.5 Gy in 15 fractions or 20 Gy in 5 fractions. Those with multiple metastases were randomly assigned to 1 of 4 regimens, 30 Gy in 10 fractions, 15 Gy in 5 fractions, 20 Gy in 5 fractions, or 25 Gy in 5 fractions. Response was assessed using a quantitative measure of pain, based on severity and frequency of pain, as well as frequency of pain medication usage. Overall, 54% of patients obtained complete relief, and 89% of patients experienced at least minimal relief. There were no significant differences between any of the treatment arms in terms of degree or duration of pain relief. Of note, patients with higher pain scores prior to treatment were less likely to respond. Also, patients who completed their treatment as planned had a significantly higher rate of complete response than patients who did not complete treatment. Patients with metastatic breast or prostate cancer responded at significantly higher rates than those with lung or other primary cancers. The authors also noted that regardless of the fractionation schedule, pain relief was first noted within the first 4 weeks of treatment, although complete relief was first reported later than 4 weeks in 50% of patients.

In a re-examination of the data at a later date, the biologically effective dose (BED) was calculated for the different treatment regimens.[7] Linear regression analyses of pain response and freedom from retreatment as a function of BED suggested that regimens with a higher BED resulted in improved pain relief and decreased retreatment rates.

In a move from investigating different multiple fraction regimens, the British Bone Pain Trial Working Party conducted a prospective randomized controlled trial comparing a single fraction of 8 Gy with multiple fraction regimens of 20 Gy in 5 fractions or 30 Gy in 10 fractions.[5] Pain relief, as measured by pain severity and analgesic requirements on self-assessment questionnaires, was the primary endpoint. There were no statistically significant differences in the degree of pain relief or in the time to improvement or increase in pain at any time up to 12 months from randomization. The retreatment rate was twice as high after 8 Gy, consistent with other studies.

Dose and fractionation were again investigated in RTOG 9714, in which 898 patients with bone metastases of breast or prostate cancer primaries were randomized to receive EBRT of 8 Gy in 1 fraction versus 30 Gy in 10 fractions.[2] Complete and partial pain response rates at 3 months were equivalent, with pain complete response/partial response rates of 15%/50% for 8 Gy and 18%/48% for 30 Gy. Although patients receiving 30 Gy experienced more acute toxicity (17% vs 10%), those who received 8 Gy had higher retreatment rates (18% vs 9%). This may have been confounded, however, by greater comfort in retreating after 8 Gy on the part of treating physicians. A subsequent subset analysis of patients with painful vertebral bone metastases demonstrated the same results, namely equivalent efficacy with higher acute toxicity for patients receiving 30 Gy (20% vs 10%) and higher retreatment rates for those receiving 8 Gy (15% vs 5%).[3]

A similar investigation was conducted in the Dutch Bone Metastasis Study, which randomized patients with painful bone metastases to 8 Gy in 1 fraction or 24 Gy in 6 fractions.[6] The difference in pain response, defined as a decrease of at least 2 points on a 10-point scale compared with the initial pain score, was not significant. Secondary endpoints of pain medication usage, quality of life, and adverse effects were also equivalent between the 2 groups. As seen in other studies, the retreatment rate was higher in the single fraction arm.

An updated meta-analysis of palliative radiotherapy trials for bone metastases included 25 randomized controlled trials comparing single-fraction versus multiple-fraction radiotherapy.[4] Overall and complete pain response rates were equivalent. However, retreatment rates were 2.6 times higher for single-fraction radiotherapy. Another meta-analysis also reported a similarly high increase in retreatment rates for single-fraction radiotherapy (21.5% vs 7.4%).[8] In addition, the pathologic fracture rate was twice as high for single-fraction radiotherapy, although the rates were low regardless of fractionation (3% vs 1.6%).

Dose

Single-fraction radiotherapy is most commonly administered as an 8 Gy fraction. Studies have investigated doses ranging from 4 Gy to 10 Gy, although few studies have compared single-fraction regimens. A meta-analysis reported that in those studies that did compare 8 Gy versus lower doses of 4 or 6 Gy, the 8 Gy regimen resulted in superior pain response rates.[9] Only 1 study has investigated the use of 10 Gy in 1 fraction; in that study, patients were randomly assigned to receive 10 Gy in 1 fraction versus 22.5 Gy in 5 fractions.[10] Patients who received 10 Gy had a high complete response rate of 39%, although still lower than the complete response rate of 42% for the patients in the fractionated group. There was no difference in the rate of acute toxicity (fatigue, nausea, or vomiting) between the 2 groups.

Factors Influencing Response

For patients with limited survival, the question of fractionation may be even more relevant. Based on a subanalysis of the Dutch Bone Metastasis Study, pain responded to EBRT in about half of patients who survived up to 12 weeks regardless of fractionation.[11] For those patients, therefore, a single fraction of radiation may be recommended.

Even for patients with a more favorable prognosis, a single fraction may be as effective as multiple-fraction radiotherapy. In another subanalysis of the Dutch Bone Metastasis Study, in those 320 patients who survived more than 1 year, responses were equivalent between the 2 groups (87% after 8 Gy and 85% after 24 Gy).[12] Duration of response and progression rates were also noted to be similar.

Age has not been shown to predict for a different pain response to palliative radiotherapy. When patients in the Dutch Bone Metastasis Study were grouped into 3 age cohorts (<65, 65–74, and ≥75 years), all patients responded similarly to the 2 different fractionation schedules.[13]

Tumor histology may affect the overall response to palliative radiation. In 1 study, patients with a tumor histology other than breast or prostate had a shorter duration of pain relief, with the respective mean duration of pain relief for prostate, breast, and miscellaneous tumors (mostly nonsmall lung cancer [NSCLC]) of 74, 65, and 39 weeks.[14] However, on multivariate analysis, there was no difference noted for the effect of different dose/fractionation schedules on pain relief in patients with different tumor types.

Spinal Cord Compression

When pain is associated with a bone metastasis in the spinal column causing spinal cord compression in surgical candidates (ie, radio-resistant tumors in a single site of the spine, low comorbidities, prognosis of >6 months, spinal instability, neurologic compromise), decompressive surgery followed by postoperative radiotherapy in multiple fractions has been shown to be more effective than multiple-fraction radiotherapy alone in terms of neurologic function and survival.[15] For nonsurgical candidates, radiotherapy alone may be used. A retrospective study of 5 radiotherapy schedules, 8 Gy in a single fraction, 20 Gy in 5 fractions, 30 Gy in 10 fractions, 37.5 Gy in 15 fractions, and 40 Gy in 20 fractions, reported no significant differences for functional outcome between single-fraction and any of the multiple-fraction radiation schedules.[16] However, the 3 more protracted schedules did result in statistically significant lower rates of in-field recurrence. Therefore, for patients with poor predicted survival, 8 Gy in a single fraction may be considered, while patients with a more favorable prognosis may benefit from 30 Gy in 10 fractions. Another consideration is SBRT, which will be discussed further.

Summary of External Beam Radiation Therapy

EBRT has been demonstrated in numerous studies to be an effective way to treat pain in the setting of bone metastases. Most patients will derive as much benefit from a single fraction of radiation as from a multiple-fraction course. Given the consistently higher retreatment rates seen for single-fraction radiotherapy across many studies, for those patients with oligometastatic disease and an otherwise favorable prognosis, a more protracted course may be considered in order to produce a more durable response.

STEREOTACTIC BODY RADIATION THERAPY

As discussed previously, EBRT is often used to treat painful bone metastases, but with conventional techniques, the amount of dose that can be delivered is limited by surrounding normal tissue (ie, the spinal cord). In order to overcome this challenge, SBRT can be used in select patients. SBRT is a highly focused form of radiation designed to deliver high doses to targets while sparing normal surrounding tissue. It is performed using daily image guidance to deliver radiation precisely to the target. This section will focus on the local control benefits of SBRT, toxicity, patient selection, and dose/fractionation. Although SBRT can be used to treat many sites of metastases, here the focus will be primarily on SBRT to the spine.

Local Control

One of the proposed benefits of SBRT over conventional radiation is improved local control due to the higher equivalent doses of radiation that can be delivered. Multiple studies have shown local control rates of 80% to 90% at 1 year with SBRT.[17–21] In a phase 1/2 trial of SBRT for previously unirradiated spine metastases,[20] 61 patients with 63 noncervical spine tumors received SBRT between 2005 and 2010. With a median follow-up of 20 months, the 18-month local control rate was 88%, and no differences were noted in local control with respect to tumor histology of radiation dose. The study also assessed neurologic deterioration and found that with SBRT, the rate of 18-month freedom from neurologic deterioration was 82%. A multi-institution analysis confirmed these local control rates, retrospectively assessing 387 spinal metastases treated at 8 centers in the United States, Canada, and Germany. Local control at 2 years was 83.9%.[22] This study found that on multivariate analysis, an interval between primary diagnosis of cancer and SBRT of no more than 30 months and a histology of NSCLC, renal cell cancer, melanoma, or "other," were correlated with a worse local control rate.

Toxicity

Theoretically, by using a more conformal and focused radiation technique, SBRT can reduce toxicity to normal surrounding structures. Several studies have confirmed this theory for the spinal cord, showing a less than 5% risk of radiation myelopathy with SBRT.[23] However, there remains a considerable risk of vertebral compression fracture, which is the most common toxicity seen with SBRT to the spine. In a systematic review addressing complications with SBRT for spinal metastases, the overall risk of vertebral compression fracture was found to be 13.7%.[23] In another study of 594 tumors treated with spine SBRT, multivariate analysis showed that a pre-existing vertebral compression fracture, a solitary metastasis, and a prescription dose of 38.4 Gy or higher were predictive of a new or progressive vertebral compression fracture.[24]

Candidates for Stereotactic Body Radiation Therapy

SBRT is most often recommended for 3 situations: oligometastatic tumors, repeat irradiation, and radiation-resistant tumors.

Oligometastatic tumors

Although definitions vary, oligometastatic disease is typically defined as having fewer than 4 metastatic lesions. Patients with oligometastatic disease are thought to have improved outcomes compared with those with more widely metastatic disease, with median survivals greater than 1 to 2 years.[25,26] For these patients, more aggressive treatment has been proposed. In a phase 2 study of 49 patients with 3 or fewer metastatic sites, patients were randomized to local consolidative therapy to all metastatic lesions or maintenance therapy (including observation).[27] With a median follow-up of about 12 months, median progression-free survival was 11.9 months for the local ablative therapy group versus 3.9 months for the maintenance therapy group. There was no significant difference in adverse events between the 2 groups. In these patients with longer expected overall survivals, local recurrences after radiation for spine metastases are a real possibility and may be associated with significant morbidity, such as cord compression and compression fractures.[28] In these cases, sites of metastases would ideally be treated with a goal of long-term local control. In a prospective study of patients with 5 or fewer oligometastatic lesions, the 2-year local control rate with SBRT was 67%, and the 4-year local control rate was 60%.[25] These long-term local control rates highlight the rationale for SBRT in patients with oligometastatic disease.

Repeat irradiation

Repeat irradiation is a prime indication for SBRT because of the dose limitations of the spinal cord. With conventional radiation techniques, it is difficult to deliver enough dose with repeat irradiation while still sparing the spinal cord from reaching its tolerance dose. In a meta-analysis of repeat irradiation for painful bone metastases, pain response after repeat irradiation was seen in only about 58% of patients.[29] However, because of the steep gradient of dose with SBRT, it is possible to deliver higher doses to the lesion while limiting the dose to the spinal cord. Multiple studies have shown a 1 year local control rate of 70% to 80% in patients receiving repeat irradiation with SBRT.[30,31] Pain control after SBRT in patients receiving repeat irradiation has been shown to occur in 65% to 81% of patients.[32] Rates of toxicity remain low, with rates of myelopathy ranging from 0% to 2%.[21,31,33]

Radio-resistant histologies

SBRT may also have a role to play in the treatment of metastases from radio-resistant tumors. Numerous animal studies have found renal cell carcinoma and melanoma to be relatively resistant to radiation.[34–36] One study of 107 patients with renal cell metastases at 150 sites found that higher biologically equivalent doses were associated with a higher rate of response to palliative radiation.[37] SBRT has been proposed as a strategy of achieving this higher BED, ideally to improve response and control in these patients. In a study assessing SBRT in the treatment of spinal metastases from renal cell carcinoma, the 1-year tumor progression-free survival rate was 82.1%, and 52% of patients were pain free at 12 months after SBRT.[38] Similarly, a study assessing SBRT in patients treated with SBRT for metastatic melanoma found a metastasis control rate of 94% at 1 year with a complete response achieved in 90% of patients.[39]

Dose and Fractionation

Dose and fractionation schemes vary for SBRT, but typically 1 to 5 fractions are used, with total doses ranging from 18 to 30 Gy. Example schemes include 18 Gy in a single fraction, 30 Gy in 5 fractions, and 27 Gy in 3 fractions. No data currently exist to suggest the ideal dose/fractionation regimen.

Summary of Stereotactic Body Radiation Therapy

SBRT is a highly focused form of radiation that can deliver high doses to target tissue while sparing surrounding normal tissues. It has demonstrated high local control rates when used to treat the spine with minimal toxicity to the spinal cord, although it is associated with a higher risk of vertebral compression fractures. It is primarily indicated in patients with oligometastatic disease, patients requiring retreatment, and patients with radioresistant histologies, such as renal cell carcinoma or melanoma. Dose and fractionation vary, and there are no data to suggest the ideal regimen. Ongoing studies will be aimed at comparing SBRT directly to conventional EBRT.

RADIOPHARMACEUTICALS

Although external beam radiation techniques, including SBRT, have had success for localized pain caused by bone metastases, patients often present with diffuse bone metastases, for which external beam radiation alone is not adequate. Radionuclides, including beta-emitters such as Strontium-89 (^{89}Sr) and Samarium-153 (^{153}Sa), and alpha-emitters such as Radium-223 (^{223}Ra), are promising treatments for pain caused by diffuse bone metastases, as these preferentially target these sites by either inherent calcium-mimetic properties (^{223}Ra, ^{89}Sr) or chelation with ligands that have a high affinity for calcium (^{153}Sm). Research on these radionuclides has thus far been limited primarily to castrate-resistant metastatic prostate cancer. This section will review both beta-emitters and alpha-emitters, their use in patients with metastatic prostate cancer and bone metastases, and their associated toxicities.

Beta-Emitters

Beta-emitters such as ^{89}Sr and ^{153}Sm have been shown to palliate pain, but at the cost of myelosuppression. In a phase 3 randomized controlled trial, 152 men with hormone-refractory prostate cancer and painful bone metastases were randomized to either radioactive ^{153}Sm or placebo (nonradioactive ^{152}Sm).[40] The study showed statistically significant improvement in analgesic consumption and pain with radioactive ^{153}Sm. Pain showed improvement as early as weeks 1 and 2. In another phase 3 randomized placebo control trial, 126 patients with prostate cancer and painful bone metastases were randomized to EBRT alone versus EBRT with ^{89}Sr.[41] There was a statistically significant decrease in analgesic use among patients receiving ^{89}Sr, and a decrease in the number of new painful metastases (58.7% of patients in the ^{153}Sm group vs 34% in the placebo group were free of new painful metastases at 3 months, P<.002), as well as improvement in quality of life. Additionally, more patients in the treatment arm had a greater than 50% reduction in alkaline phosphatase and prostate specific antigen (PSA) over the first 4 months. There was no statistically significant difference in overall survival. In both studies, the primary toxicity was hematological. Both ^{153}Sm and ^{89}Sr demonstrated an increase in thrombocytopenia and leukopenia compared with placebo. With ^{89}Sr + EBRT, there was a 10.4% risk of grade 3 leukopenia compared with a 0% risk with EBRT alone and a 22.4% risk of grade 3 thrombocytopenia, compared with a 1.7% risk with EBRT alone. With ^{153}Sm, there was a 5% risk of grade 3 leukopenia compared with a 0% risk with placebo and a 3% risk of thrombocytopenia compared with a 0% risk with placebo.

Alpha-Emitters

^{223}Ra, an alpha-emitter, has been shown to improve both pain and overall survival without the added myelosuppression seen with beta-emitters. In the ALSYMPCA study, a phase 3 randomized, placebo-controlled trial, 921 patients with castrate-resistant prostate cancer and bone metastases who had received, were not eligible to receive, or declined docetaxel chemotherapy, were randomized to 6 injections of ^{223}Ra versus placebo.[42] The study found a statistically significant improvement in survival with ^{223}Ra. Median survival was 14.9 months in the ^{223}Ra arm versus 11.3 months in the placebo arm, with a 30% reduction in the risk of death in the ^{223}Ra arm. ^{223}Ra was also found to confer statistically significant benefits in time to first symptomatic skeletal event, time to increase in total alkaline phosphatase level, time to increase in PSA level, and quality of life. The number of patients experiencing adverse events was lower in the ^{223}Ra group, and, specifically, there was no statistically significant difference in hematologic adverse events between the 2 groups.

Summary of Radionuclides

Radionuclides are a promising tool to treat bone pain, particularly in patients with castrate-resistant metastatic prostate cancer. Although the beta-emitters ^{153}Sm and ^{89}Sr have shown benefits in pain palliation, they are also associated with myelosuppression. Both are US Food and Drug Administration (FDA) approved for the treatment of pain associated with bone metastases. ^{223}Ra, an alpha-emitter, has demonstrated not only benefits in quality of life, but also improvements in overall survival, without an increase in myelosuppression. ^{223}Ra is approved by the FDA for treatment of patients with castrate-resistant prostate cancer, symptomatic bone metastases, and no known visceral metastatic disease. Future studies will focus on the proper sequencing of ^{223}Ra with other treatments, as well as its use in histologies other than prostate cancer.

REFERENCES

1. Tong D, Gillick L, Hendrickson FR. The palliation of symptomatic osseous metastases: final results of the study by the radiation therapy oncology group. Cancer 1982;50:893–9.

2. Hartsell WF, Scott CB, Bruner DW, et al. Randomized trial of short- versus long-course radiotherapy for palliation of painful bone metastases. J Natl Cancer Ist 2005;97:798–804.

3. Howell DD, James JL, Hartsell WF, et al. Single-fraction radiotherapy versus multifraction radiotherapy for palliation of painful vertebral bone metastases-equivalent efficacy, less toxicity, more convenient: a subset analysis of Radiation Therapy Oncology Group trial 97-14. Cancer 2013;119(4):888–96.

4. Chow E, Zeng L, Salvo N, et al. Update on the systematic review of palliative radiotherapy trials for bone metastases. Clin Oncol 2012;24(2):112–24.

5. 8 Gy single fraction radiotherapy for the treatment of metastatic skeletal pain: randomized comparison with a multifraction schedule over 12 months of patient follow-up. Bone Pain Trial Working Party. Radiother Oncol 1999;52(2):111–21.

6. Steenland E, Leer JW, van Houwelingen H, et al. The effect of a single fraction compared to multiple fractions on painful bone metastases: a global analysis of the dutch bone metastasis study. Radiother Oncol 1999;52(2):101–9.

7. Usuki KY, Milano MT, David M, et al. Metastatic disease: bone, spinal cord, brain, liver, and lung. Clinical Radiation Oncology 2016;432–48.

8. Sze WM, Shelley M, Held I, et al. Palliation of metastatic bone pain: single fraction versus multifraction radiotherapy – a systematic review of the randomised trials. Cochrane Database Syst Rev 2004;(2):CD004721.

9. Chow R, Hoskin P, Hollenberg D, et al. Efficacy of single fraction conventional radiation therapy for painful uncomplicated bone metastases: a systematic review and meta-analysis. Ann Palliat Med 2017;6(2):125–42.

10. Gaze MN, Kelly CG, Kerr CR, et al. Pain relief and quality of life following radiotherapy for bone metastases: a randomised trial of two fractionation schedules. Radiother Oncol 1997;45(2):109–16.

11. Meeuse JJ, van der Linden YM, van Tienhoven G, et al. Efficacy of radiotherapy for painful bone metastases during the last 12 weeks of life: results from the Dutch Bone Metastasis Study. Cancer 2010;116(11):2716–25.

12. Van der Linden YM, Steenland E, van Houwelingen HC, et al. Patients with a favourable prognosis are equally palliated with single and multiple fraction radiotherapy: results on survival in the Dutch Bone Metastasis Study. Radiother Oncol 2006;78(3):245–53.

13. Westhoff PG, de Graeff A, Reyners AK, et al. Effect of age on response to palliative radiotherapy and quality of life on patients with painful bone metastases. Radiother Oncol 2014;111(2):264–9.

14. Arcangeli G, Giovinazzo G, Saracino B, et al. Radiation therapy in the management of symptomatic bone metastases: the effect of total dose and histology on pain relief and response duration. Int J Radiat Oncol Biol Phys 1998;42(5):1119–26.

15. Patchell RA, Tibbs PA, Regine WF. Direct decompressive surgical resection in the treatment of spinal cord compression caused by metastatic cancer: a randomised trial. Lancet 2005;366:643–8.

16. Rades D, Stalpers LJ, Veninga T, et al. Evaluation of five radiation schedules and prognostic factors for metastatic spinal cord compression. J Clin Oncol 2005;23(15):3366–75.

17. Ahmed KA, Stauder MC, Miller RC, et al. Stereotactic body radiation therapy in spinal metastases. Int J Radiat Oncol Biol Phys 2012;82:e803–9.

18. Bishop AJ, Tao R, Rebueno NC, et al. Outcomes for spine stereotactic body radiation therapy and an analysis of predictors of local recurrence. Int J Radiat Oncol Biol Phys 2015;92:1016–26.

19. Finnigan R, Burmeister B, Barry T, et al. Technique and early clinical outcomes for spinal and paraspinal tumours treated with stereotactic body radiotherapy. J Clin Neurosci 2015;22:1258–63.

20. Garg AK, Shiu AS, Yang J, et al. Phase 1/2 trial of single-session stereotactic body radiotherapy for previously unirradiated spinal metastases. Cancer 2012; 118:5069–77.
21. Garg AK, Wang XS, Shiu AS, et al. Prospective evaluation of spinal reirradiation by using stereotactic body radiation therapy: The University of Texas MD Anderson Cancer Center experience. Cancer 2011;117:3509–16.
22. Guckenberger M, Mantel F, Gerszten PC, et al. Safety and efficacy of stereotactic body radiotherapy as primary treatment for vertebral metastases: a multi-institutional analysis. Radiat Oncol 2014;9:226.
23. Husain ZA, Sahgal A, De Salles A, et al. Stereotactic body radiotherapy for de novo spinal metastases: systematic review. J Neurosurg Spine 2017;27(3): 295–302.
24. Jawad MS, Fahim DK, Gerszten PC, et al. Vertebral compression fractures after stereotactic body radiation therapy: a large, multi-institutional, multinational evaluation. J Neurosurg Spine 2016;24:928–36.
25. Milano MT, Katz AW, Muhs AG, et al. A prospective pilot study of curative-intent stereotactic body radiation therapy in patients with 5 or fewer oligometastatic lesions. Cancer 2008;112:650–8.
26. Tree AC, Khoo VS, Eeles RA, et al. Stereotactic body radiotherapy for oligometastases. Lancet Oncol 2013;14:e28–37.
27. Gomez DR, Blumenschein GR Jr, Lee JJ, et al. Local consolidative therapy versus maintenance therapy or observation for patients with oligometastatic non-small-cell lung cancer without progression after first-line systemic therapy: a multicentre, randomised, controlled, phase 2 study. Lancet Oncol 2016;17:1672–82.
28. Lam TC, Uno H, Krishnan M, et al. Adverse outcomes after palliative radiation therapy for uncomplicated spine metastases: role of spinal instability and single-fraction radiation therapy. Int J Radiat Oncol Biol Phys 2015;93:373–81.
29. Huisman M, van den Bosch MA, Wijlemans JW, et al. Effectiveness of reirradiation for painful bone metastases: a systematic review and meta-analysis. Int J Radiat Oncol Biol Phys 2012;84:8–14.
30. Chang UK, Cho WI, Kim MS, et al. Local tumor control after retreatment of spinal metastasis using stereotactic body radiotherapy; comparison with initial treatment group. Acta Oncol 2012;51:589–95.
31. Choi CY, Adler JR, Gibbs IC, et al. Stereotactic radiosurgery for treatment of spinal metastases recurring in close proximity to previously irradiated spinal cord. Int J Radiat Oncol Biol Phys 2010;78:499–506.
32. Myrehaug S, Sahgal A, Hayashi M, et al. Reirradiation spine stereotactic body radiation therapy for spinal metastases: systematic review. J Neurosurg Spine 2017;27(4):428–35.
33. Mahadevan A, Floyd S, Wong E, et al. Stereotactic body radiotherapy reirradiation for recurrent epidural spinal metastases. Int J Radiat Oncol Biol Phys 2011;81:1500–5.
34. Barranco SC, Romsdahl MM, Humphrey RM. The radiation response of human malignant melanoma cells grown in vitro. Cancer Res 1971;31:830–3.
35. Deschavanne PJ, Fertil B. A review of human cell radiosensitivity in vitro. Int J Radiat Oncol Biol Phys 1996;34:251–66.
36. Dewey DL. The radiosensitivity of melanoma cells in culture. Br J Radiol 1971;44: 816–7.
37. DiBiase SJ, Valicenti RK, Schultz D, et al. Palliative irradiation for focally symptomatic metastatic renal cell carcinoma: support for dose escalation based on a biological model. J Urol 1997;158:746–9.

38. Nguyen QN, Shiu AS, Rhines LD, et al. Management of spinal metastases from renal cell carcinoma using stereotactic body radiotherapy. Int J Radiat Oncol Biol Phys 2010;76:1185–92.

39. Youland RS, Packard AT, Blanchard MJ, et al. 18F-FDG PET response and clinical outcomes after stereotactic body radiation therapy for metastatic melanoma. Adv Radiat Oncol 2017;2:204–10.

40. Sartor O, Reid RH, Hoskin PJ, et al. Samarium-153-Lexidronam complex for treatment of painful bone metastases in hormone-refractory prostate cancer. Urology 2004;63:940–5.

41. Porter AT, McEwan AJ, Powe JE, et al. Results of a randomized phase-III trial to evaluate the efficacy of strontium-89 adjuvant to local field external beam irradiation in the management of endocrine resistant metastatic prostate cancer. Int J Radiat Oncol Biol Phys 1993;25:805–13.

42. Parker C, Nilsson S, Heinrich D, et al. Alpha emitter radium-223 and survival in metastatic prostate cancer. N Engl J Med 2013;369:213–23.

Rehabilitation Medicine Approaches to Pain Management

Andrea L. Cheville, MD, MSCE[a],*, Sean R. Smith, MD[b],
Jeffrey R. Basford, MD, PhD[a]

KEYWORDS

- Rehabilitation • Movement-associated pain • Musculoskeletal pain • Orthotics
- Therapeutic exercise • Modalities

KEY POINTS

- Pain arising from musculoskeletal structures is prevalent, functionally devastating, and often refractory to conventional analgesic approaches but is significantly mitigated through rehabilitative approaches.
- Rehabilitative approaches modulate nociception, stabilize and unload painful structures, influence pain perception, and alleviate soft tissue musculotendinous pain.
- Conventional strategies for managing musculoskeletal pain, such as massage, orthotics, and therapeutic exercise, among others, are effective even among patients in the advanced stages of cancer and hematologic conditions, but their use warrants consideration of prognosis, patient resources and preferences, and functional/medical comorbidities.

INTRODUCTION

Pain is a principal driver of disablement and other negative outcomes among patients with hematologic disorders and malignancies. In addition to its adverse effects on the patient, uncontrolled pain radically increases the direct costs of care and results an increased use of the health care system and unplanned hospitalizations and emergency department visits. Analgesics have long been the mainstay of cancer pain management. Unfortunately, despite the use of the World Health Organization Pain

The authors do not have any commercial or financial conflicts of interest. No federal, institutional, or commercial funding sources were used in the preparation of this article.
[a] Department of Physical Medicine and Rehabilitation, Mayo Clinic, 200 First Street Southwest, Rochester, MN 55905, USA; [b] Department of Physical Medicine and Rehabilitation, University of Michigan, University of Michigan Health System, Burlington Building, 325 East Eisenhower Parkway, Ann Arbor, MI 48108, USA
* Corresponding author.
E-mail address: Cheville.andrea@mayo.edu

Hematol Oncol Clin N Am 32 (2018) 469–482
https://doi.org/10.1016/j.hoc.2018.02.001
0889-8588/18/© 2018 Elsevier Inc. All rights reserved.

hemonc.theclinics.com

Ladder, a huge expansion in the number agents available, and the increased use of interventional procedures, many patients fail to achieve adequate control of their pain.

Several factors limit the effectiveness of current modalities. Among these are poorly tolerated side effects; prohibitive cost; and, often, limited efficacy. Although all pain is limiting, pain from bone metastases by impeding movement and weight bearing is uniquely damaging given its profound effects on patients' mobility and activities.

Although it has been integrated into the management of cancer and/or hematologic conditions in only a limited fashion, rehabilitation medicine, has developed strategies that reduce musculoskeletal pain in general and targeted approaches to alleviate movement-related pain. A more systematic integration of its services and approaches into the management of hematology/oncology patients with painful conditions offers several important benefits. First, physical approaches have the potential to reduce pain intensity, particularly of musculoskeletal origin, and thereby lessen patients' dependence on analgesics and interventional procedures. Second, the use of stabilizing and deweighting devices can protect painful structures and thereby enhance patients' comfort, independence, and quality of life. Third, physical therapists (PTs) and occupational therapists (OTs) can work with patients to develop individualized strategies for essential activities (eg, transferring from a bed to a wheelchair) in ways that minimize exacerbation of their pain. Fourth, tailored exercise programs have been shown in diverse cancer and hematologic populations to not only alleviate some types of pain, but also to improve other common, distressing symptoms, such as disturbed sleep and fatigue that may exacerbate pain.

Rehabilitation approaches generally serve as adjuncts to conventional pain management strategies. Although few, with the exceptions of mobility aids and bracing, have a strong evidence base or history of robust use in palliative settings, extensive experience and face validity in other clinical contexts argues that the integration of rehabilitation services should, at a minimum, be considered for patients with refractory pain in light of (1) their potential to lessen the pain; (2) the proven benefits of therapeutic exercise on mobility, symptom burden, and independence; and (3) their limited side effects.

Rehabilitation approaches are grouped into the following categories which, in turn, provide structure for this article: (1) modulating nociception, (2) stabilizing and unloading painful structures, (3) influencing pain perception, and (4) alleviating soft tissue musculotendinous pain. This latter section is included because of benign pain related to the overloading or maladaptive use of muscles that occurs with the loss of skeletal muscle mass, a common feature of late-stage cancers and many hematologic conditions. This article reviews each of these categories and offers examples to illustrate their clinical application. Many applications focus on minimizing movement-associated pain and permitting the patient to remain as functional and independent as possible despite the persistence of pain.

MODULATION OF NOCICEPTIVE INPUT

Rehabilitation uses two approaches to lessen the effects of nociceptive input on pain perception. The first, the use of heat and cold, dates back thousands of years. The second uses low or moderate levels of sensory input to reduce or modulate nociceptive input. The concept, which was introduced by Melzack and Wall[1] in the 1960s, has been termed the "gate theory of pain" and posits that cells in the spinal cord's substantia gelatinosa inhibit the perception of pain by lessening the passage of nociceptive information to the brain in the presence of benign sensory afferent signals. The theory and the approach's effectiveness have been challenged but not disproved despite more than 50 years of research.

Heat and Cold

Heat and cold exert clinically significant effects on the body. Metabolic and enzymatic processes may be markedly accelerated or slowed by temperature changes on the order of 3°C to 7°C altering, among other things, nerve conduction, blood flow/perfusion, and collagen stiffness.[2–5] Effects are local or systemic: immersion of the body at robust but tolerable temperatures can alter core temperatures by 0.3°C to 0.4°C with local heating or cooling effects being even more pronounced.[6] Ice massage over the knee can reduce intra-articular temperatures by 6°C,[7] and agents, such as hot paraffin and diathermy, although now less commonly used, can significantly increase local skin and intra-articular temperatures.[7] Although the heating agents differ, most gain their benefits by producing analgesia and hyperemia or by reducing muscle tone. Cold, although reducing perfusion, also is used for its analgesic and tone-reducing capabilities.

Heat and cold alter a variety of physiologic processes. Their main use, however, has been primarily for analgesia, commonly as adjuncts to exercise and mobilization.[8–11] Heating pads, ice packs, and ice massage are used even in immobilized patients. There are few relative contraindications to their use, but the most significant is sensory or motor impairments that render a patient unable to detect tissue injury or respond to discomfort from thermal modalities.

Electrical Stimulation

Electrical stimulation has a wide number of uses that range from muscle re-education, to strengthening, pain control, and even the healing of bony fractures. This discussion is restricted to its analgesic applications.

Transcutaneous electrical nerve stimulation

Transcutaneous electronic nerve stimulation (TENS) is one of the most thoroughly studied and widespread of the modalities used to modulate nociception. Its introduction offered a noninvasive means to provide the afferent sensory stimuli posited by the "gate theory" as necessary to block nociceptive signals.[1] A few successful trials ensured its acceptance. This acceptance and use have not, however, resulted in a full characterization of its best applications or the complete characterization of how it achieves its effects.

TENS units are typically small and consist of a power source, one or more sets of electrodes, and a programable signal generator. These devices can produce a variety of stimuli with currents generally less than 100 mA, pulse rates ranging from a few to 200 Hz, and pulse widths of from 10 to a few hundred microseconds. Varying stimulation parameters are chosen to increase their effectiveness, improve comfort, and lessen tachyphylaxis.

Electrodes may be located over the painful area, but the stimulation of afferent nerves, acupuncture points, and other locations is often assessed. Stimulation settings are similarly idiosyncratic. Two options are the most commonly used. The first ("low intensity" or "conventional" TENS) uses barely perceptible levels of stimulation at frequencies of about 40 to 90 Hz. The second is more nociceptive in nature and uses low, 1- to 8-Hz, frequencies in association with more intense and mildly uncomfortable stimulation levels.

Therapeutic responses are not guaranteed and difficult to predict. TENS studies range in quality from well-designed, prospective, randomized, controlled investigations to, particularly in the earlier days, small and poorly blinded trials. Even today, comparisons of TENS with other treatment approaches are rarer than desired.

Several studies in the 1970s and 1980s focused on postoperative incisional and labor pain with the finding that TENS usage resulted in benefits comparable with limited amounts of analgesics including narcotics.[12–14]

Research over the subsequent years has had mixed results with more recent evidence-based clinical guidelines and systematic reviews finding no or insufficient evidence that TENS was more effective than sham treatment in reducing acute or amputation-related pain. Findings for low back and osteoarthritic pain are also mixed but somewhat more promising, particularly if treatment session durations are extended.[15,16] In summary, support for TENS use remains equivocal, although it must be noted that the reviews typically include a disclaimer that the strength of their conclusions are limited by heterogeneities in study design, parameter choice, and study quality.

Research in the effectiveness of TENS in cancer or hematologically related pain *per se* has been limited. As a result, although there are suggestions that TENS is capable of improving movement/weightbearing-associated cancer pain, a recent Cochrane review found little or evidenced-based support for cancer-related pain[17] with the notation that treatment was well tolerated but that the evidence was too limited to recommend the use of TENS in this context.

TENS has a long history of use and an exemplary safety record. Side effects tend to be mild and restricted to skin irritation and mild discomfort. Concerns about interference with the function of cardiac pacemakers are reasonable but these devices seem resistant to TENS. Nevertheless, it seems reasonable to avoid their use on the thorax of people with pacemakers or near the epiglottis, carotid sinus, or the low back/abdomen of women during pregnancy.

The question arises: Why does TENS continue to be prescribed and accepted by patients despite the limited evidence base? Several reasons seem pertinent. The first is that patients often note benefit over periods of long-term follow-up (eg, a year) and they may benefit from a lasting placebo effect despite teaching that placebo benefits lessen with time. Second, although systematic reviews typically find limited evidence of effectiveness, study heterogeneity prevents them from concluding that treatment is ineffective. Third, treatment is safe and side effects minimal. Fourth, efficacy in neuropathic and nociceptive pain (most patients with cancer experience a mixture of both[18,19]) is anecdotally and weakly empirically supported by reductions in patient pain ratings. Fifth, a TENS evaluation is easily included as an adjunct to a physical therapy program without limiting the PT focus on proven beneficial efforts, such as transfer training and strengthening. Sixth, the prolonged use of TENS for periods of a year seems to be beneficial for some patients. In summary, a good candidate for TENS might be someone with a moderate level of localized pain that is poorly controlled by conventional means and is either intolerant of, or wishes to avoid, analgesic medications.

Counterstimulation and desensitization techniques

Although TENS receives a great deal of attention, there are other longer standing rehabilitation approaches to lessen pain. Desensitization techniques, for example, involve the gradual increase in sensory input (eg, stroking, temperature changes, or gradually increased movement) of a painful/allodynic limb, such as may occur in complex regional and neuropathic pain. Other physical approaches, such as the compression wrapping of a painful, edematous limb, can reduce pain while also controlling edema and facilitating the use of the limb.

BONE PAIN AND STABILIZATION

Cancer, whether or not associated with metastatic bone involvement, is often associated with limitations in the body's or a limb's ability to carry out the activities essential to daily life. Bone pain in the face of metastatic cancer is a prominent concern. For example, a cervical vertebra with metastatic involvement may produce disabling and episodically severe pain because the neck not only supports the weight of the head but also its positioning in space. Uninvolved musculoskeletal elements, whether caused by muscle wasting or imbalanced/unaccustomed forces from systemic effects of cancer or its treatment,[20,21] also can be affected. Virtually any distorting force, such as radiation-induced soft tissue contractures and fibrosis, pectoralis muscle tension from breast implants, or lessened core strength following abdominal surgery, can produce abnormal and painful forces on otherwise intact musculoskeletal elements.

Four approaches are used to stabilize or reduce the forces placed on painful bony or connective tissues: (1) load displacement, (2) improving the ability of intact structures to carry out their tasks, (3) immobilization, and (4) using compensatory techniques to carry out painful activities. The information in the following sections is organized by therapeutic approach similar to the manner in which a therapy prescription is structured. More than a single modality is often used.

Assistive Devices for Mobility and Activities of Daily Living Performance

A wide range of devices to assist patients with safe and independent mobility is available. Those pictured in **Fig. 1** include a single point cane, a quad cane, a hemi-walker, and a rolling walker. Each has its unique requirements and its strengths and weaknesses. The need for the guidance of a PT and the importance of professionally supervised trials and fitting cannot be overstated if patients are to use and incorporate these devices effectively into their lives. Mechanized or electrical assistive devices may be required to substitute for entire activities if pain renders their performance intolerable. For example, a Hoyer lift or lesser variant, scooter, wheelchair, or even a stairway elevator permits a patient to maintain a modified form of independence far longer than is otherwise possible. Several reports have quantified the off-loading achieved by various mobility assistive devices and found it to exceed 30% or more in the case of a cane alone.[22]

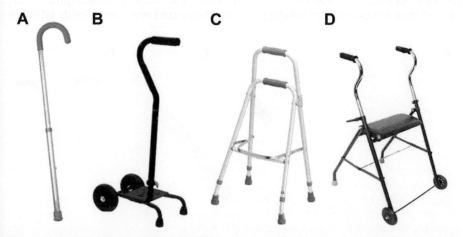

A   **B**   **C**   **D**

Fig. 1. (A–D) Assistive devices for mobility.

A wide array of assistive devices is available that can assist patients in maintaining their level of activity and protect vulnerable or painful structures from activities of daily living–related forces. **Fig. 2** shows a by no means inclusive list of simple possibilities, such as a zipper pull, dressing stick, button aid, and sock aid. It should be noted that an OT consultation is essential in all but the simplest situations because these therapists are knowledgeable about the available options, can teach compensatory strategies, and are trained in evaluating and instructing patients and their caregivers in their correct use. Although the efficacy of assistive devices for activities of daily living has not been well assessed in cancer and hematologic disorders, extensive clinical experience in stroke and other conditions (eg, the use of elastic shoe laces and a long-handled shoe horn permitting a patient to dress independently despite an inability to bend forward) supports their use.

Compensatory Strategies

Compensatory strategies deserve a more detailed review. In particular, although their pain-relieving benefits arise as do that of orthotics and assistive devices from the reduction of forces on weak and/or painful structures, there are important distinctions that should be kept in mind.

Daily activities consist of a combination of coordinated movements that PTs and OTs are trained in isolating and devising alternative, "compensatory," strategies to avoid triggering pain during their performance while still allowing the individual to carry out important tasks. Activities that can benefit from this approach vary widely and can range from propelling or transferring into or out of a wheelchair to dressing and being able to use a restroom without assistance. Home visits were once an effective way for a therapist to assess a patient's need. They have become increasingly rare because of reimbursement issues, but the use of cellphone photographs and videos have proven surprisingly effective in dealing with architectural barriers, choosing durable medical equipment, and home modifications.

Therapeutic Exercise

Muscles are dynamic and often provide the most effective means of stabilizing and immobilizing painful structures. The use of muscles in this manner, often termed dynamic stabilization, has been a mainstay in the treatment of low back and knee pain for years. As a result, therapeutic exercises aimed at enhancing the strength and stamina of muscles capable of splinting a painful body part are a remarkably effective

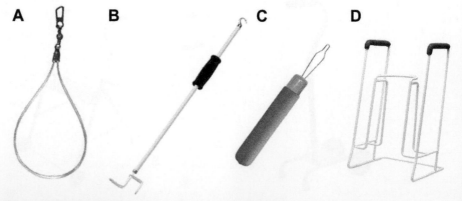

Fig. 2. (*A–D*) Assistive devices for activities of daily living.

adjunct to conventional analgesia. Further consideration of the translation of the techniques of sports and musculoskeletal medicine into the realm of palliative rehabilitation seems warranted given the benefits of unloading painful areas and mobilizing the patient with metastatic disease.[23] Core strengthening exercises have been shown to not only be safe in patients with osseous vertebral metastases, but also improve bone density when performed concurrent with palliative radiation therapy.

Although conceptually simple, therapeutic exercises should be chosen and implemented by a PT with the skills and time to identify the painful structures and movements and to design a strengthening program that can effectively splint or constrain the movement of a pain-generating structure. Frequently, patients are more tolerant of isometric contractions that avoid pain-producing changes in muscle or joint positioning. Common examples of their use to stabilize pain-generating bony structures include strengthening of the abdominal and hip abductor muscles to deweight painful vertebrae and hip joints, respectively.

Before patients with bony metastases perform therapeutic exercise, it is important that a physician evaluate them to determine the proper exercise program given their disease status, burden, and goals. Physiatrists and other specialists, such as surgeons specializing in spine care, can assess the stability of metastatic lesions based on the patient's symptoms, the physical examination, and radiographic findings.

Orthotics

Orthotics come in multiple forms but, fundamentally, all are used to stabilize, protect, and unload compromised musculoskeletal structures. Stabilization is probably the most common application of orthotics and devices that range from those that may immobilize a single joint, such as a wrist or ankle orthosis, to a molded thoracolumbar-sacral orthotic designed to limit the motion of a significant portion of the spine. Most orthotics are static but some are more complex and involve dynamic and even electronically assisted motion. Most are commercially available, whereas others may need to be fabricated by a therapist or orthotist. Those used in the palliative setting are, in large part, designed to stabilize the cervical, truncal, and lumbar spine.

Spinal braces are often ordered by an orthopedic or spinal surgeon to counteract dangerous or painful spinal instability. Custom or modular molded body jackets ("clam shell" braces) are most effective[24] but suffer from high cost and poor patient tolerance. Comfort is never ideal, but can often be improved by having the orthotist revisit to trim the orthotic (particularly in the groin and under the arms) once the patient has been up and about and has had a chance to isolate the pressure points. When possible, off-the-shelf commercially available semirigid braces are a less restricting alternative.[25]

These orthotics are designed to address instability at different levels of the spine. Extension thoraco-lumbo-sacral orthotics, such as the CASH & Jewett braces (https://www.allardusa.com/), are widely available and generally better tolerated than their molded counterparts. These devices are often referred to as "three-point braces" because they apply pressure at two anterior points (the upper and lower trunk) and at a third point on the midback. A significant benefit is that they can be assessed on a trial basis without the need to commit the patient first to an expensive custom fabrication. Although these devices do limit spinal flexion (by far the most common need in metastatic disease),[26] they do little to reduce spinal extension.

Lumbosacral orthoses (LSOs) are most effective at the L3–L4 and L4–L5 levels and are, for the most part, variations on the abdominal corset that may have variably rigid struts. The off-the-shelf Bell-Horn brace (**Fig. 3**), for example, is a lightweight LSO that is representative of many similar braces. Like abdominal binders, the Bell-Horn and

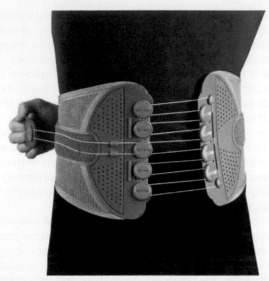

Fig. 3. Off-the-shelf Bell-Horn back brace. (*Courtesy of* DJO Global, Vista, CA.)

other LSOs are believed to alleviate pain by deweighting the spine through compression of the abdominal contents to generate a load-bearing fluid column.[25] This sounds potentially uncomfortable, but LSOs are generally well tolerated and may gain some of their benefits by simply providing a "movement reminder" and warmth to the lumbar musculature. An advantage of most LSOs is that they are easily trialed before purchase and may have drawstrings to facilitate easier donning and adjustment.

Cervical orthoses range in their ability to provide support from the more rigid immobilization of a halo brace through a range of commercially available orthoses extending from the Miami J and Philadelphia collars to the limited capabilities of a soft cervical collar.[27] All are variably uncomfortable and if pain control, rather than stabilization, is the goal of use, a trial of several alternatives may be warranted.

Once the need for an orthotic is determined (and in the case of a spinal instability, established by the surgeon) its ordering and fitting are straightforward and within the practice scope of most PTs. Patients can, in simpler situations, be directed to go to an orthotist or order one online after being instructed in the name and nature of the device they need. Larger medical centers often have arrangements with orthotists that permit the patient to be easily fitted in the hospital and outpatient clinic settings.

Positioning

The use of pillows, adaptive equipment, and home modifications is remarkably effective in maintaining a patient's comfort and protecting their vulnerable skin and soft tissue areas. Careful instruction is necessary because professional and other caregivers often receive little information in their use. For example, pillows are used to reduce pressure on compromised muscles and tissue and support the arms of people with treated head and neck cancers. **Fig. 4** illustrates a range of inexpensive and commercially available positioning options.

Laser Therapy

Laser therapy (also known as photobiomodulation) has been used since the late 1960s to treat pain and a wide variety of soft tissue injuries. Although lasers

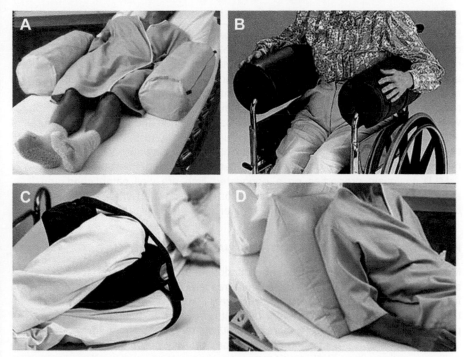

Fig. 4. (*A–D*) Positioning devices. (*Courtesy of* TIDI Products, LLC.)

continue to be used, they have largely been replaced by superluminous diodes that share their ability to produce monochromatic light. Treatment, regardless of the light source, tends to involve 30-mW to 150-mW or greater devices delivering intensities of 2 to 4 J/cm^2. The approach is considered "athermal" (hence the older "cold laser" terminology) because they do not significantly raise tissue temperatures. Support for their use is based on findings that irradiation at these intensities can, among other things, modulate cellar processes and DNA synthesis. Multiple devices are available and typically have been approved by the Food and Drug Administration as an adjunct to pain treatment because of their similarity to heat lamps.

Clinical benefits, in distinction to laboratory-based cellular findings, have proven more difficult to establish. As a result, although several systematic reviews find variably strong evidence of treatment benefit in complex regional pain[28] and a variety of localized soft tissue musculoskeletal disorders[29,30] more generalized involvement, such as myofascial pain, may be more resistant. Mucositis has received some attention in the photobiomodulation community. Reports tend to be positive and a 2010 Cochrane review found that there was limited evidence that light therapy could reduce the severity of mucositis and lessen the need for analgesia.[31] The benefits of light therapy versus other approaches is unknown.

Safety

These devices are typically used at very low power. Therefore, safety other than the need to exhibit reasonable restraint and for the patient and the therapist to wear safety goggles, has not been a concern.

Manual Lymphatic Drainage for Interstitial Fluid Congestion

Manual lymphatic drainage (MLD), also known as lymphatic or Vodder massage, requires highly trained and experienced therapists capable of administering a complex regimen. Specific stroking maneuvers, orientations, pressures, and sequences, applied in a carefully choreographed manner, are essential to the transport of lymph and the effective clearance of fluid and potentially inflammatory and nociceptive macromolecules.[32] Gentle and rhythmic stretching of the skin is used to direct lymph toward intact lymph vessels and nodes. Massage is gentle and limited to pressures of around 30 to 45 mm Hg. Treatment is begun proximally to the involved region with the mobilized fluids directed toward functioning lymphatic vessels and nodes. Treatments gradually progress distally to the most distal areas of involvement.

MLD analgesic properties on a congested limb are well established and it is, accordingly, being applied to other painful conditions in which lymphedema is thought to play a role.[33,34] MLD is well tolerated, even by patients with significant allodynia.

REHABILITATION APPROACHES TO THE MANAGEMENT OF MUSCULOSKELETAL PAIN

Most analgesic modalities used in rehabilitation medicine are directed toward soft tissue and musculoskeletal pain. These structures may become pain generators through four primary mechanisms: (1) direct involvement by disease processes (eg, tumor infiltration), (2) changes resulting from treatment or muscle wasting, (3) exacerbation of pre-existing conditions, and (4) increased muscle tone because of items 2 and 3.

Exacerbation of a pre-existing condition or pain may be the most common in the palliative setting, although this, as far as we can ascertain, has never been epidemiologically confirmed. It should be noted that although the listing that follows isolates individual approaches, two or more may be combined into a single treatment program.

Rest, Ice, Compression, and Elevation

Rest, ice, compression, and elevation, although somewhat controversial, continues to be widely used because of its effectiveness and safety in controlling acute inflammation. Acute musculoskeletal pain with a clear precipitating factor, such as trauma, warrants a trial. Techniques vary from regular placement and removal of cold wraps for a day or two (when tolerated) to a more aggressive twice daily immersion of the affected body part in an ice water slurry.

Injections

Therapeutic injections are designed to deliver high concentrations of an analgesic or anti-inflammatory agent to a localized area with a goal of minimizing systemic effects. Although a large number of agents are used, steroids and local anesthetics, often in combination, remain the most common. Ultrasound guidance is increasingly used to optimize localization. In some cases, such as nerve blocks, ultrasound may be more effective than traditional landmark guided techniques; in others, especially when lipophilic agents are used, it may not be. Inflamed tendons, bursae, and synovium are the most common targets. The role of botulinum toxin in treating myofascial pain and other musculoskeletal pain sources remains unclear but intriguing.[35]

The long-term benefits of musculoskeletal injections seem to be less pronounced than PT alone, although the onset of their benefits tends to be more rapid. In lateral epicondylitis,[36] for example, although injections produce near-term anti-inflammatory benefits, a rebound of symptoms may follow.[37] Given this, it may be that for patients with slowly progressive diseases, PT in conjunction with, or independent of, an injection, may offer a greater benefit than an injection alone. Those in the late stages need near-term relief and may not survive to enjoy the more sustained benefits of PT.

Injections involving steroids are safe, although cumulative long-term detrimental effects may exist; an individual joint should receive at most three in a given year. Many physicians perform these procedures, although specialists should be consulted for difficult to reach sites, when the pain generator is infiltrated by or adjacent to cancer, or when unconventional approaches are needed.

Myofascial Release Techniques and Trigger Points

Myofascial pain is frequently located in the upper back and affects millions of people.[38,39] It is associated with tenderness on palpation, areas of increased tone ("taut bands"), and smaller areas of tenderness ("trigger points") that when subjected to pressure, generate stereotypical patterns of referred pain. Although its nature is becoming clearer with research, its cause remains unknown. Massage, often accompanied with heat, and muscle tension release techniques and relaxation exercises are central to treatment. The relative benefits of injecting a local anesthetic, botulinum toxin, steroids, or simply using a bare needle to stimulate the bands or trigger points remains unclear. However, because benefits have been found for the use of even small gauge (>30) needles, these may be preferred for the initial invasive trial.

Therapeutic Exercise

It cannot be emphasized too strongly that therapeutic exercise is central to the treatment of muscle-related pain whether of myofascial origin or related to overuse. The latter occurs frequently in advanced disease. It may not be possible to reverse the effects of the precipitating event, but the intensity and chronicity of the forces can generally be improved through judicious use of therapeutic exercise. Evaluation by a physician or therapist familiar with complex musculoskeletal pain syndromes, whether myofascial or other causes, offers the best chance of developing an effective and appropriately individualized exercise program.

When conducted properly, therapeutic exercise can have profound benefits with few side effects. For example, patients with breast cancer experience lower pain levels with directed exercise for a variety of conditions, including post-treatment shoulder pain[40] and aromatase inhibitor arthralgias.[41] Additionally, exercise seems to be effective and well-tolerated even during acute pain in chemotherapy.[42] The reasons for this are multifactorial. First, exercise can directly stretch painful, tight muscles, such as the pectoralis major and serratus anterior, and strengthen antagonist muscles to prevent reinjury. Exercise also increases trophic factors to heal muscles and reduce deleterious inflammation. Finally, a structured exercise program empowers patients to understand better what generates and alleviates their pain, potentially reducing the severity of future pain flares.

Overuse injuries are among the most common in cancer survivors, because initial oncologic treatment may lead to deconditioning and a possibly painful re-entry into physical activity. In fact, most cancer survivors do not meet recommended exercise guidelines and reduce their overall activity even after cancer treatment is complete.[43] Furthermore, certain conditions that require long-term corticosteroid use as treatment (eg, multiple myeloma, graft-versus-host disease, symptomatic metastatic disease) can weaken muscles through the destruction of type 2 fibers and lead to tendinopathies.[44] In this event, the proper application of therapeutic exercise, such as eccentric strengthening of the affected muscle and stretching antagonist muscles, can lead to long-term relief and prevent further injury. Eccentric strengthening is the contraction of the muscle during lengthening, and induces small tears in the tendon leading to a proinflammatory response to strengthen the structure. Expert evaluation is recommended, however, because the timeframe for recovery may be long and sometimes painful, and adjunctive treatments, such as corticosteroid injections, tenodesis, and modalities described previously may be required.

Safety must be considered before starting an exercise program in certain conditions, such as bone metastases, and a physician with expertise in the neuromusculoskeletal system, such as a physiatrist, can evaluate a patient before beginning a program and tailor treatment plans specific to the patient's needs. Up to 90% of patients with cancer have comorbid conditions that potentially interfere with an exercise program, including peripheral neuropathy, steroid myopathy, cognitive dysfunction following chemotherapy, and more.[45] Controlling the symptoms from these conditions, if present, is essential to a successful exercise program.

Beyond pain, the benefits of exercise in cancer survivors are numerous, and it should be a mainstay of treatment along the care continuum. It has been shown consistently to have positive benefits on body composition, physical function, psychological well-being, body mass index, peak oxygen consumption, and quality of life.[46] If a patient is having difficulty exercising because of pain or for any other reason, undergoing supervised, focused physical or occupational therapy may be necessary to facilitate long-term patient-directed exercise. If needed, a physiatrist can coordinate therapy and diagnose and treat other pain generators and symptoms inhibiting patients from exercising.

SUMMARY

Rehabilitation medicine offers a range of pain management approaches. Rehabilitative approach may be particularly helpful for patients with refractory movement-associated pain who do not wish to, or cannot, tolerate pharmacoanalgesia.

REFERENCES

1. Melzack R, Wall PD. Pain mechanisms: a new theory. Science 1965;150(3699): 971–9.
2. Knight KL. Cryotherapy: theory, technique and physiology. 1st edition. Chattanooga (TN): Chattanooga Corporation; 1985.
3. Guyton AC. Textbook of medical physiology. 7th edition. Philadelphia: WB Saunders; 1986.
4. Denys EH. AAEM minimonograph #14: the influence of temperature in clinical neurophysiology. Muscle Nerve 1991;14:795–811.
5. Lehmann JF, Silverman DR, Baum BR, et al. Temperature distributions in the human thigh, produced by infrared, hot pack and microwave applications. Arch Phys Med Rehabil 1966;47:291–9.
6. Doering TJ, Aaslid R, Steuernagel B, et al. Cerebral autoregulation during whole-body hypothermia and hyperthermia. Am J Phys Med Rehabil 1999;78(1):33–8.
7. Oosterveld FG, Rasker JJ. Effects of local heat and cold treatment of surface and articular temperature of arthritic knees. Arthritis Rheum 1994;31(11):1578–82.
8. Chou R, Huffman LH. Nonpharmacologic therapies for acute and chronic low back pain: a review of the evidence for an American Pain Society/American College of Physicians clinical practice guideline. Ann Intern Med 2007;147(7): 492–504 [Summary for patients in Ann Intern Med 2007;147(7):I45; PMID: 17909203].
9. French SD, Cameron M, Walker BF, et al. Superficial heat or cold for low back pain. Cochrane Database Syst Rev 2006;(1):CD004750.

10. Lin YH. Effects of thermal therapy in improving the passive range of knee motion: comparison of cold and superficial heat applications. Clin Rehabil 2003;17(6): 618–23.

11. Brosseau L, Robinson V, Pelland L, et al. Efficacy of thermotherapy for rheumatoid arthritis: a meta-analysis. Phys Ther Rev 2002;7(1):5–15.

12. Philadelphia Panel. Philadelphia panel evidence-based clinical practice guidelines on selected rehabilitation interventions for knee pain. Phys Ther 2001; 81(10):1675–700.

13. Chen L, Tang J, White PF, et al. The effect of location of transcutaneous electrical nerve stimulation on postoperative opioid analgesic requirement: acupoint versus nonacupoint stimulation. Anesth Analg 1998;87(5):1129–34.

14. Hamza MA, White PF, Ahmed HE, et al. Effect of the frequency of transcutaneous electrical nerve stimulation on the postoperative opioid analgesic requirement and recovery profile. Anesthesiology 1999;91(5):1232–8.

15. Pengel HM, Maher CG, Refshauge KM, et al. Systematic review of conservative interventions for subacute low back pain. Clin Rehabil 2002;16(8):811–20.

16. Cheing GL, Tsui AY, Lo SK, et al. Optimal stimulation duration of tens in the management of osteoarthritic knee pain. J Rehabil Med 2003;35(2):62–8.

17. Hurlow A, Bennett MI, Robb KA, et al. Transcutaneous electric nerve stimulation (TENS) for cancer pain in adults. Cochrane Database Syst Rev 2012;(3):CD006276.

18. Caraceni A, Portenoy RK. An international survey of cancer pain characteristics and syndromes. IASP Task Force on Cancer Pain. International Association for the Study of Pain. Pain 1999;82(3):263–74.

19. Zech DF, Grond S, Lynch J, et al. Validation of World Health Organization Guidelines for cancer pain relief: a 10-year prospective study. Pain 1995;63(1):65–76.

20. Cheville AL, Tchou J. Barriers to rehabilitation following surgery for primary breast cancer. J Surg Oncol 2007;95(5):409–18.

21. Stubblefield MD. Radiation fibrosis syndrome: neuromuscular and musculoskeletal complications in cancer survivors. PM R 2011;3(11):1041–54.

22. Blount WP. Don't throw away the cane. J Bone Joint Surg Am 1956;38-A(3): 695–708.

23. Cheville AL, Kollasch J, Vandenberg J, et al. A home-based exercise program to improve function, fatigue, and sleep quality in patients with stage IV lung and colorectal cancer: a randomized controlled trial. J Pain Symptom Manage 2012;45(5):811–21.

24. Vander Kooi D, Abad G, Basford JR, et al. Lumbar spine stabilization with a thoracolumbosacral orthosis: evaluation with video fluoroscopy. Spine (Phila Pa 1976) 2004;29(1):100–4.

25. Utter A, Anderson ML, Cunniff JG, et al. Video fluoroscopic analysis of the effects of three commonly-prescribed off-the-shelf orthoses on vertebral motion. Spine (Phila Pa 1976). 2010;35(12):E525–9.

26. Rose PS, Buchowski JM. Metastatic disease in the thoracic and lumbar spine: evaluation and management. J Am Acad Orthop Surg 2011;19(1):37–48.

27. Sandler AJ, Dvorak J, Humke T, et al. The effectiveness of various cervical orthoses. An in vivo comparison of the mechanical stability provided by several widely used models. Spine (Phila Pa 1976). 1996;21(14):1624–9.

28. Smart KM, Wand BM, O'Connell NE. Physiotherapy for pain and disability in adults with complex regional pain syndrome (CRPS) types I and II. Cochrane Database Syst Rev 2016;2:CD010853.

29. Jain TK, Sharma NK. The effectiveness of physiotherapeutic interventions in treatment of frozen shoulder/adhesive capsulitis: a systematic review. J Back Musculoskeletal Rehabil 2014;27(3):247–73.
30. Dingemanse R, Randsdorp M, Koes BW, et al. Evidence for the effectiveness of electrophysical modalities for treatment of medial and lateral epicondylitis: a systematic review. Br J Sports Med 2014;48(12):957–65.
31. Clarkson JE, Worthington HV, Furness S, et al. Interventions for treating oral mucositis for patients with cancer receiving treatment. Cochrane Database Syst Rev 2010;(8):CD001973.
32. Casley-Smith JR, Casley-Smith JR. The pathophysiology of lymphedema and the action of benzo-pyrones in reducing it. Lymphology 1988;21(3):190–4.
33. Ebert JR, Joss B, Jardine B, et al. Randomized trial investigating the efficacy of manual lymphatic drainage to improve early outcome after total knee arthroplasty. Arch Phys Med Rehabil 2013;94(11):2103–11.
34. Ekici G, Bakar Y, Akbayrak T, et al. Comparison of manual lymph drainage therapy and connective tissue massage in women with fibromyalgia: a randomized controlled trial. J Manipulative Physiol Ther 2009;32(2):127–33.
35. Soares A, Andriolo RB, Atallah AN, et al. Botulinum toxin for myofascial pain syndromes in adults. Cochrane Database Syst Rev 2012;(4):CD007533.
36. Coombes BK, Bisset L, Brooks P, et al. Effect of corticosteroid injection, physiotherapy, or both on clinical outcomes in patients with unilateral lateral epicondylalgia: a randomized controlled trial. JAMA 2013;309(5):461–9.
37. Bisset L, Beller E, Jull G, et al. Mobilisation with movement and exercise, corticosteroid injection, or wait and see for tennis elbow: randomised trial. BMJ 2006;333(7575):939.
38. Alvarez DJ, Rockwell PG. Trigger points: diagnosis and management. Am Fam Physician 2002;65(4):653–60.
39. Gerwin RD. Classification, epidemiology, and natural history of myofascial pain syndrome. Curr Pain Headache Rep 2001;5(5):412–20.
40. Cantarero-Villanueva I, Fernandez-Lao C, Fernandez-de-Las-Penas C, et al. Effectiveness of water physical therapy on pain, pressure pain sensitivity, and myofascial trigger points in breast cancer survivors: a randomized, controlled clinical trial. Pain Med 2012;13(11):1509–19.
41. Irwin ML, Cartmel B, Gross CP, et al. Randomized exercise trial of aromatase inhibitor-induced arthralgia in breast cancer survivors. J Clin Oncol 2015;33(10):1104–11.
42. Andersen C, Rorth M, Ejlertsen B, et al. Exercise despite pain–breast cancer patient experiences of muscle and joint pain during adjuvant chemotherapy and concurrent participation in an exercise intervention. Eur J Cancer Care (Engl) 2014;23(5):653–67.
43. Sabatino SA, Coates RJ, Uhler RJ, et al. Provider counseling about health behaviors among cancer survivors in the United States. J Clin Oncol 2007;25(15):2100–6.
44. Pereira RM, Freire de Carvalho J. Glucocorticoid-induced myopathy. Joint Bone Spine 2011;78(1):41–4.
45. Brown JC, Ko EM, Schmitz KH. Development of a risk-screening tool for cancer survivors to participate in unsupervised moderate- to vigorous-intensity exercise: results from a survey study. PM R 2015;7(2):113–22.
46. Fong DY, Ho JW, Hui BP, et al. Physical activity for cancer survivors: meta-analysis of randomised controlled trials. BMJ 2012;344:e70.

Psychological Treatment

Thomas B. Strouse, MD[a],*, Brenda Bursch, PhD[b]

KEYWORDS

- Cancer • Pain • Psychological • Cognitive behavioral • Hypnosis • Relaxation

KEY POINTS

- Pain, coping challenges, psychological distress, and psychiatric disorders are highly prevalent during cancer treatment and its sequelae.
- Cognitive behavioral approaches that include relaxation skills and/or hypnotherapy have strong research support for pain reduction among cancer patients.
- Research results support the value of integrating behavioral health interventions into cancer treatment settings.

INTRODUCTION

Psychological distress and pain associated with cancer and its treatment can create a toxic dyad, with each potentially exacerbating the other in a cyclical manner. The biopsychosocial model defines symptoms as the product of biological, psychological, and social subsystems interacting at multiple levels.[1] Psychological factors shown to contribute to pain range from personality traits (eg, passive and dependent coping styles, low self-efficacy, attentional control, and the tendency to catastrophize in response to stressors) to emotional state factors (such as anxiety, depression, trauma symptoms, uncertainty, helplessness, hopelessness, and anger). Beliefs about the cause or consequences of pain can also contribute to the pain experience. Such factors can represent longstanding, precancer patterns, or can emerge for the first time during the stresses of diagnosis, treatment, and survivorship.

Pain, coping challenges, psychological distress, and psychiatric disorders are highly prevalent during cancer treatment and its sequelae. Research has revealed that 53% of patients will report significant pain symptoms at some point during or after cancer treatment.[2] Mood disorders are found in 20% to 30% of patients engaged in active disease-modifying treatment and in up to 40% of those in survivorship.[3] It is likely that treatments

Disclosure Statement: Neither author has a conflict to disclose.
a Resnick Neuropsychiatric Hospital at UCLA, UCLA Department of Psychiatry, David Geffen School of Medicine, 757 Westwood Plaza, Room 4230B, Los Angeles, CA 90095, USA;
b Pediatric Psychiatry Consultation Liaison Service, David Geffen School of Medicine at UCLA, 760 Westwood Plaza, Semel 48-241, Los Angeles, CA 90024-1759, USA
* Corresponding author:
E-mail address: TStrouse@mednet.ucla.edu

Hematol Oncol Clin N Am 32 (2018) 483–491
https://doi.org/10.1016/j.hoc.2018.01.010
0889-8588/18/© 2018 Elsevier Inc. All rights reserved.

hemonc.theclinics.com

that improve depression symptoms have a greater impact on cancer-related pain that the converse, although this is a complicated interplay.[4] Patients whose mental health screener results exceed routine distress screening thresholds should be referred for a diagnostic evaluation by a social worker, psychologist, or psychiatrist with the aim of facilitating access to evidence-based treatment for any diagnosed disorders. Recent work indicates significantly higher rates of opioid prescriptions in cancer survivors compared with age-matched controls, providing another perspective on the prevalence of chronic pain and the possibility of comorbid behavioral disorders, including opioid dependency, among some individuals in that population.[5]

In their comprehensive 2012 meta-analysis of psychosocial interventions for cancer pain, Gorin and colleagues[6] reviewed 37 studies containing 4199 patients. They found a weighted average effect size of psychological interventions on pain severity of 0.34 (P<.001), and an effect size of psychological interventions on pain interference of 0.40 (P<.001). These moderate-size results support the value of integrating behavioral health expertise and interventions into cancer treatment settings,[7] particularly in an era in which concerns about opioid abuse are creating increased caution among patients and prescribing clinicians.

DIAGNOSTIC AND INITIAL TREATMENT PHASE

For many individuals, receiving a new cancer diagnosis and engaging in initial diagnostic testing and treatment can be overwhelming and traumatic experiences. A new cancer diagnosis can also reactivate distress and trauma-related symptoms in those with a trauma history, including prior medical trauma, childhood abuse, domestic violence, military service, high trauma-exposure occupations, and/or other sources of high stress or trauma.[8,9] Even when pain has been one of the presenting symptoms that led to a cancer diagnosis, many factors can conspire to lead to inadequate attention to cancer pain and its management at that early juncture. From the patient side, those factors may include fears that pain correlates with disease severity or recurrence risk, concerns that pain complaints will create an impression of weakness or will distract the oncologist from the war against the disease, wishes to avoid appearing to be seeking drugs for pain management, or beliefs that cancer pain cannot be managed.[10,11] It seems reasonable to consider these factors as elemental to psychological approaches to helping patients get better cancer pain control.

Although clinician attitudes and health system-imposed obstacles are not the focus of this article, it would be a major omission not to acknowledge their importance as potential obstructing or facilitating factors. In the face of a national opioid misuse epidemic and mounting pressures on prescribers to minimize or avoid opioid prescriptions entirely, physicians have retreated from the decade of pain and pain as the fifth vital sign almost to a don't ask, don't tell modus operandi. Particularly for patients with cancer pain, this can be another kind of malignancy. The national opioid abuse problem, and the sometimes sensationalistic press it generates, has the potential to drive many cancer pain patients underground, exploiting their baseline fears and making it easier to disavow the pain problem until it cannot be ignored. Clinician discomfort with opioid prescribing can easily become a confounding factor. When this happens, the unnecessary suffering that results is unfortunate and may contribute to worse medical outcomes.[12]

In light of the challenges related to opioid management of cancer pain, the strong and enduring evidence that psychological interventions are effective in reducing pain during the early phases of cancer diagnosis and treatment has become even more relevant. **Table 1** presents the best-studied interventions and the supporting science for those in the early phases of cancer diagnosis and treatment.

Those interventions include various forms of cognitive behavioral therapy (CBT), psychoeducational approaches, hypnosis, mindfulness meditation, and/or relaxation with imagery. The reader will note some overlap among the identified interventions. Differing experimental models, and a tendency to blend or customize techniques to patient populations, may reduce specificity and reproducibility of at least some of the reported results. Outcomes measures also vary.

CBT, which was developed to treat depressive and anxiety disorders, has been studied with attention to its effect on both those symptoms and to overall quality of life in cancer patients, but rarely on pain. CBT focuses on developing personal coping strategies that target solving current problems and changing unhelpful patterns in cognitions, behaviors, and emotional regulation. Originally designed to treat depression, it is now used for several mental health conditions.[29] CBT is often provided in a limited (8–12 sessions) series of treatments focused on skills attainment and practice in executing them. Tatrow and colleagues[13] concluded in a meta-analysis that CBT reduced both distress and pain in women with breast cancer. Work by Syrjala led to similar conclusions, although her team's work included imagery, making it more difficult to draw specific conclusions about CBT alone.[17]

Psychoeducational approaches, which tend to be group-based interventions, focus on skills for responding to disease-related problems and teaching problem-solving strategies for coping with cancer, information sharing that generally includes providing patients with knowledge about treatments, symptoms, resources and services, and relaxation techniques. Such approaches have been demonstrated to be effective in improving locus of control, perceptions of self-efficacy, and to reduce symptom burden, including pain (see **Table 1**).[13–28]

Hypnosis has been demonstrated to be effective in reducing distress and pain in cancer patient populations, lowering costs, hastening recovery, and simplifying

Table 1
Psychological interventions for cancer patients during diagnosis and treatment

Intervention	Results	References
CBT, including psychoeducation and relaxation	Across cancer diagnoses, CBT with relaxation and imagery reduces distress and pain among various cancer diagnosis	Tatrow & Montgomery,[13] 2006 Syrjala et al,[14] 1992 Osborn et al,[15] 2006 Hart et al,[16] 2012 Syrjala et al,[17] 1995
Hypnosis	Across cancer diagnoses, reduces distress and multiple types of pain, including procedural/surgical pain and adverse effects, such as mucositis	Carlson et al,[18] 2017 Montgomery et al,[19] 2013 Syrjala et al,[52] 2002
Mindfulness meditation	No positive evidence to date for pain	Carlson et al,[18] 2017
Psychoeducation, including CBT components	Reduces pain	Butler et al,[20] 2009 Bennett et al,[21] 2009 Marie et al,[22] 2013 Goodwin et al,[23] 2001 Spiegel and Bloom,[24] 1983 Fawzy et al,[25] 1993
Relaxation with imagery	Reduces pain	Carlson et al,[18] 2017 Sheinfeld et al,[26] 2012 Johannsen et al,[27] 2013 Kwekkeboom et al,[28] 2010

procedural sedation needed for various diagnostic and treatment procedures (see **Table 1**).[13–28] It appears to work for children and adults, and can help with mucositis pain, pain associated with blood draws, bone marrow biopsies, lumbar punctures, breast biopsies, and other painful interventions. Hypnotherapy offers patients a means of finding an altered state of consciousness by focusing one's attention under the guidance of the hypnotherapist while in a state of deep relaxation. Patients are typically guided to imagine competing sensory input (eg, visual, auditory, tactile, olfactory) and thus experience reduced awareness of aversive environmental factors or symptoms, such as procedure-related pain. It is ideally performed by a trained and certified hypnotherapist who may have a background in nursing, social work, internal medicine, psychology, psychiatry, or other fields.

Mindfulness meditation (MM)[30] and relaxation with imagery are categories sometimes difficult to distinguish from one another and have been frequently studied together. MM is reviewed in depth in Hess' article, "Mindfulness Based Interventions for Hematology and Oncology Patients with Pain," in this issue. Relaxation training with or without imagery tends to focus on directing patients to reduce skeletal muscle tension through guided awareness and directions. Research strongly supports a mediating effect on cancer pain.

Post-treatment and Survivorship

In 2006, the National Institutes of Health established an Office of Cancer Survivorship. Among its many important tasks, this entity was charged with helping to improve basic knowledge about survivorship, as well as to advance recognition and management of common symptoms and disorders. Chief among those common symptoms is pain and its treatment. **Table 2** presents the best-studied interventions and the supporting science for cancer survivors.

As Syrjala and colleagues[7] have pointed out, clinical trials knowledge about survivor pain remains scarce. Women who are breast cancer survivors comprise the largest share of patients in the evidence base. Between 20% and 40% of such patients report some element of chronic pain.[34] Efforts to elaborate treatment guidelines for these patients are now available for public review and use,[35,36] but they tend to reflect expert consensus rather than a large clinical trials evidence base.

The behavioral intervention of exercise continues to be validated as a helpful tonic for a range of survivorship burdens, including pain.[37] Often exercise/physical activity is performed as part of a more comprehensive post-treatment rehabilitation program that includes one or more psychological or behavioral interventions. For example, the combination of physical activity and a CBT regimen was shown to both reduce pain and improve quality of life[38] in women who had completed treatment for breast cancer.

Table 2
Psychological interventions for cancer survivors with pain

Intervention	Results	References
CBT, with additional intervention (eg, yoga)	Preliminary evidence suggests effectiveness in reducing pain	Robb et al,[31] 2006
Hypnosis among breast cancer survivors	Preliminary evidence suggests effectiveness in reducing pain	Porter and Higginson,[32] 2004
Meditation	Limited data suggest no clear effect	Lengacher et al,[33] 2009

A YMCA-based community program showed wide-ranging improvements in pain, quality of life, and well-being.[39] Meanwhile, there has been interesting recent progress in Web-based or personal device-based telecommunities and structured rehabilitation efforts[40,41] (see Andrea L. Cheville and colleagues' article, "Rehabilitation Medicine Approaches to Pain Management," in this issue).

Studies of CBT interventions for post-treatment/survivorship pain are unavailable. The recently completed SWORD trial,[42] a structured CBT intervention targeting fear of cancer recurrence, showed efficacy for anxiety reduction, but did not measure impacts on pain or other physical symptoms. Nevertheless, given the relationship between anxiety and pain and the efficacy of CBT for pain in other populations, it is anticipated that future research may reveal that CBT assists with both anxiety and pain.

Hypnosis for pain in cancer survivors is an important and emerging area of study. An 8-patient pilot showed trends toward relief of chronic pain, fatigue, hot flashes, and sleep difficulties in breast cancer survivors.[43] A recent meta-analysis confirms optimism that hypnosis is generally helpful in reducing pain in cancer survivors.[44]

The data on meditation in survivors focuses less on pain than on other important and common symptoms such as insomnia and fatigue. The evidence currently does not directly support pain relief associated with meditation practices.[33]

RECURRENCE, PROGRESSION, AND END OF LIFE

For most patients and families, recurrence and progression are particularly stressful times. Distress tends to worsen pain by increasing central nervous system arousal and decreasing the effective use of coping skills. Thus, strategies designed to reduce distress may also reduce pain. Patients and families naturally fear unrelieved pain in advanced disease.[32] Data suggest that pain is both highly prevalent, present in as many as 90% of patients,[45] and more severe[46] in patients with progressive illness.

In these clinical circumstances, the data tend to commingle the beneficial effects of CBT, hypnosis, and meditation strategies. Clinicians and research investigators alike, seeking commonsense ways to reduce suffering in the face of stressful and often chaotic clinical pressures, may utilize a pragmatic toolkit approach to pain and distress management. Often this leads to a skills-focused plan in which patients are taught self-regulatory techniques that encompass varying blends of CBT, relaxation, imagery, hypnosis, and/or other elements. A meta-analysis of the evidence showed that these kinds of approaches reduce pain and pain-related interference with daily functioning,[26] even in patients with advanced disease and complex symptoms.

Efforts have also been made to assess elements of skills-building and self-regulation as individual treatment modalities. For example, a comprehensive and scholarly overview performed by Montgomery and colleagues[19] reports that hypnosis has reliable and robust pain reduction effects across age groups and cancer diagnoses, including among those with advanced disease.[14] Hypnosis as a preprocedure intervention helps reduce requirements for pharmacologic sedation and may reduce costs and improve the patient experience.[47] This modality has been shown to be effective for procedures as simple as blood draws and as complex as bone marrow biopsy or lumbar puncture.

A series of thematically related studies performed at different institutions outlined the positive impacts of structured psychoeducational group interventions for persons with metastatic disease.[20,23–25] Typically, these groups meet for a predetermined number of structured sessions. Each session includes a relaxation intervention, a specific skills-attainment module, a didactic disease-related information element, and a social support opportunity. In addition to showing a positive effect on symptom burden, some of these interventions also confer an extended survival benefit, possibly mediated through immune factors.

A new line of investigation on the impact of structured social networking (often digital/e-community based) on various cancer-related symptoms builds on these early models of psychoeducational groups. Preliminary evidence[48] suggests that, after 12 weeks, depression and fatigue scores are significantly improved in those randomized to active intervention versus a wait list. Pain outcomes were not reported, but may be included in future research efforts.

Table 3 presents the best-studied interventions and the supporting science for cancer patients with recurrence, progression and/or terminal disease.

DISCUSSION

Cancer pain remains an important problem across the entire scope of a cancer patient's illness trajectory. There is no scientific or ethical controversy about the importance of skilled surveillance and competent intervention when cancer pain is present. Among the range of psychological and behavioral interventions for cancer pain, there is moderate-to-strong evidence for efficacy and utility. Although data that would allow optimal matching of specific interventions to specific individuals are lacking, the array of available interventions serves to increase patient choice and control over treatment approaches. Patients often have strong beliefs and values that guide their decisions and lead them to seek out specific pain therapies. It is one of the many important clinical duties of the pain/palliative care consultant to understand those beliefs and values and to assist patients and families to make the most informed choices possible.

Psychological and behavioral interventions for cancer pain can be delivered as solo treatments, or they can be integrated into a more comprehensive and interdisciplinary approach. Those additional modalities might include pharmacologic therapies, physical therapy or exercise, rehabilitative strategies, interventional analgesic techniques, neuromodulation approaches (TENS, Scrambler), disease-modifying therapies (whether cure-focused or palliative), and a variety of other complementary treatments and modalities discussed in this special issue.

Finally, it is crucial to point out that most cancer treatment settings still fall short when it comes to providing patient access to basic palliative care and supportive oncology services. The 2015 National Report Card for Palliative Care[49] suggests that there remains significant variance around the United States. Unfortunately, in those hospitals and health systems where palliative care teams are available, there is no way to know how many include individuals with competencies and the time to provide the evidence-based behavioral interventions that are the subject of this review. Even the National Comprehensive Cancer Network guidelines, which outline

Table 3 Psychological interventions in advanced illness or end of life		
Intervention	Results	References
CBT, with relaxation, imagery, meditation	When part of skills training, reduces pain and pain-related interference	Sheinfeld et al,[26] 2012
Hypnosis in a group format among breast cancer patients	Reduces pain	Johannsen et al,[27] 2013 Butler et al,[20] 2009 Goodwin et al,[23] 2001 Spiegel and Bloom,[24] 1983

de minimis components of a palliative care interdisciplinary team, do not mandate a behavioral health expert (eg, psychologist).[50] Similarly, recently published American Cancer Society guidelines pertaining to integrative therapies during and after breast cancer treatment do not address the scope of professional disciplines to be included in comprehensive care.[51] In an era of emphasis on patient-centered outcomes and cost containment, available data suggest this is a significant omission.

REFERENCES

1. Engel GL. The need for a new medical model: a challenge for biomedicine. Science 1977;196:129–36.
2. Van den Beuken-van Everdingen M. Chronic pain in cancer survivors: a growing issue. J Pain Palliat Care Pharmacother 2012;26:385–7.
3. Mitchell AJ, Chan M, Bhatti H. Prevalence of depression, anxiety, and adjustment disorders in oncological, hematological and palliative-care settings: a meta-analysis of 94 interview-based studies. Lancet Oncol 2011;12:160–74.
4. Wang HL, Kroenke K, Wu J, et al. Predictors of cancer-related pain improvement over time. Psychosom Med 2012;74:642–7.
5. Sutradadhar R, Lokku A, Barbera L. Cancer survivorship and opioid prescribing rates: a population-based matched cohort study among individuals with and without a history of cancer. Cancer 2017;123(21):4286–93.
6. Gorin SS, Krebs P, Badr H, et al. Meta-analysis of psychosocial interventions to reduce pain in patients with cancer. J Clin Oncol 2012;30(5):539–47.
7. Syrjala K, Jensen MP, Mendoza ME, et al. Psychological and behavioral approaches to cancer pain management. J Clin Oncol 2014;32:1703–11.
8. Arnaboldi P, Riva S, Crico C, et al. A systematic literature review exploring the prevalence of post-traumatic stress disorder and the role played by stress and traumatic stress in breast cancer diagnosis and trajectory. Breast Cancer (Dove Med Press) 2017;9:473–85.
9. Baider L, Goldzweig G, Ever-Hadani P, et al. Psychological distress and coping in breast cancer patients and healthy women whose parents survived the Holocaust. Psychooncology 2006;15(7):635–46.
10. Ward SE, Goldberg NM, Miller-Mccauley V, et al. Patient-related barriers to management of cancer pain. Pain 1993;52:319–24.
11. Pargeon KL, Halley BJ. Barriers to effective cancer pain management: a review of the literature. J Pain Symptom Manage 1999;18:358–68.
12. Janjan N. Improving cancer pain control with NCCN guideline-based analgesic administration: a patient-centered outcome. J Natl Compr Canc Netw 2014; 12(9):1243–9.
13. Tatrow K, Montgomery GH. Cognitive behavioral therapy techniques for distress and pain in breast cancer patients: a meta-analysis. J Behav Med 2006;29: 17–27.
14. Syrjala KL, Cummings C, Donaldson GW. Hypnosis or cognitive behavioral training for the reduction of pain and nausea during cancer treatment: a controlled clinical trial. Pain 1992;48:137–46.
15. Osborn RL, Demoncada AC, Feurestein M. Psychosocial Interventions for depression, anxiety, and quality of life in cancer survivors: meta-analyses. Int J Psychiatry Med 2006;36:13–34.
16. Hart SL, Hoyt MA, Diefenbach M, et al. Meta-analysis of efficacy of interventions for elevated depressive s ymptom sin adults diagnosed with cancer. J Natl Cancer Inst 2012;104:990–1004.

17. Syrjala KL, Donaldson GW, Davis MW. Relaxation and imagery and cognitive=behavioral training reduce pain during cancer treatment. Pain 1995;63:189–98.
18. Carlson LE, Zelinski E, Toivonen K, et al. Mind-body therapies in cancer: what is the latest evidence? Curr Oncol Rep 2017;19:67.
19. Montgomery GH, Schnur JB, Kravitz K. Hypnosis for cancer care: over 200 years young. CA Cancer J Clin 2013;63:31–44.
20. Butler LD, Koopman C, Neri E, et al. Effects of supportive-expressive group therapy on pain in women with metastatic breast cancer. Health Psychol 2009;28:579–87.
21. Bennett MI, Bagnall AM, Jose Closs S. How effective are patient-based educational interventions in the management of cancer pain? Systematic review and meta-analysis. Pain 2009;143:192–9.
22. Marie N, Luckett T, Davidson PM, et al. Optimal patient education for cancer pain: a systematic review and theory-based meta-analysis. Support Care Cancer 2013; 21:3529–37.
23. Goodwin PJ, Leszcz M, Ennis M, et al. The effect of group psychosocial support on survival in metastatic breast cancer. N Engl J Med 2001;345:1719–26.
24. Spiegel D, Bloom JR. Group therapy and hypnosis reduce metastatic breast carcinoma pain. Psychosom Med 1983;45:333–9.
25. Fawzy FI, Fawzy NW, Hyun CS, et al. Malignant melanoma. Effects of an early structured psychiatric intervention, coping, and affective state on recurrence and survival 6 years later. Arch Gen Psychiatry 1993;50(9):681–9.
26. Sheinfeld X, Gorin S, Krebs P, et al. Meta-analysis for psychosocial interventions to reduce pain in patients with cancer. J Clin Oncol 2012;30:539–47.
27. Johannsen M, Farver I, Beck N, et al. The efficacy of psychosocial intervention for pain in breast cancer patients and survivors: a systematic review and meta-analysis. Breast Cancer Res Treat 2013;138:675–90.
28. Kwekkeboom KL, Cherwin CH, Lee JW, et al. Mind-body treatments for the pain-fatigue-sleep disturbance symptom cluster in persons with cancer. J Pain Symptom Manage 2010;39:126–38.
29. CBT definition. Available at: https://en.wikipedia.org/wiki/Cognitive_behavioral_therapy. Accessed November 14, 2017.
30. Kabat-Zinn J. Available at: https://www.mindful.org/jon-kabat-zinn-defining-mindfulness/. Accessed October 10, 2017.
31. Robb KA, Williams JE, Duvivier V, et al. A pain management program for chronic cancer-treatment-related pain: a preliminary study. J Pain 2006;7:82–90.
32. Porter J, Higginson IJ. Pain experienced by lung cancer patients: a review of prevalence, causes, and pathophysiology. Lung Cancer 2004;43:247–57.
33. Lengacher CA, Johnson-Mallard V, Post-White J. Randomized controlled trial of mindfulness-based stress-reduction (MBSR) for survivors of breast cancer. Psychooncology 2009;18:1261–72.
34. Lu Q, Krull KR, Eisenring LW. Pain in long-term adult survivors of childhood cancers and their siblings. A report from the Childhood Cancer Survivor Study. Pain 2011;152:2616–24.
35. Dy S, Isenberg SM, Al Hamayel NA. Palliative care for cancer survivors. Med Clin North Am 2017;101(6):1181–96.
36. National Comprehensive Cancer Network: NCCN Guidelines for Survivorship. Available at: www.ncc.org/professionals/pphysician_gis/f_guidelines.asp. Accessed November 15, 2017.
37. National Comprehensive Cancer Network. Available at: https://www.nccn.org/professionals/physician_gls/pdf/survivorship.pdf. Accessed November 15, 2017.

38. Basen-Engquist K, Taylor CL, Rosenblum C. Randomized pilot test of a lifestyle physical activity intervention for breast cancer survivors. Patient Educ Couns 2006;64:225–34.
39. Rajott EJ, Yi JC, Baker KS, et al. Community-based exercise program effectiveness and safety for cancer survivors. J Cancer Surviv 2012;6:219–28.
40. Baseman J, Revere D, Baldwin LM. A mobile breast cancer survivorship care app: pilot study. JMIR Cancer 2017;3(2):e14.
41. Ritvo P, Obadia M, Santa Mina D, et al. Smartphone-enabled health coaching intervention (iMOVE) to promote long-term maintenance of physical activity in breast cancer survivors: protocol for a feasibility pilot randomized controlled trial. JMIR Res Protoc 2017;6(8):e165.
42. van de Wal M, Thewes B, Gielissen M, et al. Efficacy of blended cognitive behavior therapy for high fear of recurrence in breast, prostate, and colorectal cancer survivors: the SWORD study, a randomized controlled trial. J Clin Oncol 2017;35(19):2173–83.
43. Jensen MP, Gralow JR, Braden A, et al. Hypnosis for symptom management in women with breast cancer: a pilot study. Int J Clin Exp Hypn 2012;60(2):135–59.
44. Cramer H, Lauche R, Paul A, et al. Hypnosis in breast cancer care: a systematic review of randomized controlled trials. Integr Cancer Ther 2015;14(1):5–15.
45. Teunissen SC, Wesker W, Kruitwagen C, et al. Symptom prevalence in patients with incurable cancer: a systematic review. J Pain Symptom Manage 2007; 34(1):94–104.
46. Zeppetella G. Breakthrough pain in cancer patients. Clin Oncol 2011;23:393–8.
47. Potié A, Roelants F, Pospiech A, et al. Hypnosis in the perioperative management of breast cancer surgery: clinical benefits and potential implications. Anesthesiol Res Pract 2016;2016:2942416.
48. Owen JE, O'Carroll Bantum E, Pagano IS, et al. Randomized trial of a social networking intervention for cancer-related distress. Ann Behav Med 2017;51(5): 661–72.
49. Morrison RS, Meier DE. State-by-State Report Card on Access to Palliative Care in Our Nation's Hospitals. Available at: https://reportcard.capc.org/wp-content/uploads/2015/08/reportcard-2015-table-a.pdf. Accessed November 1, 2017.
50. Dans M, Smith T. NCCN Clinical Practice Guidelines in Oncology: Palliative Care. Available at: https://www.nccn.org/professionals/physician_gls/PDF/palliative.pdf. Accessed November 1, 2017.
51. Greenlee H, DuPont-Reyes MJ, Balneaves LG, et al. Clinical practice guidelines on the evidence-based use of integrative therapies during and after breast cancer treatment. CA Cancer J Clin 2017;17(67):194–232.
52. Fann JR, Roth-Roemer S, Syrjala K, et al. Delirium in Patients Undergoing Hematopoietic Stem Cell Transplantation. Cancer 2002;95:1971–81.

Mindfulness-Based Interventions for Hematology and Oncology Patients with Pain

Denise Hess, MDiv, LMFT

KEYWORDS

- Mindfulness • Mindfulness-based interventions • Pain • Cancer pain
- Pain catastrophizing

KEY POINTS

- Pain is a reality for approximately 40% of patients with cancer after treatment, for 55% during treatment, and for 66% of patients with terminal disease. Opioids are the treatment of choice for cancer-related pain.
- Pain is a constellation of physical sensations that can negatively impact cognitive and emotional states. The whole person experience of pain has been called "total pain."
- Total pain may not respond to pharmacologic interventions and may pave the way for the onset of suffering whereby suffering is defined as physical pain accompanied by negative cognitive interpretations.
- Mindfulness-based interventions provide an alternate interpretive framework for pain and suffering and may lessen a patient's experience of pain.
- Mindfulness-based interventions have potential to modify a patient's relationship to pain, reducing pain catastrophizing, and enhancing patient reported overall well-being.

INTRODUCTION

In a systematic review and meta-analysis of 122 research articles on cancer pain prevalence, pain was found to be a reality for 39.3% of patients with cancer after curative treatment, 55.0% during anticancer treatment, 66.4% in advanced, metastatic, or terminal disease, and 50.7% in all cancer stages.[1] Fifty-two of the 122 studies that measured pain intensity found that 38% of patients with cancer report moderate to severe pain.[1] In addition, patients with cancer report that pain is an intolerable aspect of their cancer that profoundly affects their quality of life.[2,3]

Ms D. Hess has no commercial or financial conflicts of interest to disclose and no funding sources to declare.
Supportive Care Coalition, Providence St. Joseph Health, 18530 Northwest Cornell Road, Suite 101, Hillsboro, OR 97124, USA
E-mail address: denise.hess@providence.org

Hematol Oncol Clin N Am 32 (2018) 493–504
https://doi.org/10.1016/j.hoc.2018.01.013
0889-8588/18/© 2018 Elsevier Inc. All rights reserved.

Since the seminal work of Dame Cicely Saunders and her introduction of the "total pain" concept, cancer pain has been conceptualized and treated as a multidimensional, individual experience encompassing body, mind, and spirit.[4] Following this logic, research on cancer pain commonly uses validated self-report pain measurement tools that assess a person's physical and affective experience of pain.[5,6] Nevertheless, cancer pain is regularly treated with opioids alone presumably under the assumption that if the physical pain is ameliorated, the emotional and behavioral symptoms will also resolve.

Clinical experience, however, often proves the above assumption false. As palliative care physician Michael Kearney has noted, there are types of pain not amenable to pharmacologic intervention.[7] Grief is one such example. Grieving people often report physical symptoms that may not respond to pharmacologic or nonpharmacologic interventions and instead yield only to the salve of time. For clinicians used to exercising their skills to provide symptom relief, complex types of pain like grief can become an exercise in clinical humility in the face of suffering that persists (**Fig. 1**).[8]

Considering grief as a type of pain raises the question about the difference between pain and suffering. In both the research literature and common parlance, the terms are often conflated or used interchangeably. Pain and suffering are assumed to be synonyms for identical subjective experiences.

However, as Cassell has carefully articulated, pain and suffering are two distinct entities:

> *Suffering occurs when an impending destruction of the person is perceived; it continues until the threat of disintegration has passed or until the integrity of the person can be restored in some other manner. It follows, then, that although suffering often occurs in the presence of acute pain, shortness of breath, or other bodily symptoms, suffering extends beyond the physical. Most generally, suffering can be defined as the state of severe distress associated with events that threaten the intactness of the person.[9]*

This distinction is key to uncoupling the corresponding value judgments often placed on pain and suffering. Pain and suffering are most often portrayed as unambiguously negative experiences that must be assessed, addressed, and eliminated. However, what if pain, or more specifically the suffering that may arise from pain, is agnostic? Contrast the pain of a woman in childbirth versus the pain of a woman waiting for a kidney stone to pass. Both are experiencing intense physical sensations in response to a foreign body's attempted exit. It can be imagined although both women

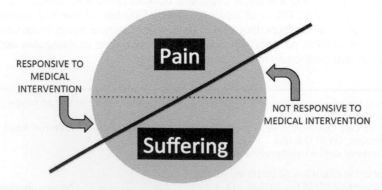

Fig. 1. Pain that is not responsive to medical intervention.

are looking forward to the exit of the foreign body with great anticipation, each may be narrating the experience of their pain within vastly differing cognitive frameworks. The birthing woman's pain might not be experienced as suffering because of her belief that her pain is time limited, purposeful, and for a greater good. The unfortunate kidney stone victim's pain might more easily become suffering if the pain is believed to be out of control, without clear beginning or end, or purposeless.

This uncoupling of pain and suffering is elucidated by Papadatou,[10] "Suffering is neither invariably evil nor invariably good (ie, always leading to growth or some desired end). Suffering just is; it is painful, yet integral to our human existence," and summarized in the oft-quoted anonymous saying, "pain is inevitable, suffering is optional." According to this point of view, addressing pain requires first understanding the nature of the suffering that may or may not accompany the pain. If pain is a constellation of physical sensations and suffering is the negative interpretation of those sensations, then theoretically, reframing one's interpretation of pain could lessen both pain and suffering (Fig. 2).

Practices to uncouple and reframe pain and suffering undergird mindfulness-based interventions (MBIs) for cancer-related pain. Pain, as the research endorses, is a reality for at least half of patients with cancer before, during, or after treatment. Opioids, the current treatment of choice, address the physical aspects of pain, yet may or may not address the suffering that often accompanies pain. MBIs do not claim to provide analgesic effects, but do purport to provide a framework for changing one's relationship to the highly individual, complex, subjective experience of pain. Subsequently, suffering becomes an optional not obligatory experience through greater awareness of the cognitive and emotional processes that create suffering. If pain plus negative

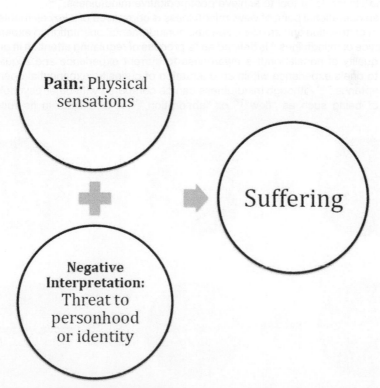

Fig. 2. The uncoupling of pain and suffering.

interpretation equals suffering, then altering one's interpretations can reduce or eliminate suffering (**Fig. 3**).

DISCUSSION
Mindfulness-Based Interventions

MBIs are a collection of practices gleaned from the Mindfulness-Based Stress Reduction (MBSR) program started in 1979 by Jon Kabat-Zinn[11] at the University of Massachusetts. Based on a 2500-year-old Buddhist tradition, secular MBSR courses were originally conceived as an 8-week classroom-based introduction to MBIs (body scan, sitting meditation, mindful movement/hatha yoga, walking meditation, and lovingkindness/metta meditation) for chronic pain patients who were not helped by traditional medical treatments. Since then, MBSR has been shown to benefit people with numerous physical and psychological diagnoses from psoriasis to severe depression, irritable bowel to addictions. Similarly, MBSR principles are foundational to many other mindfulness-based programs, such as Mindfulness-based Cognitive Therapy for anxiety and depression, Acceptance and Commitment Therapy for a variety of psychological disorders, and Dialectical Behavioral Therapy for addiction and personality disorders.[12–14]

Mindfulness has been defined numerous ways. Kabat-Zinn and colleagues[11] at the MBSR clinics define mindfulness as "paying attention on purpose in the present moment, non-judgmentally...being awake, and owning your moments as best you can, and as often as you can." Ellen Langer,[15] an early mindfulness researcher, defines mindfulness in contrast to mindlessness, "to be mindful is to be present, noticing all the wonders that we didn't realize were right in front of us." Meditation, often conflated with mindfulness, is "a tool to achieve postmeditative mindfulness."[15]

From an operational point of view, mindfulness is composed of 2 key elements: self-regulation of attention and an open, curious, nonjudgmental orientation to experience. The practice of m(indfulness) is defined as "a process of regulating attention in order to bring a quality of nonelaborative awareness to current experience and a quality of relating to one's experience within an orientation of curiosity, experiential openness, and acceptance."[16] Although mindfulness can be compared with other psychological modes of being such as "flow"[17] or "absorption,"[18] it is distinct in its focus on

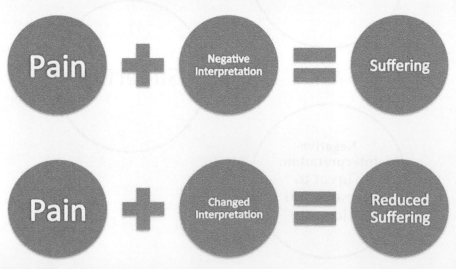

Fig. 3. MBIs and interpretive frameworks.

increasing insight into one's own habitual patterns of perceiving and relating to present-moment experience.

Because mindfulness is a particular way of relating to one's inner and outer experience, mindfulness can be cultivated via various techniques and actions. Mindfulness meditation is most often the activity of choice for cultivating greater mindfulness. In contrast to other forms of meditation designed to increase concentration or achieve deep states of relaxation, mindfulness meditation is a focused application of self-regulation and present-moment orientation skills.

For example, consider these instructions for sitting meditation:

The client maintains an upright sitting posture, either in a chair or cross-legged on the floor and attempts to maintain attention on a particular focus, most commonly the somatic sensation of his or her own breathing. Whenever attention wanders from the breath to inevitable thoughts and feelings that arise, the client will simply take notice of them and then let them go as attention is returned to the breath. This process is repeated each time that attention wanders away from the breath. As sitting meditation is practiced, there is an emphasis on simply taking notice of whatever the mind happens to wander to and accepting each object without making judgments about it or elaborating on its implications, additional meanings, or need for action.[16]

Sitting meditation is only one of several tools used to enhance mindfulness; the body scan practice, walking meditation, and lovingkindness meditation are a few other commonly taught mindfulness practices. By acknowledging that meditation practices are only as effective as their ability to influence thoughts, emotions, and behaviors while not formally meditating, there are many informal meditation practices designed to promote a mindful attitude toward all activities of daily living.[19] For purposes of research, MBIs refer to the collection of practices, skills, and mindsets that enhance moment-to-moment mindful modes of being.

Mindfulness-Based Cognitive Psychotherapy

Although not primarily directed at pain reduction, there are also several psychologically based interventions that use mindfulness to reframe a person's relationship to the symptoms of depression, anxiety, and addictive disorders. Mindfulness-Based Cognitive Therapy is an 8-week psychotherapist-facilitated group therapy that incorporates mindfulness meditation with cognitive behavioral therapy–based interventions to reframe the patterns of negative thinking that often accompany and exacerbate psychological suffering.[12] Based in Relational Frame Theory, Acceptance and Commitment Therapy incorporates mindfulness practices such as present-moment awareness and cognitive defusion to lessen psychological pain and increase psychological flexibility.[20] Examples of Acceptance and Commitment Therapy cognitive defusion techniques are described in **Table 1**.[21]

Mindfulness-Based Interventions and Chronic Pain

Several key studies have investigated the effect of MBIs on chronic pain with mixed results.

Kabat-Zinn and colleagues[22–24] conducted several key studies investigating the effect of MBIs with chronic pain patients. Using a pretest and posttest assessment methodology, patients treated with an 8-week MBSR course versus treatment as usual (TAU) showed greater improvement in pain scores, although this effect seemed to diminish at the 6-month follow-up assessment.

Based on review of 10 studies, Chiesa and Serretti[25] concluded that MBIs could have nonspecific beneficial effects on mood, coping, and pain symptoms in chronic

Table 1
Acceptance and commitment therapy cognitive defusion techniques

Technique	Description
The mind	Treat "the mind" as an external event, almost as a separate person
Mental appreciation	Thank your mind; show aesthetic appreciation for its products
Cubbyholing	Label private events as to kind or function in a back channel communication
"I'm having the thought that…"	Include category labels in descriptions of private events
Commitment to openness	Ask if the content is acceptable when negative content shows up
Just noticing	Use the language of observation (eg, noticing) when talking about thoughts
Open mindfulness	Watching thoughts as external objects without use or involvement
Focused mindfulness	Direct attention to nonliteral dimensions of experience

Adapted from Hayes SC. Cognitive defusion (deliteralization). Association for Contextual Behavioral Science (ACBS). Available at: https://contextualscience.org/cognitive_defusion_deliteralization. Accessed August 21, 2017; with permission.

pain patients, but that the studies often suffered from small sample sizes, lack of randomization, and the use of nonspecific control groups.[25] They discouraged generalizing their findings due to small sample size and lack of standard randomized, controlled trial (RCT) protocols in the extant body of research in this area.

Veehof and colleagues[26] conducted a meta-analysis of both controlled and uncontrolled studies on the use of MBIs with chronic pain patients and found small effect sizes for both pain and depression. Veehof concluded that although MBIs for chronic pain can be good alternatives, they are not superior to other psychologically based treatments such as cognitive behavioral therapy for pain.

In a controlled study comparing MBIs to massage therapy to TAU in patients with chronic musculoskeletal pain, Plews-Ogan and colleagues[27] observed that massage therapy was more effective than MBIs for sustained pain relief, whereas MBIs had more long-term efficacy for psychological symptoms.

In a summary article reviewing the effectiveness of MBIs on pain, Carlson[28] found mixed results, many of which are cited above, and recommended additional RCTs of MBIs and chronic pain before affirming their value as a stand-alone treatment modality.[28]

Mindfulness-Based Interventions and Cancer Pain

Most relevant to this article is a recent study investigating the relationship between pain intensity and pain catastrophizing in patients with cancer. Poulin and colleagues[29] conducted a cross-sectional survey with 76 cancer survivors who were at least 1-year posttreatment and reporting symptoms of chronic neuropathic pain for more than 3 months. They found that higher scores on the Five Facets Mindfulness Questionnaire were negatively correlated with patient-reported pain intensity, pain catastrophizing, and overall pain interference with activities of daily life. They suggest the mechanism described in **Fig. 4**.

Poulin and colleagues[29] suggest that mindfulness interrupts the fear avoidance cycle of pain via the 5 facets of mindfulness:

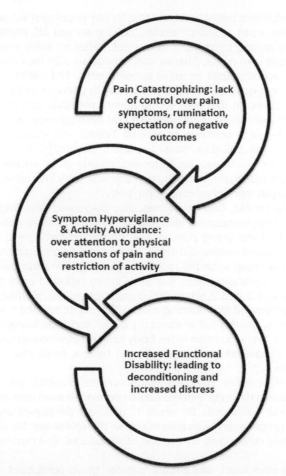

Fig. 4. Fear avoidance model of disability in chronic pain.

- Observing
- Describing
- Acting with awareness
- Nonjudging of inner experience
- Nonreactivity to inner experience

It should also be noted that study participants with higher scores on the Five Facet Mindfulness Questionnaire also reported higher levels of health-related quality of life and lower incidence of depression.

Mindfulness: State or Trait?

Studies on mindfulness as discussed above raise the following question: if MBIs can change a patient's relationship to pain via a cultivation of moment-to-moment, nonjudgmental, noncatastrophizing awareness, why don't all patients respond equally well to these techniques?

Consider the following composite case examples:

Sharon is a 54-year-old, Caucasian woman diagnosed with stage IV pancreatic cancer. She is not a surgical candidate and is currently receiving gemcitabine. She was referred to an outpatient palliative care clinic by her oncologist for pain that Sharon described as, "like a belt of sharp needles, pulsing on and off, starting from my left rib and wrapping around to my right side waist." After an initial assessment by the outpatient palliative care nurse, Sharon was scheduled with the clinic palliative care physician and psychotherapist for initial appointments. The palliative care physician recommended a low-dose Methadone regimen with Dilaudid for breakthrough pain. Sharon told the physician that she "would never, ever take pain medications" after watching a family member become addicted and eventually die from an opioid overdose. Sharon planned to continue as-needed Tylenol and acupuncture. During her appointment with the palliative care outpatient psychotherapist, Sharon readily agreed to attend a clinic-based, facilitator-led, weekly group on mindfulness-based approaches to pain management stating that she was "very interested in feeling better without having to put more chemicals in my body."

Robert is a 62-year-old, Caucasian man, also diagnosed with stage IV pancreatic cancer and receiving gemcitabine, also referred to the outpatient palliative care clinic by his oncologist for increasing pain. Unlike Sharon, Robert agreed to the palliative care physician's recommended low-dose opioid medication regimen and signed up for the mindfulness group upon the recommendation of the clinic psychotherapist.

At the end of the 8-week group, Sue and Robert reported quite different experiences. During weeks 1 and 2, when group participants are oriented to mindfulness and given the assignment of practicing a daily, 30-minute mindful body scan, Robert reported on week 3, "feeling better about my body" and "less worried about my cancer." Sue reported, "I tried to listen to the body scan meditation recording and I just got restless, once I almost felt like I was going to have a panic attack. I stopped the recording right away."

Although experiences like Sue's are not uncommon in participants new to mindfulness practices, Sue's difficulty with the course continued even after several modifications in the course homework. By week 7, Sue had developed an affinity for the "lovingkindness practice" and was able to spend 10 minutes per day sitting still quietly wishing herself and others well. By the end of the course, Sue reported no change in her pain levels.

Robert, on the other hand, was a more "typical" group participant. Although he did struggle to find 45 minutes per day to complete the course homework, he reported finding most benefit from the sitting meditation practice. By the end of the course, Robert and the outpatient palliative care physician were able to taper and then discontinue his opioid medication. At the 3-month follow-up, Robert continued to report manageable pain levels without any use of opioids.

As indicated in the mindfulness research discussed above, Sue and Richard's respective experiences are mirrored in current research trends. It seems that MBIs are no "quick fix" and neither are they guaranteed to reduce patient-reported pain. Instead, MBIs have an indeterminate effect on physical pain, seeming to be effective with some patients and not with others. It is highly likely that there are many mechanisms at play that account for these differences in patient outcomes, some of which may be the patient's preexisting psychological well-being, health, and resilience.

Mindfulness and Pain Catastrophizing

A study by Elvery and colleagues[30] proposes that patients' pain catastrophizing is the most robust determinant of patient's responsiveness, or lack thereof, to MBIs. Elvery and colleagues state that although mindful awareness and nonjudgmental acceptance of pain are indeed factors in patient-reported pain levels, it is the degree to which patients engage in excessive catastrophic thoughts about their pain that is the strongest mediator of perceived pain intensity.

Fig. 5 outlines the cognitive emotional processes involved in changing one's relationship to pain through mindfulness practices. At the top right and left of the diagram are the 2 most common reactive responses to pain that lead to suffering:

- Avoidance: pushing painful sensations from awareness through distraction, blame, numbing (as in use of alcohol, recreational drugs, or misuse of prescription medications), repression, or denial may provide temporary relief but only serve to exacerbate suffering.

Or

- Fusion: cognitively and emotionally merging with pain through catastrophizing (my pain will only get worse and never stop), personalizing (why is this happening to me? what did I do to deserve this?), all-or-nothing thinking (pain is all bad and the absence of pain is all good), negative filtering (difficulty recalling absences or lessening of pain), and "shoulds" (I should feel better by now).

Both of these reactive responses constitute resistance to pain based on negative interpretations of the body's physical sensations. Both avoidance of and fusion with pain circumvent present-moment, nonjudgmental awareness of pain initiating pain-suffering response since "what we resist persists."

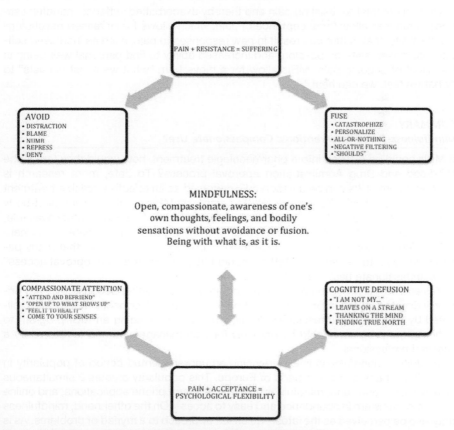

Fig. 5. Reframing pain with mindfulness: "what we resist persists."

Fig. 5 also illustrates a mindfulness-based, open, nonjudgmental awareness of painful sensations in the body without resistance through avoidance or fusion. Pain is acknowledged as it is, held in compassionate attention as it is, and is not denied, avoided, catastrophized, or personalized. Pain is what it is. Pain can be attended and befriended. When painful sensations arise, one can open to it, lean into it, turn toward the immediate sensory experience to explore the contours, the natural rise and fall, and the changing landscape of pain.

This openness is enhanced and sustained by mindfulness-based cognitive defusion practices, such as those referenced in **Table 1** and summarized in **Fig. 5**. Thoughts about one's pain can be acknowledged, compassionately attended to, and even accepted as one learns to separate the direct experience of pain from cognitive interpretations of the pain.

The following practices are skillful strategies to lessen both pain and suffering:

- Acknowledging the distinction between the sensations of pain and often negative or catastrophizing thoughts about pain
- Noticing that negative thoughts about pain are passing phenomenon like leaves on a stream
- Recognizing thoughts as a creation of the mind
- Reengaging with one's deepest purpose, values, and meaning in the midst of pain

Thus, in contrast to resisting pain and thereby exacerbating suffering, mindfulness-based practices allow for acceptance of pain, which allows for increased psychological flexibility, that in turn can result in new responses to pain, such as increased self-care, increased self-compassion, and increased ability to find personal well-being in the midst of ongoing pain. MBIs allow for a move from "what we resist persists" to "what we feel, we can heal."

SUMMARY
Mindfulness-Based Interventions: Compassionate Use?

If MBIs could be distilled into a pharmacologic treatment, how would they fare in the US Food and Drug Administration approval process? To date, more research is needed before MBIs can be unreservedly endorsed as an effective, reliable treatment of cancer-related pain. Specifically, RCTs comparing MBIs to other similar mind-body interventions and to TAU are needed to verify the efficacy of MBIs over other available, well-researched interventions. More research is needed to determine when and where MBIs might be contraindicated. Nevertheless, in the meantime, given that many patients do seem to benefit from MBIs, should MBIs be granted "preapproval access" or "compassionate use" status?

Yes and no. All MBI programs are not created equally, either because they are primarily directed at self-improvement not pain management or because they are facilitated by unlicensed professionals. Thus, when recommending an MBI program to patients, the program should be primarily for pain management and facilitated by a licensed professional.

In addition, mindfulness is experiencing an unprecedented period of popularity in the United States and some parts of Europe. This popularity creates 2 simultaneous issues. On the one hand, mindfulness programs, smart phone applications, and online study programs are in abundance and easy to access. On the other hand, mindfulness may also be perceived as the latest "quick fix" approach to a myriad of problems. As is clear from the discussion above, MBIs are not a quick fix for cancer pain.

Last, in the current setting of outcome-based health care, MBIs are likely to become an integrated component of cancer pain treatment to the degree that they reduce patient opioid use and emergency hospitalizations. As has been demonstrated in the discussion above, current research has yet to demonstrate such outcomes.

REFERENCES

1. van den Beuken-van Everdingen M, Hochstenbach L, Joosten E, et al. Update on prevalence of pain in patients with cancer: systematic review and meta-analysis. J Pain Symptom Manage 2016;51(6):1070–90.
2. Breivik H, Cherny N, Collett B, et al. Cancer-related pain: a pan-European survey of prevalence, treatment, and patient attitudes. Ann Oncol 2009;20(8):1420–33.
3. Kroenke K, Theobald D, Wu J, et al. The association of depression and pain with health-related quality of life, disability, and health care use in cancer patients. J Pain Symptom Management 2010;40(3):327–41.
4. Clark D. 'Total pain', disciplinary power and the body in the work of Cicely Saunders, 1958-1967. Soc Sci Med 1999;49(6):727–36.
5. Melzack R. The short-form McGill pain questionnaire. Pain 1987;30(2):191–7.
6. Cleeland CS, Ryan KM. Pain assessment: global use of the Brief Pain Inventory. Ann Acad Med Singapore 1994;23(2):129–38.
7. Kearney M. A place of healing: working with nature and soul at the end of life. New Orleans (LA): Spring Journal; 2009.
8. Byock I. When suffering persists.... J Palliat Care 1994;10(2):8–13.
9. Cassell E. The nature of suffering and the goals of medicine. London: Oxford University Press; 2004. p. 32.
10. Papadatou D. In the face of death. New York: Springer Publishing; 2009. p. 119.
11. Kabat-Zinn J. Full catastrophe living: using the wisdom of your body and mind to face stress, pain and illness. New York: Delacourt; 1990.
12. Segal ZV, Williams MG, Teasdale JD. Mindfulness-based cognitive therapy for depression: a new approach to preventing relapse. New York: The Guilford Press; 2002.
13. Hayes SC, Luoma JB, Bond FW, et al. Acceptance and commitment therapy: model, processes and outcomes. Behav Res Ther 2006;44(1):1–25.
14. Linehan MM. DBT skills training manual. 2nd edition. New York: The Guilford Press; 2015.
15. Langer E. Mindfulness: 25th anniversary edition. Boston: A Merloyd Lawrence Book; 2014. p. xxv.
16. Bishop SR, Lau M, Shapiro S, et al. Mindfulness: a proposed operational definition. Clin Psychol Sci Pract 2004;11(3):230–41.
17. Csikszentmihalyi M. Finding flow: the psychology of engagement with everyday life. New York: Basic Books; 1997.
18. Tellegen A, Atkinson G. Openness to absorption and self-altering experiences: a trait related to hypnotic susceptibility. J Abnorm Psychol 1974;83:268–77.
19. Bays JC. How to train a wild elephant: and other adventures in mindfulness. Boston: Shambala Publications; 2011.
20. Hayes SC, Strosahl KG, Wilson KG. Acceptance and commitment therapy: an experiential approach to behavior change. New York: Guilford Press; 1996.
21. Hayes SC. Cognitive defusion (deliteralization). Association for Contextual Behavioral Science. Available at: https://contextualscience.org/cognitive_defusion_deliteralization. Accessed August 21, 2017.

22. Kabat-Zinn J. An outpatient program in behavioral medicine for chronic pain patients based on the practice of mindfulness meditation: theoretical considerations and preliminary results. Gen Hosp Psychiatry 1982;4(1):33–47.

23. Kabat-Zinn J, Lipworth L, Burney R. The clinical use of mindfulness meditation for the self-regulation of chronic pain. J Behav Med 1985;8(2):163–90.

24. Kabat-Zinn J, Lipworth L, Burney R, et al. Four-year follow-up of a meditation-based program for the self-regulation of chronic pain: treatment outcomes and compliance. Clin J Pain 1986;2(3):159–73.

25. Chiesa A, Serretti A. Mindfulness-based interventions for chronic pain: a systematic review of the evidence. J Altern Complement Med 2011;17(1):83–93.

26. Veehof MM, Oskam MJ, Schreurs KM, et al. Acceptance-based interventions for the treatment of chronic pain: a systematic review and meta-analysis. Pain 2011; 152(3):533–42.

27. Plews-Ogan M, Owens JE, Goodman M, et al. A pilot study evaluating mindfulness-based stress reduction and massage for the management of chronic pain. J Gen Intern Med 2005;20(12):1136–8.

28. Carlson LE. Mindfulness-based interventions for physical conditions: a narrative review evaluating levels of evidence. ISRN Psychiatry 2012;2012:651583.

29. Poulin P, Romanow H, Wilson K, et al. The relationship between mindfulness, pain intensity, pain catastrophizing, depression, and quality of life among cancer survivors living with chronic neuropathic pain. Support Care Cancer 2016;24(10): 4167–75.

30. Elvery N, Jensen M, Ehde D, et al. Pain catastrophizing, mindfulness, and pain acceptance: what's the difference? Clin J Pain 2017;33(6):485–95.

Spiritual Considerations

Christina M. Puchalski, MD, OCDS[a],*, Stephen D.W. King, PhD[b],
Betty R. Ferrell, RN, PhD, MA, FPCN, CHPN[c]

KEYWORDS

- Spirituality • Spiritual distress • Existential distress • Spiritual well-being

KEY POINTS

- Spiritual or existential distress is highly prevalent in patients with cancer and can impact the overall management of distress.
- It is critical that all members of the team screen for spiritual or existential distress.
- Spiritual or existential distress can be treated by compassionate listening, referral to appropriate resources, and especially by working closely with certified chaplains or spiritual care professionals.
- Consensus-based models have identified recommendations and tools for assessing and treating spiritual distress by all members of the team.

INTRODUCTION

The experiences of patients with cancer—from diagnosis through treatment, survivorship, and death—encompass many aspects of their lives—physical, social, emotional, and spiritual.[1] From the moment of diagnosis, patients' lives are changed forever, with the diagnosis often triggering questions of meaning and purpose, as well as finding hope and fulfillment.[2,3] Scientific advances have resulted in longer life for patients with cancer, many of whom are now considered survivors. With more than 15 million cancer survivors in the United States today,[4] a cancer diagnosis raises questions about living well with the disease through treatment and survivorship, rather than planning for imminent death. With an estimate that 39% of people born today will be diagnosed with cancer during their lifetime,[4] the National Cancer Institute and other

Disclosure: None of the authors has any commercial or financial conflicts of interest.
[a] Department of Medicine and Health Sciences, Health Leadership and Management, The George Washington Institute for Spirituality & Health, The George Washington University School of Medicine & Health Sciences, The George Washington University School of Public Health, MFA-GWU Supportive and Palliative Care Clinic, 2600 Virginia Avenue, Northwest, Suite 300, Washington, DC 20037, USA; [b] Chaplaincy, Child Life, Seattle Cancer Care Alliance, PO Box 19023, Mail Stop K-231, Seattle, WA 98109, USA; [c] Division of Nursing Research and Education, Department of Population Sciences, City of Hope Medical Center, 1500 East Duarte Road, Duarte, CA 91010, USA
* Corresponding author.
E-mail address: cpuchals@gwu.edu

cancer organizations are shifting their focus to longevity and quality of life across the continuum of cancer care. Quality of life for patients with cancer has been shown to encompass the spiritual as well as the physical and psychosocial domains of care, with spiritual well-being found to be as significant as physical well-being.[5,6] The concept of quality of life is recognized as encompassing spirituality, with increasing recognition that this includes religious support as well as existential aspects of spirituality related to meaning or purpose in life.[7–9]

A diagnosis of cancer, especially when the patient is in pain, raises spirituality-related questions and concerns, both existential and religious.[10,11] The uncertainties and myriad decisions may raise spirituality-related issues more often in persons diagnosed with cancer than with other long-term illnesses. Studies show that individuals may have increased levels of spiritual distress and clinical depression after a cancer diagnosis, and at the end of active treatment when predictable routines end.[12,13]

SPIRITUALITY

Spirituality is defined as a way people find meaning and purpose and how they experience their connectedness to self, others, and the significant or the sacred.[7,14] Spirituality is seen as a universal human characteristic, one's relationship with the transcendent, expressed through one's attitudes, habits, and practices. Religion, one expression of spirituality, is a set of organized beliefs about God shared within a community of people.[15–17] Having a strong sense of spirituality helps patients to adjust to and cope with an illness, including cancer, and to find meaning and peace. Spirituality may help a patient to define wellness during cancer treatment and survivorship, despite fatigue or pain, and may assist patients in finding a sense of health in the midst of disease.[3,12]

Other studies have shown that spiritual well-being in patients with cancer has been associated with lower levels of depression, better quality of life near death, and protection against end-of-life despair, and a desire for hastened death.[2,12,15] Patients with cancer report their spirituality helped them to find hope, gratitude, and positivity in their cancer experience, and that their spirituality is a source of strength that helps them to cope, find meaning in their lives, and make sense of the cancer experience as they recover from treatment.[18–20] Spiritual well-being has been associated with lower levels of distress and greater quality of life across life expectancy prognoses, and as a source of strength. Religion helps people with spiritual suffering by offering them historical understandings of suffering and ways to reframe their distress. Rituals and spiritual practices may help people to cope with cancer-related pain and suffering, including physical pain and psychosocial or spiritual suffering, and with facing dying or experiencing anticipatory grief.[19]

Numerous studies have reported that spirituality and/or religion may be important to patients with cancer and may influence medical decision making. Patients with cancer often consider spirituality to be at least somewhat important in their treatment decisions, and frequently of extreme importance. Patients report that belief in God is an important factor in decision making about treatment, often more so than the efficacy of treatment.[21–23]

SPIRITUAL DISTRESS: A CLINICAL DIAGNOSIS?

Spirituality impacts coping, decision making, and quality of life, but may also be a source or contributor to distress. Examples of spiritual distress are listed in **Table 1**. Spiritual suffering may influence how a person experiences and expresses pain, with a spiritual intervention as effective as a medical intervention in pain management. Untreated spiritual suffering may worsen the pain experience.[11] For some patients

Table 1
Spiritual concerns

Spiritual Concerns	Key Feature From History
Lack of meaning and purpose	Lack of meaning Concerns about afterlife Questions about the existence and meaning of suffering
Despair/hopelessness	Despair as absolute hopelessness No hope or value of life
Not being remembered	Separated from community No sense of relatedness
Guilt/shame	Feeling that one has done something wrong or evil Feeling the one is bad or evil
Anger at God/others	Displace anger toward religious representatives or others Inability to forgive
Abandonment by God/others	Lack of love, loneliness
Feeling out of control	Deep sense of lack of control over physical and mental function
Spiritual or existential suffering	Loss of faith or meaning
Reconciliation	Need for forgiveness or reconciliation from self or others
Grief/loss	The feeling and process associated the loss of person, health, relationship

with cancer, spiritual suffering/distress may be of greater concern than physical symptoms. Patients with cancer report feelings of anger and diminished self-esteem, which may be spirituality related. Patients with cancer express spiritual needs, which often change across the trajectory of disease. Patients with cancer with low levels of spiritual well-being often express hopelessness and a desire for a hastened death, and may have more frequent follow-up visits.[2] Thus, identifying spiritual distress can have important implications for health outcomes, including an improved quality of life for patients.

The National Comprehensive Cancer Network identifies spiritual distress that may extend along the continuum of care from "common, normal feelings of vulnerability, sadness, and fear, to problems that become disabling such as depression, anxiety, panic, social isolation, and existential spiritual crises."[11] Studies show that spirituality is an integral component of cancer care, with an intrinsic significance to caring for and respecting patients as whole persons.[24] The Joint Commission requires spiritual assessments. The National Consensus Project and National Quality Forum identify spiritual, religious, and existential aspects of care as 1 of 8 domains of quality palliative and hospice care.[25]

ATTENDING TO PATIENT SPIRITUAL ISSUES

Attending to the psychosocial–spiritual needs as well as the physical needs of patients with cancer across the continuum of care is important, both from the perspective of patient desire and the benefits to patients' quality of life.[8,26] Clinician inquiry into patients' spirituality is also important in terms of building trust with the patient, as well as ensuring treatment plans are congruent with patients' beliefs and values. Not addressing spirituality could result in poorer outcomes, increased noncompliance with the treatment plan, and failure to help the patient find effective coping mechanisms.[27]

Attending to an individual's spiritual distress and/or spiritual resources of strength correlates with quality of life across the trajectory of the cancer experience.[28–31] Inquiring about the spirituality of a patient with cancer also correlates with a whole-person health care model that shifts care from a focus on disease cure to one that addresses how an individual patient with cancer defines wellness in the context of the disease experience. Wellness, defined by the World Health Organization, is the "dynamic state of complete physical, mental, spiritual, and social well-being and not merely the absence of disease or infirmity."[32] Thus, spiritual well-being is a determinant of whole health and, by extension, quality of life.

THE WHOLE PERSON ASSESSMENT AND TREATMENT PLAN

To standardize and institutionalize spirituality as a component of whole-patient care, the biopsychosocial–spiritual model must be integrated across the continuum of care for patients with cancer. The biopsychosocial–spiritual model recognizes the distinct dimensions—biological, psychological, social, and spiritual—of a person and the fact that no dimension can be left out when caring for the whole person.[32] For the same reason that current practice includes psychosocial inquiries, spiritual inquiry also is needed in recognition that each person's history and illness is unique and will affect all dimensions of that person in unique ways.[11]

Based on several national and international consensus conferences, a model for implementing this whole person assessment and treatment plan for interprofessional spiritual care was created (**Box 1**). This model integrates dignity-centered and compassionate care into the biopsychosocial framework. These conferences also developed a consensus-based definition of spirituality:

Spirituality is a dynamic and intrinsic aspect of humanity through which persons seek ultimate meaning, purpose, transcendence, and experience relationship to

---

Box 1
Recommendations for interprofessional spiritual care

- All health care professionals should be trained in doing a spiritual screening or history as part of their routine history and evaluation.

- Spiritual screenings, histories, and assessments should be communicated and documented in patient records (eg, charts, computerized databases, and shared with the interprofessional health care team).

- Follow-up spiritual histories or assessments should be conducted for all patients whose medical, psychosocial, or spiritual condition changes, and as part of routine follow-up in a medical history.

- A spiritual issue becomes a diagnosis if the following criteria are met: (1) the spiritual issue leads to distress or suffering (eg, lack of meaning, conflicted religious beliefs, inability to forgive); (2) the spiritual issue is the cause of a psychological or physical diagnosis such as depression, anxiety, or acute or chronic pain (eg, severe meaninglessness that leads to depression or suicidality, guilt that leads to chronic physical pain); and (3) the spiritual issue is a secondary cause or affects the presenting psychological or physical diagnosis (eg, hypertension is difficult to control because the patient refuses to take medications because of his or her religious beliefs).

- Treatment or care plans should include but not be limited to referral to chaplains, spiritual directors, pastoral counselors, and other spiritual care providers including clergy or faith community healers for spiritual counseling; development of spiritual goals; meaning-oriented therapy; mind–body interventions; rituals, spiritual practices; and contemplative interventions.

self, family, others, community, society, nature, and the significant or sacred. Spirituality is expressed through beliefs, values, traditions and practices.[14]

The basis of this model is that spiritual care is essential for professional clinical practice. In this model, chaplains serve as spiritual care specialists, with the nonchaplain clinicians providing generalist spiritual care. Thus, all clinicians should address patients' spirituality, identify and treat spiritual distress, and support spiritual resources of strength. In-depth spiritual counseling and exploration should be referred to the trained chaplain.[14,16]

As with other aspects of oncology care, this multidisciplinary collaboration is important when it comes to addressing spirituality. All members of the multidisciplinary team interact with patients, including responding to and addressing all dimensions of patient care: spiritual, religious, and existential as well as the physical, psychological, and social. Each of these components of care provides insight into the patient's suffering and his or her ability to manage that suffering. It is important to note that, when patients complain of pain, they may actually have complex or "total pain" originating from physical, emotional, social, and/or spiritual distress, which they express as a complaint of pain. Teams occur in inpatient as well as outpatient clinical settings and in communities, such as neighborhood community support settings, nursing home, continuum of care facilities, and senior communities.

COMMUNICATION AND ASSESSMENT OF SPIRITUAL DISTRESS

The first step in communicating about spiritual issues is to recognize spiritual themes that patients bring up, such as meaning, hope, relationships, religious beliefs, and values. Inherent to this aspect of spiritual care is the practice of compassionate presence, which can be characterized as being fully present with another as a witness to the patient's suffering. Being present means creating a safe space where the patient can share what matters most for that patient, what is that patient's greatest concerns and deepest suffering. One component is assessment and treatment of spiritual distress.[11] The other is the provision of compassionate presence to the patient and the family. The experience of compassionate presence by the clinician to the patient may result in a sense of healing by the patient within the context of the relationship with the clinician, even when the disease becomes refractory to medical care. This outcome was described by the consensus conference as the concept of a transformational healing relationship. Healing may be finding meaning, hope, or a sense of coherence in the midst of their illness.[7]

Once the health care provider hears the spiritual themes of the patients, they can begin asking open-ended questions to invite patients to share their inner story. The clinician can listen for how important the patient's spirituality is in their lives and whether the patient's spirituality impacts his or her health, and listen also for themes of suffering or spiritual distress. Important components in the implementation of spiritual care include a spiritual screening and history for the nonchaplain clinicians and a full spiritual assessment by a board-certified chaplain.[24,33]

Spiritual Screening

Spiritual screening usually is performed at the time of an initial intake by any clinician, whether it is at an outpatient, inpatient, or nursing facility, or even during admission into home hospice. The primary objectives of the spiritual screen are to:

- Assess for spiritual emergencies; and
- Identify patients who may benefit from an in-depth spiritual assessment.

Spiritual screening need not be an overly complicated task and may necessitate only a few simple questions incorporated into initial screening, such as, "How important is religion and spirituality in your coping?" If a patient responds that they are important, then a follow-up question could be, "How well are those resources working for you at this time?" If the patient describes difficulty with coping and/or that spiritual or religious resources are not working well for him or her, a referral to a trained chaplain is advised.[24]

Spiritual History

As with other components of the medical history, a spiritual history is important for clinicians to take, especially during the initial consultation. The goal is to understand better how a patient's spiritual needs and resources may complement or complicate the patient's overall care. A spiritual history typically is asked in the context of a comprehensive social history. Targeted questions are used to invite the patient to share his or her spiritual and/or religious beliefs, and to help guide the patient to explore questions of meaning. The questions are not meant as checklists, but as guides to help the clinician invite the patient to share his or her beliefs, hopes, fears, and concerns. Ultimately, for clinicians, the spiritual history can serve the following goals:

- To better understand the patient's beliefs and values;
- To identify spiritual themes and assess for spiritual distress (meaninglessness, hopelessness, etc) and spiritual resources of strength (hope, meaning and purpose, resiliency, spiritual community);
- To connect with the patient in a deeper and more profound way;
- To empower the patient to find inner resources of healing and acceptance; and
- To identify spiritual and religious beliefs that might affect health care decision making.

Finally, the spiritual history serves as a primary opportunity to identify patients who may benefit from referral to chaplains or other resources. An example of a spiritual history is the FICA spiritual history tool,[34] which was initially developed by a focus group of primary care physicians. It is validated, widely used, and integrated into some medical health records. The format of the tool is presented in **Table 2**.

Spiritual Assessment

For patients who the clinician feels would benefit from a more in-depth conversation with a chaplain, referral for a more formal spiritual assessment is advised.[34] The chaplain will conduct an in-depth, extensive, ongoing conversation that can be performed with patients from any religious or spiritual tradition and belief system. The primary objectives are to:

- Develop a relationship with the patient in a clinical setting;
- Identify spiritual issues and confirm, elaborate, or make a spiritual diagnosis; and
- Develop a spiritual care plan that can be shared with the treatment team.

The aim is to understand the patient's needs and resources by first listening to the patient's story. There is no specified set of questions. That is, the assessment strategy is a process without a defined script, which is necessary because the content area itself is not amenable to a formulaic structure. As a result, it requires extensive training, which is part of the certification process for professional chaplains.

Table 2 The FICA spiritual history tool	
F– Faith and Belief	• Do you consider yourself spiritual or religious? or • Do you have spiritual beliefs that help you cope with stress? • If the patient responds "No," the clinician might ask, "What gives your life meaning?" Sometimes patients respond with answers such as family, career, or nature.
I – Importance	• What importance does your faith or belief have in our life? • Have your beliefs influenced how you take care of yourself in this illness? • What role do your beliefs play in regaining your health
C – Community	• Are you part of a spiritual or religious community? • Is this of support to you and how? • Is there a group of people you really love or who are important to you? Communities such as churches, temples, and mosques, or a group of like-minded friends can serve as strong support systems for some patients.
A – Address in Care/Assessment	• How would you like me, your health care provider, to address these issues in your health care? • Use this category to assess for spiritual distress.

From Puchalski CM, Ferrell B. Making healthcare whole: integrating spirituality into patient care. West Conshohocken (PA): Templeton Press; 2010; with permission.

TREATMENT PLAN

Once spiritual distress or issues are identified, they need to be addressed as part of the assessment and treatment plan. Clinicians can also document the patient's spiritual and psychosocial resources of strength and note those in the assessment and plans.

PAIN AND SPIRITUALITY: INTERVENTIONS

Patients are spiritual beings whose spirituality is often accentuated in a health care crisis such as confronting cancer, cancer pain, and its treatment.[19] The trajectory of spiritual coping during this journey is not clear given the limited longitudinal studies. Furthermore, there have been limited randomized controlled trials to test interventions for spiritual care for patients with cancer. This section focuses on positive spiritual coping, spiritual struggle, studies of chaplain visits, and meditation as an intervention.

POSITIVE COPING

Some patients have primarily positive types of spiritual coping, that is, the spiritual coping is characterized by having a secure relationship with the sacred, others, and self around spiritual issues,[35] and by having helpful spiritual resources. For these patients, it is important to nurture the strengths and positive resources of their spirituality. Health care providers may intervene by being attentive to what they observe as potential resources, for example, sacred texts (eg, the Qu'ran), nature-based poetry, spiritual music (eg, gospel music, or nonreligious music), spiritual symbols in the room (Buddha, stones) or in what the patient is wearing (eg, yarmulke), language used (eg, "I pray every day"), and inspirations on the wall (eg, "The Lord is my Shepherd," or a painting of nature, or poetry) and inquiring about these as potential sources of strength and comfort. Health care staff can encourage their patients in using those resources that have been helpful to them and offer to contact persons or communities that provide them support, for example, faith-specific communities or practices (eg, blessing from a Latter Day Saint elder) or a professional chaplain, spiritual director, meditation teachers, or other person.[36] Praying may be a coping strategy in response to pain (and suffering) that is a positive intervention for the patient. Encouraging the patient to tap into the practices that are important to them could be beneficial. Religious, cultural, or personal beliefs can give meaning and purpose (ie, opportunity for growth) to pain and suffering, thereby reducing the suffering and lessening the intensity of the pain experienced. Thus, engaging patients with cancer who are in pain around their beliefs, whether religious, humanist, or cultural, is an important intervention by health care providers.[37,38]

SPIRITUAL STRUGGLE

However, not all spirituality is secure; rather, often one has conflict with spirituality. Conflicts with what one holds sacred (eg, Higher Power, God), with others regarding spiritual beliefs or practices, and within oneself (eg, doubts, struggle with meaning, guilt or values conflict) are common. Studies indicate that about 50% of patients with cancer have a spiritual struggle to a degree that is positively associated with poorer emotional and quality of life outcomes.[35] The associations of spiritual struggle and pain are inconclusive in studies given the different results and the limited number of longitudinal studies.[38] Nonetheless, even without physical pain, spiritual struggle by definition implies struggle and potential spiritual pain. For example, certain religious beliefs can induce guilt ("If I prayed harder, I would be cured"), create false hopes ("God will heal me even though the doctors say I have a few weeks to live"), and lead one to believe that the cancer and/or pain are God's will and thereby exacerbate pain.

Other beliefs can also cause distress, for example, feeling that one has worked hard to live a natural healthy life but now, despite that, has cancer. These ultimately are "why me" questions for which there is no answer or solution. Health care providers can listen to these struggles and explore how the patient is addressing them (and with whom) in what is sometimes referred to as compassionate presence—listing to the patient's spiritual pain with compassion and without judgment. Often patients will come to a deeper understanding of their suffering and achieve peace over time in the presence of others who can listen in this way. For patients in which this type of intervention is not sufficient or where the suffering is immense or has overtones of complicated religious or other beliefs, referral to professional chaplains is very helpful. Using their theological, counseling, and clinical training, chaplains can help the patient to move toward spiritual healing.[39]

There are several ways chaplains can help with spiritual struggle, including a representative role, talk therapy, introduction, ritual, and reframing. Chaplains often play a "representative" role with patients, that is, patients may experience them as representing God or the spiritual community. If the chaplain is attentive and caring, the patient's negative experience of God or spiritual community may change in a more positive direction, which can help to improve the spiritual struggle. Further, having someone with whom to talk about and talk through their struggles can help to ease or resolve the struggle. Chaplains can also provide guidance that helps a patient to reconnect with and begin to resolve struggles with her or his spiritual community. For example, when the formal spiritual community is missed, the patient can be helped to connect with a clergy person or shaman, for example, years after a very hurtful experience with another individual in that community.[38,40] Chaplains may also provide a ritual that helps the patient to release their hurt and begin to heal. Finally, chaplains have the sensitivity and expertise to explore patients' beliefs and then help patients to reframe (collaboratively talking together, which leads to a reinterpretation) their beliefs in ways that are congruent with their experience while easing the source of the struggle.[39]

MEDITATION

Another methodology used by health care providers, including chaplains, is to educate about or lead the patient in meditation. The patient's spiritual beliefs may inform the content of the meditation used by the chaplain, for example, whether or not spiritual language is used in the meditation. In a review of studies on the effects of mindfulness-based stress reduction on chronic pain, Baer[41] in general found that chronic pain patients who used mindfulness-based stress reduction experienced improvements in ratings of pain, with many of the improvements continuing through a follow-up evaluation (see Denise Hess' article, "Mindfulness Based Interventions for Hematology and Oncology Patients with Pain," in this issue). Furthermore, Wachholtz and Pargament[42] have demonstrated that the content of the meditation makes a difference. They studied 80 patients with intense migraines comparing 4 interventions longitudinally with 3 time periods: using a spiritual phrase (eg, "God is peace"), an internal secular phrase (eg, "I am happy"), an external secular phrase (eg, "Sunshine is warm"), and progressive relaxation technique in a control group.[42] Compared with the other 3 interventions, the people using the spiritual phrase reported less pain, greater pain tolerance, and better existential well-being, and other beneficial outcomes.

CASE STUDY

Leslie was a 45-year-old white woman with leukemia (acute myelogenous leukemia) being treated with an allogeneic stem cell transplant. She had a partner, a 12-year-old son, and a 7-year-old daughter. She had been trying to keep the children's lives normal, so had them stay close to home. Her sister, partner, and children were only able to visit about 1 weekend per month, being separated by hundreds of miles during the treatment. Leslie described herself as spiritual but not religious. She had a spiritual practice of meditation that had provided some meaning for her in the past. Her primary reasons for wanting chaplaincy care were to talk about her existential distress, her fears regarding dying and death, the emotional pain associated with this existential distress, and grief surrounding these fears.

Leslie contracted graft-versus-host disease as a complication from the transplant that required hospitalization for about 10 weeks. Early in the hospital stay, her oncologist identified existential distress and anxiety and referred Leslie to the chaplain. Chaplain Donna had regular inpatient visits with her once or twice per week during those weeks. They met initially because Leslie was struggling with anxiety when starting the transplant, sharing the fear that she might never see her children again if the transplant went poorly and she died. Donna established rapport and trust with Leslie and she conveyed her distressing fears to the chaplain.

After talking about these fears and assessing Donna's spiritual and existential distress and resources, which included learning about the patient's interest in and valuing of meditation, the chaplain and Leslie agreed to explore different types of meditation that might benefit Leslie. Donna started with a guided meditation that walked Leslie through an experience of going blind. The next time they met, she

Table 3 Whole person assessment and treatment plan	
	Leslie was a 45-year-old white woman with leukemia (acute myelogenous leukemia) being treated with an allogeneic stem cell transplant with mild graft-versus-host disease (rash on upper extremities), existential distress, no depression, but with insomnia and fatigue, and worried about effects of her illness on her family.
Physical	Continue with current plan, corticosteroid cream as per dermatology; insomnia likely from worrying about her health and mortality, fatigue from medication side effects, encouraged gentle activity as tolerated.
Emotional	Anxiety related to her diagnosis, being separated from her family.
Social	Concern re effects of her illness on her family and has had trouble sharing those concerns with family. Will refer to social worker for family meeting.
Spiritual	Existential distress, affecting her quality of life including worsening anxiety and insomnia. Supportive care, referral to chaplain for more in-depth spiritual counseling, encouraged use of meditation.

guided Leslie through a meditation that walked her through Leslie's own death. The chaplain also offered other guided meditations, for example, breathing, loving, and kindness. After the meditations, they talked through whatever feelings these exercises brought up. Their plan was to collaboratively and actively work on what Jon O'Donohue calls "befriending death."[43] The chaplain facilitated exploration around fears of death and in life, the two of them working actively to engage death as a companion instead of an enemy. A lot of the work involved the chaplain engaging in deep listening and then encouraging Leslie to be gentle with herself, to help her see what she could let go of emotionally and what she could make room for. The chaplain also suggested ways the oncologist could address Leslie's distress; the chaplain wrote her findings and recommendations in the patient's chart so that the rest of the patient team could better support Leslie. The oncologist also documented her findings in a whole-person assessment and treatment plan shown in **Table 3**.

The initial outcomes included Leslie's having "small victories" of "conquering fears of death." At 1 visit in particular, she told the chaplain that she had let go of her fear of death. The chaplain helped Leslie to explore what had helped her let it go. However, because these things generally ebb and flow, at the next visit, some of the fears returned. Donna encouraged Leslie to let the "befriending" be a process that is not linear. Leslie's greatest areas of growth were acknowledging the deep pain and grief that had accumulated during treatment and being kind to herself saying, "I really have been through so much." She continued to face her fears and wanted to talk about her feelings and attitudes around death. She also felt empowered to share these feelings with the oncologist and found it helpful to be able to discuss her existential distress at her visits with the oncologist and rest of the team.

SUMMARY

From the moment of diagnosis of cancer, through treatment, survivorship, recurrence, and dying, patients with cancer, especially those with pain, are faced with spiritual issues that may cause spiritual distress or may help them as they face their illness. Spirituality can be a powerful positive force in helping patients to reframe their illness, find greater meaning in life, decrease their suffering, and recognize what is ultimately important and of value to them. Unresolved spiritual distress, however, can lead to poorer quality of life and poorer health outcomes. It is, therefore, critical that oncologists and other clinicians address the spiritual issues of the patient as part of every assessment, diagnose and treat spiritual distress and integrate patient spiritual resources of strength into the patient treatment plan. Working with certified chaplains or spiritual care professionals is essential to attending to patient spiritual issues. But every member of the health care team must be responsible for attending to all dimensions of a patients' suffering: the spiritual as well as the psychosocial and physical suffering.

ACKNOWLEDGMENTS

The authors acknowledge Deanna Drake, BCC, the chaplain mentioned in this article, and Ellen Friedmann, JD, for her editorial assistance.

B.R. Ferrell and C.M. Puchalski acknowledge the support of the Archstone Foundation and the Fetzer Institute for their support of prior work in spirituality. Dr C.M. Puchalski also acknowledges the John Templeton Foundation and the Arthur Vining Davis Foundation for prior work in this area.

REFERENCES

1. Norris L, Walseman K, Puchalski CM. Communicating about spiritual issues with cancer patients. In: Surbone A, Zwitter M, Rajer M, et al, editors. New challenges in communication with cancer patients. Boston (MA): Springer; 2013. p. 91–103.
2. Cannon AJ, Darrington DL, Reed EC, et al. Spirituality, patients' worry, and follow-up health-care utilization among cancer survivors. J Support Oncol 2011;9(4): 141–8.
3. Skalla KA, Ferrell B. Challenges in assessing spiritual distress in survivors of cancer. Clin J Oncol Nurs 2015;19(1):99–104. Available at: http://www.ncbi.nlm.nih.gov/pubmed/25706479. Accessed September 3, 2015.
4. Miller KD, Siegel RL, Lin CC, et al. Cancer treatment and survivorship statistics, 2016. CA Cancer J Clin 2016;66(4):271–89.
5. National Cancer Institute. PDQ® spirituality in cancer care. 2016. Available at: https://www.cancer.gov/publications/pdq. Accessed October 12, 2017.
6. Hui D, de la Cruz M, Thorney S, et al. The frequency and correlates of spiritual distress among patients with advanced cancer admitted to an acute palliative care unit. Am J Hosp Palliat Care 2011;28(4):264–70.
7. Puchalski CM, Vitillo R, Hull SK, et al. Improving the spiritual dimension of whole person care: reaching national and international consensus. J Palliat Med 2014; 17(6):642–56.
8. Ferrell B, Sun V, Hurria A, et al. Interdisciplinary palliative care for patients with lung cancer. J Pain Symptom Manage 2015;50(6):758–67.
9. Salsman JM, Fitchett G, Merluzzi TV, et al. Religion, spirituality, and health outcomes in cancer: a case for a meta-analytic investigation. Cancer 2015; 121(21):3754–9. Available at: https://onlinelibrary.wiley.com/doi/full/10.1002/cncr.29349. Accessed September 3, 2015.
10. Balboni TA, Balboni M, Enzinger AC, et al. Provision of spiritual support to patients with advanced cancer by religious communities and associations with medical care at the end of life. JAMA Intern Med 2013;173(12):1109–17.
11. Holland JC, Andersen B, Breitbart WS, et al. Distress management clinical practice guidelines in oncology. J Natl Compr Canc Netw 2013;11(2):190–208.
12. Norris L, Pratt-Chapman M, Noblick JA, et al. Distress, demoralization, and depression in cancer survivorship. Psychiatr Ann 2011;41(9):433–8.

13. National Coalition for Cancer Survivorship. Long term and late effects. 2011. Available at: www.canceradvocacy.org/resources/take-charge/long-term-late-effects.html. Accessed October 12, 2017.

14. Puchalski C, Ferrell B, Virani R, et al. Improving the quality of spiritual care as a dimension of palliative care: the report of the Consensus Conference. J Palliat Med 2009;12:885–904.

15. Koenig HG, King D, Carson VB. Handbook of religion and health. 2nd edition. Oxford (United Kingdom): Oxford University Press; 2012.

16. Puchalski CM, Dorff RE, Hendi IY. Spirituality, religion, and healing in palliative care. Clin Geriatr Med 2004;20:689–714, vi–vii.

17. Nolan S, Saltmarsh P, Leget C. Spiritual care in palliative care: working towards an EAPC taskforce. Eur J Palliat Care 2011;18:86–9.

18. Alcorn SR, Balboni MJ, Prigerson HG, et al. "If God wanted me yesterday, I wouldn't be here today": religious and spiritual themes in patients' experiences of advanced cancer. J Palliat Med 2010;13:581–8.

19. Vallurupalli M, Lauderdale K, Balboni MJ, et al. The role of spirituality and religious coping in the quality of life of patients with advanced cancer receiving palliative radiation therapy. J Support Oncol 2012;10:81–7.

20. Jim HS, Pustejovsky JE, Park CL, et al. Religion, spirituality, and physical health in cancer patients: a meta-analysis. Cancer 2015;121:3760–8.

21. Salsman JM, Pustejovsky JE, Jim HS, et al. A meta-analytic approach to examining the correlation between religion/spirituality and mental health in cancer. Cancer 2015;121:3769–78.

22. Hebert R, Zdaniuk B, Schulz R, et al. Positive and negative religious coping and well-being in women with breast cancer. J Palliat Med 2009;12:537–45.

23. Winkelman WD, Lauderdale K, Balboni MJ, et al. The relationship of spiritual concerns to the quality of life of advanced cancer patients: preliminary findings. J Palliat Med 2011;14:1022–8.

24. Taylor EJ. Spiritual assessment. In: Ferrell BR, Coyle N, Paice JA, editors. Oxford textbook of palliative nursing. 4th edition. New York: Oxford University Press; 2015.

25. National Consensus Project for Quality Palliative Care. Clinical practice guidelines for quality palliative care. 3rd edition. 2013. Available at: http://www.nationalconsensusproject.org. Accessed June 28, 2016.

26. Sun V, Kim JY, Irish TL, et al. Palliative care and spiritual well-being in lung cancer patients and family caregivers. Psychooncology 2015;25:1448–55.

27. Balboni TA, Paulk ME, Balboni MJ, et al. Provision of spiritual care to patients with advanced cancer: associations with medical care and quality of life near death. J Clin Oncol 2010;28:445–52.

28. Sherman AC, Merluzzi TV, Pustejovsky JE, et al. A meta-analytic review of religious or spiritual involvement and social health among cancer patients. Cancer 2015;121:3779–88.

29. Delgado-Guay MO, Parsons HA, Hui D, et al. Spirituality, religiosity, and spiritual pain among caregivers of patients with advanced cancer. Am J Hosp Palliat Care 2013;30:455–61.

30. Johnson JR, Engelberg RA, Nielsen EL, et al. The association of spiritual care providers' activities with family members' satisfaction with care after a death in the ICU. Crit Care Med 2014;42:1991–2000.

31. Epstein-Peterson ZD, Sullivan AJ, Enzinger AC, et al. Examining forms of spiritual care provided in the advanced cancer setting. Am J Hosp Palliat Care 2015;32:750–7.

32. World Health Organization Definition of Palliative Care. Available at: http://www. who.int/cancer/palliative/definition/en. Accessed October 28, 2016.
33. Borneman T, Brown-Saltzman K. Meaning in illness. In: Ferrell BR, Coyle N, Paice JA, editors. Oxford textbook of palliative nursing. 4th edition. New York: Oxford University Press; 2015.
34. Pulchalski CM, Ferrell BF. Making healthcare whole: integrating spirituality into patient care. West Conshohocken (PA): Templeton Press; 2010.
35. Thune-Boyle ICV, Stygall J, Keshtgar MRS, et al. Religious/spiritual coping resources and their relationship with adjustment in patients newly diagnosed with breast cancer in the UK. Psycho-oncology 2013;22:646–58.
36. King S. Spirituality and medicine: an overview pertinent to medical providers. MedEdPORTAL. 2011. Available at: https://www.mededportal.org/publication/9043. Accessed October 12, 2017.
37. Pargament K, Feuille M, Burdzy D. The Brief RCOPE: current psychometric status of a short measure of religious coping. Religions 2011;2(1):51–76.
38. King SDW, Fitchett G, Murphy P, et al. Spiritual or religious struggle in hematopoietic cell transplant survivors. Psycho-oncology 2017;26(2):270–7.
39. King SDW. Facing fears and counting blessings: a case study of a chaplain's faithful companioning a cancer patient. J Health Care Chaplain 2012;18:3–22.
40. Cooper RS. Case study of a chaplain's spiritual care for a patient with advanced metastatic breast cancer. J Health Care Chaplain 2011;17:19–37.
41. Baer RA. Mindfulness training as a clinical intervention: a conceptual and empirical review. Clin Psychol Sci Pract 2003;10:125–43.
42. Wachholtz AB, Pargament KI. Migraines and meditation: does spirituality matter? J Behav Med 2008;31:351–66.
43. O'Donohue J. Anam Cara: a book of Celtic wisdom. New York: HarperCollins Publishers Inc; 2009.

Oncology Acupuncture for Chronic Pain in Cancer Survivors

A Reflection on the American Society of Clinical Oncology Chronic Pain Guideline

Weidong Lu, MB, MPH, PhD*, David S. Rosenthal, MD

KEYWORDS

- Oncology acupuncture • ASCO practice guideline • Chronic pain • Cancer survivors

KEY POINTS

- Acupuncture is recommended by the American Society of Clinical Oncology practice guideline for chronic pain in adult cancer survivors.
- Recent randomized clinical trials of acupuncture demonstrated favorable benefits for reducing chronic pain related to chemotherapy, hormonal therapy, radiotherapy and surgery.
- Oncology acupuncture is a new subspecialty of cancer supportive care.

INTRODUCTION

Cancer-related pain is one of most common but difficult to manage symptoms, whether it occurs during or after the completion of cancer treatment. It is reported that 40% to 85% of patients with cancer experience pain.[1,2] Cancer pain frequently occurs at different stages of the cancer journey: 25% in newly diagnosed patients, 33% in patients receiving anticancer treatment, and up to 75% in later stage of cancers.[2] With earlier cancer diagnosis and advances in cancer treatment, more patients are living longer. It is estimated that more than 15 million cancer survivors are currently living in the United States, which reflects an historically high survival rate.[3] However, cancer survivors often have physical, social, and emotional issues that seriously affect their quality of life. Among these issues are chronic pain, which continues to be a major medical issue.[4]

Disclosure Statement: This work is partially supported by Asia-Pacific Cancer Research Fund.
Leonard P. Zakim Center for Integrative Therapies and Healthy Living, Dana-Farber Cancer Institute, Harvard Medical School, 450 Brookline Avenue, Boston, MA 02215, USA
* Corresponding author.
E-mail address: weidong_lu@dfci.harvard.edu

Hematol Oncol Clin N Am 32 (2018) 519–533
https://doi.org/10.1016/j.hoc.2018.01.009
0889-8588/18/© 2018 Elsevier Inc. All rights reserved.

hemonc.theclinics.com

In general, cancer pain is caused by 2 major factors:

1. Tumor growth and tumor compression-related pain usually is the major cause, especially for patients with active disease; and
2. Pain related to the therapy, whether it is chemotherapy-related, hormonal therapy-related, radiation-related, stem cell transplantation–mediated, or surgery-related pain. In cancer survivors, chronic pain associated with these therapies is very relevant.

In 2016, the American Society of Clinical Oncology (ASCO) published a chronic pain related practice guideline, *Management of Chronic Pain in Survivors of Adult Cancers*.[5] It is the first ASCO guideline for chronic pain in cancer survivors. The guideline recommends that clinicians be aware of chronic pain syndromes resulting from cancer treatments, acknowledge the prevalence of these pain syndromes, the risk factors for individual patients, and know appropriate treatment options. A list of common cancer pain syndromes is presented in the guideline.[5] The guideline strongly recommends that clinicians either prescribe directly or refer patients to other professionals to provide the nonpharmacologic interventions available to mitigate chronic pain or improve pain-related outcomes. These nonpharmacologic interventions include:

1. Physical medicine and rehabilitation;
2. Integrative therapies;
3. Interventional therapies;
4. Psychological approaches; and
5. Neurostimulatory therapies.

"There is no compelling data to recommend one therapy over another," as is pointed out in the guideline. With modest strength of evidence and various methodologic limitations of these therapies, the guideline recognizes that these therapies have minimal side effects and the selection of these therapies may be based on patients and family goals, potential toxicities, ability of participation, and cost.[5]

Acupuncture, a major component of integrative therapies, along with massage and music therapy, is recommended by the ASCO guideline for chronic pain in cancer survivors. In the past 20 years, integrative oncology, a branch of integrative medicine, has emerged. It combines complementary therapies with conventional mainstream oncology care.[6-9] Clinical trial-generated evidence has shown that acupuncture is safe and effective as an adjunctive treatment for managing cancer-related symptoms.[10-12] However, despite thousands of years of practice outside of the conventional medical system, acupuncture use as an adjunctive therapy within a mainstream oncology setting presents an entirely new challenge.

Oncology acupuncture, a new breed of acupuncture, has emerged as a specialty in cancer symptom management.[13] This review focuses on randomized clinical trials of acupuncture used to treat chronic pain in cancer survivors, although some relevant clinical trials from noncancer populations and acute pain settings are also discussed. The purpose of the review is to provide randomized clinical trial-level evidence of acupuncture for specific chronic pain syndromes associated with cancer treatments, to further expand the potential clinical applications of acupuncture for this population as recommended by the ASCO, and to provide future directions for oncology acupuncture research and practice in cancer survivorship.

ACUPUNCTURE IN THE AMERICAN SOCIETY OF CLINICAL ONCOLOGY PAIN GUIDELINE: MANAGEMENT OF CHRONIC PAIN IN SURVIVORS OF ADULT CANCERS

The ASCO guideline recommending acupuncture for patients with chronic cancer pain are largely based on 3 systematic reviews,[14–16] with a metaanalysis in 2 of them.[15,16] Two of these 3 studies found positive outcomes[15,16] and 1 study deemed that evidence was insufficient[14] (**Table 1**).

An updated Cochrane systematic review investigated effectiveness of randomized clinical trials of acupuncture in treating cancer pain in adults.[14] The authors identified 5 randomized clinical trials (n = 285). The authors found that all studies had a high risk of bias from inadequate sample size[16] and concluded that there was insufficient evidence to judge whether or not acupuncture is effective in treating cancer pain in adults. However, a second systematic review published on *Journal of Clinical Oncology* identified 11 randomized clinical trials of acupuncture for cancer pain.[15] The authors found that the within-group effect size estimates for significant pain studies ranged from 1.11 to 2.10 for true acupuncture and from −0.45 to 0.45 for sham acupuncture, which suggests the magnitude of true acupuncture's effect for cancer pain falls into effect size categories from "large" to "huge," as judged by Cohen and Sawilowsky's criteria (0.8 as large, 1.20 as very large, and 2.0 as a huge effect).[17,18] A third systematic review identified 15 randomized clinical trials of acupuncture (n = 1157) from 14 medical databases.[16] It also pointed out that these trials suffered from poor methodological quality, but found better pain control in the patients with cancer when acupuncture was combined with an analgesic drug therapy than in patients who received analgesic drug therapy alone (n = 437; relative risk, 1.36; 95% confidence interval, 1.13–1.64; P = .003). A combined use of acupuncture and analgesic medications may yield favorable clinical outcomes in controlling cancer pain.

Table 1
Summary of systematic reviews on acupuncture for cancer pain cited by the American Society of Clinical Oncology pain guideline: Management of chronic pain in survivors of adult cancers

Author, Year	Types of Trials Included	No. of Trials Included	N	Key Findings
Paley et al,[14] 2015	Invasive acupuncture RCTs for pain directly related to cancer in adults	5	285	There is insufficient evidence to judge whether acupuncture is effective in treating cancer pain in adults.
Garcia et al,[15] 2013	Acupuncture RCTs involving needle insertion into acupuncture points for cancer symptoms	11	N/A	Within-group effect size estimates for significant pain studies ranged from 1.11 to 2.10 for true acupuncture and from -0.45 to 0.45 for sham acupuncture.
Choi et al,[16] 2012	Acupuncture RCTs as the sole treatment or as a part of a combination therapy for cancer pain	7	437	The effects of acupuncture combined with conventional drug therapy for pain reduction is superior as compared with conventional drug therapy alone (P = .003) with high heterogeneity (χ^2 = 19.92, P = .003, I^2 = 70%)

Abbreviations: N/A, not applicable; RCT, randomized clinical trial.

In addition, recent published randomized clinical trials suggest that acupuncture plays a special role in managing a wide range of chronic pain syndromes arising from cancer treatments, which is particularly relevant to cancer survivors. These chronic pain syndromes associated with cancer treatment include chemotherapy-related pain syndromes, hormonal therapy-related pain syndromes, radiation-related pain syndromes, and surgery-related pain syndromes. **Table 2** demonstrates that at least 1 acupuncture randomized clinical trial has been carried out in 4 of the 5 major pain syndrome categories,[5] excluding only those from stem cell transplantation–mediated graft-versus-host disease.

ACUPUNCTURE IN CHEMOTHERAPY-RELATED PAIN SYNDROMES

Published randomized clinical trials suggest that acupuncture may be an effective option in managing chemotherapy-related pain syndromes, including chemotherapy-induced peripheral neuropathy in patients with multiple myeloma[19]; chemotherapy-associated gastrointestinal distress and abdominal pain in gastric cancer,[20] and carpal tunnel syndrome.[21] **Table 3** presents the recently published clinical trials of acupuncture for these pain conditions.

Chemotherapy-induced peripheral neuropathy is a common side effect of a number of chemotherapeutic agents, including bortezomib, vinca alkaloids, taxanes, and platinum-containing regimens. Up to 76% of patients reported neuropathic symptoms after chemotherapy.[22] Although some forms of chemotherapy-induced neuropathy are reversible, permanent damage of neurologic functions can be observed. A recently published randomized clinical trial investigated effects of acupuncture plus methylcobalamin therapy versus methylcobalamin therapy alone in a group of patients with multiple myeloma (n = 104) who were treated with the proteasome inhibitor, bortezomib, and subsequently developed grade II or above chemotherapy-induced peripheral neuropathy.[19] Acupuncture was given daily for 3 days, then once every alternate day for 10 days as a treatment cycle. Each cycle was repeated every 28 days for 3 cycles (a total of 24 acupuncture sessions over 84 days). At the end of the study, 85.7% and 77.6% of patients in both groups reported decreased visual analogue scale pain scores, but the visual analogue scale pain scores in the acupuncture group decreased more significantly than those in the control group (P<.01). Other quality-of-life measures and objective measures such as nerve conduction velocity further demonstrated the superiority of acupuncture plus methylcobalamin therapy compared with methylcobalamin alone.[19]

Table 2
Summary of cancer treatment-related chronic pain syndromes for which at least 1 randomized, controlled trial was published that included acupuncture

Categories of Treatment-Related Pain Syndromes	Chemotherapy Related	Hormonal Therapy Related	Radiation Related	Surgery Related
Specific conditions	Chemotherapy-induced peripheral neuropathy Abdominal pain Carpal tunnel syndrome	Arthralgias Dyspareunia Vulvodynia	Cystitis Proctitis Postherpetic neuralgia	Postradical neck dissection pain Postthoracotomy pain Postamputation phantom pain Chronic shoulder pain Pelvic floor pain

Table 3
Acupuncture for chemotherapy-related pain syndromes

Pain Conditions	Author, Year	Study Population	Pain Intensity (0–10) at Baseline	Pain Duration at Baseline	Study Type	Interventions	N	Key Findings
Chemotherapy-induced peripheral neuropathy	Han et al,[19] 2017	Patients with multiple myeloma with grade II or greater chemotherapy-induced peripheral neuropathy after chemotherapy	5.57 ± 0.26	Postchemotherapy within 3 mo	RCT	Methylcobalamin therapy vs methylcobalamin plus MA	104	The pain was significantly alleviated in both groups, with a significantly higher decrease in the acupuncture treated group (P<.01). The patients' daily activity evaluated by Fact/GOG-Ntx questionnaires significantly improved in the Met + Acu group (P<.001).
Abdominal pain	Zhou et al,[20] 2017	Patients with gastric cancer receiving chemotherapy	N/A	During chemotherapy	RCT	Manual acupuncture vs usual care	56	The experimental group had experienced less vomiting and diarrhea, and shorter bouts of nausea and abdominal pain than the control group (P<.05).
Carpal tunnel syndrome	Maeda et al,[21] 2017	Noncancer patients with carpal tunnel syndrome	N/A	9.9 ± 8.9 y	RCT	Local EA vs distal EA vs local SA	80	All 3 acupuncture arms reduced symptom severity at end of treatment with no statistical significance among them (P = .92, P = .26, P = .26), real (local and distal) acupuncture was superior to sham at 3 mo follow-up (P = .04, P = .04, P = .04) and in producing improvements in neurophysiologic outcomes both in the local and in the brain.

Abbreviations: ACU, acupuncture; EA, electroacupuncture; Fact/GOG-NTX, Functional Assessment of Cancer Therapy/Gynecologic Oncology Group - Neurotoxicity; MA, manual acupuncture; Met, methylcobalamin; N/A, not applicable; RCT, randomized clinical trial; SA, sham acupuncture.

One high-quality randomized clinical trial (n = 90) was identified in a Cochrane systematic review.[14,23] In this study, patients with cancer with chronic neuropathic pain, including peripheral or central neuropathy, were treated with specific auricular acupuncture implants in test subjects, whereas noninvasive seeds were used in the placebo group. Study patients received acupuncture implants once a month for 2 times and then were assessed with pain measurement scales. At the end of the second month, the study group showed a significant decrease in pain intensity by 36% from baseline; there was almost no change in the placebo group (P<.0001).

ACUPUNCTURE IN HORMONAL THERAPY–RELATED PAIN SYNDROMES

Aromatase inhibitors such as exemestane (Aromasin), anastrozole (Arimidex), and letrozole (Femara) are commonly used in patients with breast cancer and ovarian cancers. However, a common side effects of aromatase inhibitors is joint pain, and in some patients dyspareunia[24] and vulvodynia.[25] A recently published systematic review with metaanalysis examined the effectiveness of acupuncture for managing aromatase inhibitor-induced arthralgia in patients with breast cancer.[26] The study included 5 randomized clinical trials (n = 181).[26–31] All trials recruited patients with stage I through III hormone receptor–positive breast cancer. All included trials categorized patients into acupuncture or sham acupuncture groups. Acupuncture was conducted once to twice per week for 6 to 8 weeks. Although the sample sizes of these trials are small, the methodological quality of the included trials is generally acceptable; 4 studies have reported acceptable methods of randomization and carried out with a double-blind method. The study found that patients with breast cancer receiving acupuncture showed a significant decrease in the Brief Pain Inventory worst pain score (weighted mean difference of −3.81; 95% confidence interval, −5.15 to −2.47) and in the Western Ontario and McMaster Universities Osteoarthritis Index pain score (weighted mean difference of −130.77; 95% confidence interval, −230.31 to −31.22) after 6 to 8 weeks of acupuncture treatment. The authors concluded that acupuncture is a safe and viable nonpharmacologic treatment that may relieve joint pain in patients with aromatase inhibitor-induced arthralgia. Additional trials with a large sample size are needed.[26] Acupuncture is also effective for dyspareunia[32] and vulvodynia[33] in noncancer populations (**Table 4**).

ACUPUNCTURE IN RADIATION-RELATED PAIN SYNDROMES

Published randomized clinical trials suggest that acupuncture may be an effective option in managing radiation-related pain syndromes, including radiation-induced cystitis and proctitis in patients with cervical and endometrial cancer undergoing radiation therapy[34] (**Table 5**). Yang and colleagues[34] published a randomized clinical trial in a Chinese language journal to investigate the effect of acupuncture on radiation-induced proctitis and radiation-induced cystitis in female patients (n = 50 and n = 44, respectively), in patients with cervical and endometrial cancer undergoing radiotherapy. In this trial, patients with cancer who underwent radiation therapy and developed symptoms of radiation-induced proctitis and radiation-induced cystitis were randomized into acupuncture versus usual care with medication treatment groups. Manual acupuncture with electrostimulation was given daily for 10 days. After 10 days of treatment, the significant effective rate, as determined by the restored normal bowel or bladder function without recurrence for at least 15 days after the completion of the treatment, was 90% versus 60% (P<.05) for patients with radiation-induced proctitis, and 77.3% versus 75% (P>.05) in patients with radiation-induced cystitis. However, patients in the acupuncture arm

Table 4
Acupuncture for hormonal therapy-related pain syndromes

Pain Conditions	Author, Year	Study Population	Pain Intensity (0–10) at Baseline	Pain Duration at Baseline	Study Type	Interventions	N	Key Findings
Arthralgias	Chen et al,[26] 2017	Breast cancer with aromatase inhibitor-induced arthralgia	5 (1.1–8.2); 6.7 ± 2.13; 4.9 ± 1.3	389 (109–1738) d; 7 (3–32) mo; 25.9 (3–56) mo	Metaanalysis and systematic review with 5 RCTs	MA vs SA or MA vs UC	181	After 6–8 wk of acupuncture treatment, significant pain reduction was found in the BPI worst pain score (WMD, −3.81; 95% CI, −5.15 to −2.47) and the WOMAC pain score (WMD, −130.77; 95% CI, −230.31 to −31.22)
Dyspareunia	Mira et al,[32] 2015	Noncancer women with deep endometriosis with pelvic pain and/or deep dyspareunia	5.95 ± 2.13	1.65 ± 2.08 y	RCT	Acupuncture-like TENS vs self-applied TENS	22	Both application types of TENS were effective for improving the evaluated types of pain. TENS provided symptomatic pain relief, with significant differences before and after chronic pelvic pain treatment (P<.0001), deep dyspareunia (P = .001), and dyschezia (P = .001).
Vulvodynia	Schlaeger et al,[33] 2015	Noncancer women with generalized vulvodynia or localized vestibulodynia	5.6 ± 1.9	5.4 ± 5.3 y	RCT	MA vs wait-list control	36	Reports of vulvar pain and dyspareunia were significantly reduced, whereas changes in the aggregate FSFI scores suggest significant improvement in sexual functioning in those receiving acupuncture vs those who did not.

Abbreviations: BPI, Brief Pain Inventory; CI, confidence interval; FSFI, Female Sexual Function Index; MA, manual acupuncture; RCT, randomized clinical trial; SA, sham acupuncture; TENS, transcutaneous electrical nerve stimulation; UC, usual care; WMD, weighted mean difference; WOMAC, Western Ontario and McMaster Universities Osteoarthritis Index.

Table 5
Acupuncture for radiation-related pain syndromes

Pain Conditions	Author, Year	Study Population	Pain Intensity (0–10) at Baseline	Pain Duration at Baseline	Study Type	Interventions	N	Key Findings
Cystitis	Yang et al,[34] 1994	Female patients with cervical cancer, endometrial cancer undergoing radiotherapy	N/A	Post recent radiation therapy	RCT	MA + EA vs UC	42	No statistical difference between acupuncture and usual care in symptom relief (P>.05), but the acupuncture group showed a significantly shorter symptomatic duration than the usual care group (P<.05).
Proctitis	Yang et al,[34] 1994	Female patients with cervical cancer, endometrial cancer undergoing radiotherapy	N/A	After recent radiation therapy	RCT	MA + EA vs UC	50	Acupuncture group showed significant symptom relief and a significantly shorter symptomatic duration than the usual care group (P<.05, P<.05)
Postherpetic neuralgia	Hui et al,[35] 2012	Noncancer patients with herpes zoster >30 d duration	7.5 ± 1.7	145 d (range, 81.0–371.5 d)	RCT, treatment vs wait-list control	Multifaceted therapy including acupuncture, neural therapy, cupping and bleeding, meditation, and Chinese herbs	59	At 3 wk after randomization (ie, after the immediate treatment group completed treatment), pain scores differed significantly (treatment = 2.3; control = 7.2; P<.001). The observed decrease in pain in the immediate treatment group was maintained at 9 wk and at long-term follow-up (1–2 y later).

Abbreviations: EA, electroacupuncture; MA, manual acupuncture; RCT, randomized clinical trial; UC, usual care.

demonstrated statistically significant shorter durations of radiation-induced proctitis and radiation-induced cystitis symptoms as compared with the usual care arm ($P<.01$, $P<.01$).[36] This trial was conducted in an acute pain setting.

Postherpetic neuralgia (PHN) may also respond to acupuncture therapy. PHN is defined as pain persisting more than 3 months from nerve damage caused by the varicella zoster virus. It is debilitating and difficult to manage. The zoster occurrence rate is about 4% in patients with breast cancer who have completed radiation therapy within 2 years, which is 3- to 5-fold higher than in the general population.[37] Other cancer therapies may also be associated with zoster and subsequent PHN. Hui and associates[35] reported a randomized clinical trial to investigate a multifaced integrative therapy, mainly consisting of acupuncture, cupping, and meditation, for PHN in a group of patients without cancer who had PHN for an average duration of 145 days. The control for this study was a wait-listed arm. The integrative therapy was provided once daily, 5 days per week for 3 weeks; the wait-list arm served as the control. At 3 weeks after randomization, the visual analogue scale pain scores differed significantly (treatment, 2.3; control, 7.2; $P<.001$), and the results were maintained for 9 weeks and at 1 to 2 years follow-up. Given the effectiveness of acupuncture in the patients without cancer, it is reasonable to recommend it for survivors of cancer with pain from PHN.

ACUPUNCTURE IN SURGICAL PAIN SYNDROMES

Published randomized clinical trials suggest that acupuncture may be an effective option in managing patients with surgical pain syndromes, including post radical neck dissection pain in patients with head and neck cancer,[36,38] postthoracotomy pain in patients with lung cancer,[39] phantom pain in postamputation patients,[40] and possibly chronic shoulder pain[41] and chronic pelvic floor pain[42] for postoperative interventions. Acupuncture for acute postoperative pain has been studied extensively.[43] **Table 6** presents the published clinical trials of acupuncture for these pain conditions.

Head and neck cancers include cancers in the nasal cavity, sinuses, lips, mouth, salivary glands, throat, or larynx. Neck dissection with chemoradiation therapy is often recommended. Although current treatment has achieved a high curative rate for head and neck cancer, significant side effects associated with surgery and chemoradiation therapy are very common, and include neck pain, xerostomia, dysphagia, and weight loss.

Pfister and colleagues[38] randomized a group of patients with head and neck cancer (n = 70) with a history of neck dissection suffering from persistent chronic pain and other symptoms into a prospective open-label randomized clinical trial of acupuncture once a week for 4 weeks versus usual care. The median time from the surgery to the study was 39 months in the acupuncture arm, which indicates long-term chronic pain in these patients. In addition to neck dissections, most patients had also received radiation therapy. The Constant-Murley Score, a composite measure of pain, function, and activities of daily living, a numerical rating scale for pain and Xerostomia Inventory were assessed at baseline and at the end of acupuncture treatment. At follow-up (2 weeks after acupuncture), the mean pain scale in the acupuncture group dropped from 5.6 to 3.6 and from 5.92 to 5.8 in the control group ($P<.001$). Both the Constant-Murley Score and Xerostomia Inventory improved in the acupuncture group ($P = .008$, $P = .02$), respectively. The results of this study suggested that the patients who underwent neck dissection with or without radiation therapy, who were still suffering from

Table 6
Acupuncture for surgical pain syndromes

Pain Conditions	Author, Year	Study Population	Pain Duration at Baseline	Pain Intensity (0–10) at Baseline	Study Type	Interventions	N	Key Findings
Postradical neck dissection pain	Pfister et al,[38] 2010	Cancer patients received neck dissection with pain and/or dysfunction in the neck and/or shoulders	39 mo (median)	5.6 ± 1.6	RCT	MA vs UC	70	Constant-Murley scores improved more in the acupuncture group (adjusted difference between groups −11.2; 95% CI, 3.0 to 19.3; P = .008), and greater improvement in xerostomia (adjusted difference in Xerostomia Inventory −5.8; 95% CI, −0.9 to −10.7; P = 0.02).
Postthoracotomy pain	Wang et al,[39] 1988	Patients received thoracotomy for intrathoracic pathologies	Day 1 after thoracotomy to day 7	10	RCT	Ear EA with vitamin B injection vs UC	36	The pulmonary function tests showed improvements in vital capacity and forced expiratory volume at 1 second on day 3.6 (P<.05), the negative inspiratory force on days 1, 3, 4, and 5, (P<.05), and the relief in coughing pain on days 1–5 by VAS (P<.05).

Pain type	Study	Population		Duration	Design	Comparison	n	Outcome
Postamputation phantom pain	Trevelyan et al,[40] 2015	Noncancer traumatic or medical amputation of a lower limb	5.44	25.63 d (range, 18.43–32.85 d)	RCT	Body acupuncture and ear acupuncture vs UC	15	Average pain intensity (raw change = 2.69) and worst pain intensity (raw change = 4.00); effect size 0.64 at day 28
Chronic shoulder pain	Molsberger et al,[41] 2010	Noncancer patients with 1-sided shoulder pain	6.6 ± 1.4	10.7 ± 9.7 mo	RCT	MA vs SA vs UC	424	Percentages of responders (≥50% decrease from baseline) at 3 mo after the end of treatment were MA 65% (95% CI, 56%–74%), SA 24% (95% CI, 9%–39%), and usual care 37% (95% CI, 24%–50%)
Pelvic floor pain	Rubi-Klein et al,[42] 2010	Noncancer women with endometriosis and surgery related to their diagnosis	7.39	7.12 y	RCT, crossover	Verum acupuncture vs nonspecific acupuncture	101	The VAS score in group 1 showed a significant decrease in pain ($P<.0001$) but not group 2 ($P = .866$). Both groups showed a highly significant result in the Pain Disability Index score ($P<.0001$).

Abbreviations: MA, manual acupuncture; RCT, randomized clinical trial; SA, sham acupuncture; UC, usual care; VAS, visual analogue pain scale.

chronic pain more than 3 years after treatment may still benefit from acupuncture treatment.

ONCOLOGY ACUPUNCTURE, AN EMERGING SUBSPECIALTY FOR CHRONIC PAIN

Patients with cancer are a unique population for acupuncture treatment. The complexity of cancer types, the multiple types of treatment options, and the various results make administrating acupuncture in patients with cancer a greater challenge than applying acupuncture in a population without cancer. In the past 20 years, emerging clinical evidence suggests that acupuncture can be recommended for symptom relief during cancer treatment, including for cancer pain management. In the United States, many cancer centers, including MD Anderson Cancer Center, Memorial Sloan-Kettering Cancer Center, and Dana-Farber Cancer Institute, provide acupuncture to patients as a part of clinical services along with conventional cancer therapy. The recommendation of acupuncture for chronic pain in survivors of cancer by the ASCO chronic pain guideline is an exciting landmark.

Oncology acupuncture as a new subspecialty of cancer supportive care is emerging in Western countries, in which specialized oncology acupuncturists provide clinical services as a member of a multidisciplinary team inside conventional cancer centers. Because of the complexity and safety concerns of an oncologic practice, oncology acupuncture is distinctly different from traditional acupuncture with the following major characteristics:

1. It operates as a clinical trial–driven, evidence-based subspecialty;
2. Its clinical practice and procedures are highly standardized;
3. It includes oncologic data acquisition (eg, laboratory and imaging data) to determine the appropriateness of acupuncture treatment;
4. It demands that the specialist possesses knowledge and skills in both general oncology and acupuncture; and
5. It also requires intense communications and coordination with other team members such as medical, surgical, radiation oncologists, palliative care, survivorship, oncological nursing, nutritionists, social workers, and other supportive care resources.

SUMMARY

The newly published ASCO *Management of Chronic Pain in Survivors of Adult Cancers* provides recommendations that encourage use of nonpharmacological interventions for cancer survivors including acupuncture. Meanwhile, patients with various chronic pain syndromes associated with cancer treatments continue to have unmet needs that require more appropriate therapies for relief. Accumulated evidence from clinical trials suggests that acupuncture has a broader role as adjunct therapy for chronic pain. Because of the complexity of cancer, chronic pain syndromes related to cancer treatments usually present as multidimensional disorders. Although acupuncture generally is safe, it is critical for clinicians who are practicing acupuncture for this population to keep an eye on not only acupuncture techniques, but also cancer history, progression, and possible recurrent diseases, especially in any patient who reports new-onset pain, to ensure the safety of patients with cancer. Therefore, oncology acupuncture requires that clinicians possess knowledge and skills in both acupuncture and allopathic oncology.[13] The current ASCO practice guidelines and its recommendations for using acupuncture for chronic pain needs to be followed and disseminated. In the near future, specialized oncology acupuncture will have an indispensable place in cancer pain management.

REFERENCES

1. Anderson KO, Richman SP, Hurley J, et al. Cancer pain management among underserved minority outpatients: perceived needs and barriers to optimal control. Cancer 2002;94(8):2295–304.
2. Goudas LC, Bloch R, Gialeli-Goudas M, et al. The epidemiology of cancer pain. Cancer Invest 2005;23(2):182–90.
3. Bluethmann SM, Mariotto AB, Rowland JH. Anticipating the "silver tsunami": prevalence trajectories and comorbidity burden among older cancer survivors in the United States. Cancer Epidemiol Biomarkers Prev 2016;25(7):1029–36.
4. Green CR, Hart-Johnson T, Loeffler DR. Cancer-related chronic pain: examining quality of life in diverse cancer survivors. Cancer 2011;117(9):1994–2003.
5. Paice JA, Lacchetti C, Bruera E. Management of chronic pain in survivors of adult cancers: ASCO Clinical Practice Guideline Summary. J Oncol Pract 2016;12(8): 757–62.
6. Running A, Seright T. Integrative oncology: managing cancer pain with complementary and alternative therapies. Curr Pain Headache Rep 2012;16(4):325–31.
7. Cassileth B. Why integrative oncology? Complementary therapies are increasingly becoming part of mainstream care. Oncology (Williston Park) 2006;20(10):1302.
8. Deng G, Cassileth BR. Integrative oncology: complementary therapies for pain, anxiety, and mood disturbance. CA Cancer J Clin 2005;55(2):109–16.
9. Rosenthal DS, Dean-Clower E. Integrative medicine in hematology/oncology: benefits, ethical considerations, and controversies. Hematology Am Soc Hematol Educ Program 2005;491–7.
10. Meng Z, Garcia MK, Hu C, et al. Randomized controlled trial of acupuncture for prevention of radiation-induced xerostomia among patients with nasopharyngeal carcinoma. Cancer 2012;118(13):3337–44.
11. Ezzo J, Vickers A, Richardson MA, et al. Acupuncture-point stimulation for chemotherapy-induced nausea and vomiting. J Clin Oncol 2005;23(28):7188–98.
12. Lu W, Dean-Clower E, Doherty-Gilman A, et al. The value of acupuncture in cancer care. Hematol Oncol Clin North Am 2008;22(4):631–48, viii.
13. Lu W, Rosenthal DS. Recent advances in oncology acupuncture and safety considerations in practice. Curr Treat Options Oncol 2010;11(3–4):141–6.
14. Paley CA, Johnson MI, Tashani OA, et al. Acupuncture for cancer pain in adults. Cochrane Database Syst Rev 2015;(10):CD007753.
15. Garcia MK, McQuade J, Haddad R, et al. Systematic review of acupuncture in cancer care: a synthesis of the evidence. J Clin Oncol 2013;31(7):952–60.
16. Choi TY, Lee MS, Kim TH, et al. Acupuncture for the treatment of cancer pain: a systematic review of randomised clinical trials. Support Care Cancer 2012;20(6): 1147–58.
17. Sawilowsky SS. New effect size rules of thumb. Journal of Modern Applied Statistical Methods 2009;8(2):597–9.
18. Cohen J. Statistical power analysis for the behavioral sciences. Hillsdale (NJ): Lawrence Erlbaum Associates; 1988. p. 2.
19. Han X, Wang L, Shi H, et al. Acupuncture combined with methylcobalamin for the treatment of chemotherapy-induced peripheral neuropathy in patients with multiple myeloma. BMC Cancer 2017;17(1):40.
20. Zhou J, Fang L, Wu WY, et al. The effect of acupuncture on chemotherapy-associated gastrointestinal symptoms in gastric cancer. Curr Oncol 2017;24(1): e1–5.

21. Maeda Y, Kim H, Kettner N, et al. Rewiring the primary somatosensory cortex in carpal tunnel syndrome with acupuncture. Brain 2017;140(4):914–27.
22. Kautio AL, Haanpaa M, Kautiainen H, et al. Burden of chemotherapy-induced neuropathy–a cross-sectional study. Support Care Cancer 2011;19(12):1991–6.
23. Alimi D, Rubino C, Pichard-Leandri E, et al. Analgesic effect of auricular acupuncture for cancer pain: a randomized, blinded, controlled trial. J Clin Oncol 2003;21(22):4120–6.
24. Derzko C, Elliott S, Lam W. Management of sexual dysfunction in postmenopausal breast cancer patients taking adjuvant aromatase inhibitor therapy. Curr Oncol 2007;14(Suppl 1):S20–40.
25. Goetsch MF. Unprovoked vestibular burning in late estrogen-deprived menopause: a case series. J Low Genit Tract Dis 2012;16(4):442–6.
26. Chen L, Lin CC, Huang TW, et al. Effect of acupuncture on aromatase inhibitor-induced arthralgia in patients with breast cancer: a meta-analysis of randomized controlled trials. Breast 2017;33:132–8.
27. Bao T, Cai L, Giles JT, et al. A dual-center randomized controlled double blind trial assessing the effect of acupuncture in reducing musculoskeletal symptoms in breast cancer patients taking aromatase inhibitors. Breast Cancer Res Treat 2013;138(1):167–74.
28. Crew K, Capodice J, Greenlee H, et al. Randomized, blinded, sham-controlled trial of acupuncture for the management of aromatase inhibitor-associated joint symptoms in women with early-stage breast cancer. J Clin Oncol 2010;28(7):1154–60.
29. Mao JJ, Farrar JT, Bruner D, et al. Electroacupuncture for fatigue, sleep, and psychological distress in breast cancer patients with aromatase inhibitor-related arthralgia: a randomized trial. Cancer 2014;120(23):3744–51.
30. Mao JJ, Xie SX, Farrar JT, et al. A randomised trial of electro-acupuncture for arthralgia related to aromatase inhibitor use. Eur J Cancer 2014;50(2):267–76.
31. Oh B, Kimble B, Costa DS, et al. Acupuncture for treatment of arthralgia secondary to aromatase inhibitor therapy in women with early breast cancer: pilot study. Acupunct Med 2013;31(3):264–71.
32. Mira TA, Giraldo PC, Yela DA, et al. Effectiveness of complementary pain treatment for women with deep endometriosis through Transcutaneous Electrical Nerve Stimulation (TENS): randomized controlled trial. Eur J Obstet Gynecol Reprod Biol 2015;194:1–6.
33. Schlaeger JM, Xu N, Mejta CL, et al. Acupuncture for the treatment of vulvodynia: a randomized wait-list controlled pilot study. J Sex Med 2015;12(4):1019–27.
34. Yang J, Chen G, Yu M, et al. Clinical study on radioproctitis and radiocystitis treated by acupuncture. Chinese Acupuncture & Moxibustion 1994;14(4):9–10.
35. Hui F, Boyle E, Vayda E, et al. A randomized controlled trial of a multifaceted integrated complementary-alternative therapy for chronic herpes zoster-related pain. Altern Med Rev 2012;17(1):57–68.
36. Deganello A, Battat N, Muratori E, et al. Acupuncture in shoulder pain and functional impairment after neck dissection: a prospective randomized pilot study. Laryngoscope 2016;126(8):1790–5.
37. Dunst J, Steil B, Furch S, et al. Herpes zoster in breast cancer patients after radiotherapy. Strahlenther Onkol 2000;176(11):513–6.
38. Pfister DG, Cassileth BR, Deng GE, et al. Acupuncture for pain and dysfunction after neck dissection: results of a randomized controlled trial. J Clin Oncol 2010;28(15):2565–70.

39. Wang FH, Chen CL, Chen MC, et al. Auricular electroacupuncture for postthoracotomy pain. Zhonghua Yi Xue Za Zhi (Taipei) 1988;41(5):349–56.
40. Trevelyan EG, Turner WA, Robinson N. Acupuncture for the treatment of phantom limb pain in lower limb amputees: study protocol for a randomized controlled feasibility trial. Trials 2015;16:158.
41. Molsberger AF, Schneider T, Gotthardt H, et al. German Randomized Acupuncture Trial for chronic shoulder pain (GRASP) - a pragmatic, controlled, patient-blinded, multi-centre trial in an outpatient care environment. Pain 2010;151(1): 146–54.
42. Rubi-Klein K, Kucera-Sliutz E, Nissel H, et al. Is acupuncture in addition to conventional medicine effective as pain treatment for endometriosis? A randomised controlled cross-over trial. Eur J Obstet Gynecol Reprod Biol 2010;153(1):90–3.
43. Sun Y, Gan TJ, Dubose J, et al. Acupuncture and related techniques for postoperative pain: a systematic review of randomized controlled trials. Br J Anaesth 2008;101(2):151–60.

Key Components of Pain Management for Children and Adults with Sickle Cell Disease

Amanda M. Brandow, DO, MS[a],*, Michael R. DeBaun, MD, MPH[b]

KEYWORDS

- Sickle cell disease • Acute pain • Chronic pain syndrome • Opioids • Depression
- Anxiety • Sleep

KEY POINTS

- The optimal management of acute pain episodes and chronic pain syndromes in sickle cell disease requires an understanding of the pharmacology principles of pain management.
- Pain management should be delivered using the biopsychosocial model, with interactions between biological, psychological, and social influences that contribute to pain addressed.
- Sickle cell disease pain management should target and keep individuals within the therapeutic window, maximizing analgesic effect and minimizing side effects.
- A complete sickle cell disease pain assessment should include screening for depression, anxiety, and sleep disturbances.

BACKGROUND OF INDIVIDUALS WITH SICKLE CELL DISEASE PAIN

Acute pain episodes are the most common complication of sickle cell disease (SCD), an inherited hemoglobinopathy affecting more than 3 million individuals worldwide.[1,2] Acute pain episodes are abrupt in onset, unpredictable, and account for the majority of health care use for SCD; however, these episodes are also frequently managed at home.[3] Acute pain episodes increase in frequency with age, and a chronic pain

Conflicts of Interest: The authors declare no competing financial interests.
Funding: National Institutes of Health, National Heart, Lung, and Blood Institute 1K23 HL114636-01A1 (A.M. Brandow).
[a] Department of Pediatrics, Section of Pediatric Hematology/Oncology, Medical College of Wisconsin, MFRC, 8701 Watertown Plank Road, Milwaukee, WI 53226, USA; [b] Department of Pediatrics, Vanderbilt University School of Medicine, Vanderbilt University Medical Center, 2200 Children's Way, Ste 11101, Nashville, TN 37232-9000, USA
* Corresponding author.
E-mail address: abrandow@mcw.edu

Hematol Oncol Clin N Am 32 (2018) 535–550
https://doi.org/10.1016/j.hoc.2018.01.014
0889-8588/18/© 2018 Elsevier Inc. All rights reserved.

hemonc.theclinics.com

syndrome evolves in 30% to 40% of adolescents and adults with SCD that significantly impairs functioning.[4,5]

Transition from Acute to Chronic Pain

The abrupt onset of acute pain episodes commonly occurs in the back, extremities, chest, and abdomen.[6] Temporally associated triggers for pain include, but are not limited to, acute infections, dehydration, asthma, cold temperatures, and the onset of menstruation; however, often no trigger is identified.[7–10] Acute pain episodes can start as early as in the first few months of life, increase in frequency with age, and can contribute to the development of a chronic pain syndrome.[3–5] The biologic basis for acute pain and the emergence of a chronic pain syndrome are likely different. Acute pain is caused by recurrent vasoocclusion from sickled erythrocytes with resultant ischemia–reperfusion injury, whereas chronic pain is likely driven by nervous system sensitization.[11] **Fig. 1** depicts the pain trajectory in individuals with SCD.

The diagnosis of a chronic pain syndrome in SCD is challenging, and includes many biologic, psychological, and sociologic risk factors. Traditionally, chronic pain is defined as pain persisting at least 3 to 6 months beyond the normal time for healing.[12] This definition often does not apply to individuals with SCD, because SCD pain develops over the lifetime. Evidence-based consensus diagnostic criteria, however, have been established for chronic pain syndrome in SCD.[13] A key component of these criteria includes: "Reports of ongoing pain on most days over the past 6 months either in a single location or multiple locations."[13]

Assessment of Individuals with Pain in Sickle Cell Disease

No objective measure can assess pain in children and adults with SCD. Thus, the cornerstone of pain management is trust between the affected individual in pain and the health care provider. Pain assessment must incorporate tools that account for the multidimensional aspects of pain. Classic pain assessments use unidimensional measures of pain intensity such as a numeric rating scale, the Wong-Baker Pain Scale, and the visual analog scale.[14,15] These scales are limited by the momentary assessment of pain and interindividual variability owing to differences in pain tolerance. Thus, the rating on a pain intensity scale should never be the sole determinant for the administration of analgesia.

Unfortunately, pain intensity scales do not assess the impact of pain on daily functioning, making them less useful for chronic pain. Instead, patient-reported outcome measures that capture multidimensional aspects of pain and the impact on functioning should be used. These tools include SCD-specific measures (PedsQL SCD Module, Adult Sickle Cell Quality of Life Measurement Information System)[16,17] and general measures (National Institutes of Health Patient-Reported Outcomes Measurement Information Systems).[18,19] Pain-specific tools with a 7- to 30-day recall period allow for assessment of pain over time and response to treatment.[16–19] Other multidimensional tools studied in SCD include, but are not limited to, the Youth Acute Pain Functional Ability Questionnaire,[20] Adolescent and Pediatric Pain Tool,[21] Brief Pain Inventory,[22] and McGill Pain Questionnaire.[23]

Assessment of SCD pain should elicit whether pain is acute, chronic, related to SCD, or all three. A clear discussion with the affected individual is required to distinguish between potential types of pain. Pain associated with "overuse syndrome," which is defined as pain from repetitive motions in daily activities, can be misunderstood and treated as acute SCD pain, chronic pain syndrome, or a prolonged acute pain episode. The temporal association of the new onset of pain

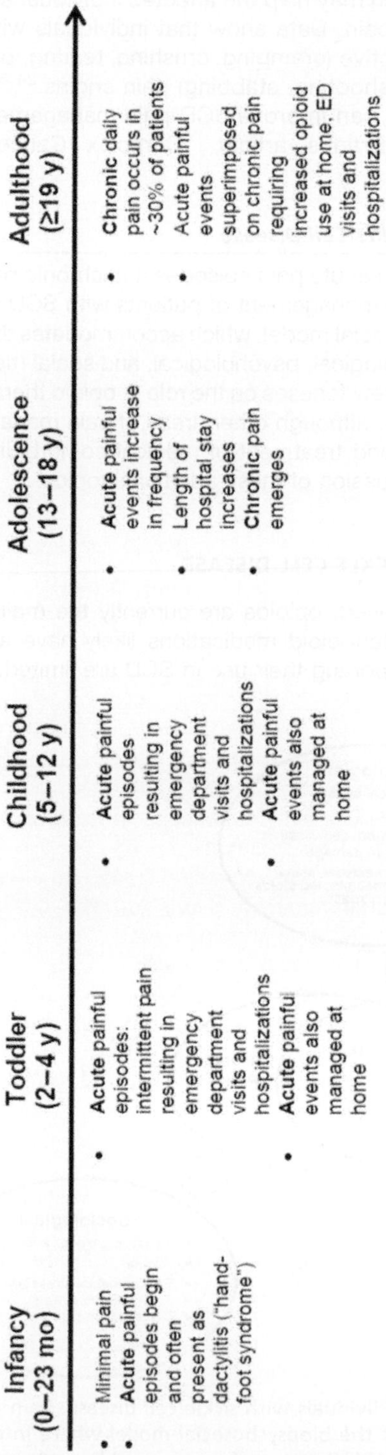

Infancy (0–23 mo)	Toddler (2–4 y)	Childhood (5–12 y)	Adolescence (13–18 y)	Adulthood (≥19 y)
• Minimal pain • **Acute painful episodes begin** and often present as dactylitis ("hand-foot syndrome")	• **Acute painful episodes:** intermittent pain resulting in emergency department visits and hospitalizations • **Acute painful events** also managed at home	• **Acute painful episodes** resulting in emergency department visits and hospitalizations • **Acute painful events** also managed at home	• **Acute painful events** increase in frequency • Length of hospital stay increases • **Chronic pain** emerges	• **Chronic daily pain** occurs in ~30% of patients • **Acute painful events** superimposed on chronic pain requiring increased opioid use at home. ED visits and hospitalizations • Increased prevalence of SCD co-morbidities (i.e., avascular necrosis, spinal compression fractures, leg ulcers, chronic kidney disease) that contribute to chronic pain syndrome

Fig. 1. Trajectory of pain experience from infancy to adulthood for individuals with sickle cell disease (SCD). ED, emergency department.

coupled with the location and type of pain may help the affected individual and provider to distinguish the etiology of the pain. Data show that individuals with SCD use descriptors suggesting both nociceptive (cramping, crushing, tearing, piercing, wrenching) and neuropathic (cold, hot, shooting, stabbing) pain origins.[24,25] Eliciting pain characteristics and descriptors can improve SCD pain management (see Regina M. Fink and Jeannine M. Brant's article, "Complex Cancer Pain Assessment," in this issue).

Treatment of Individuals with Pain in Sickle Cell Disease

Pain in SCD is complex and includes both acute pain episodes and chronic pain syndromes. We propose, therefore, that the management of patients with SCD pain be delivered in the context of the biopsychosocial model, which accommodates the complex interactions that exist among the biological, psychological, and social mediators of pain in SCD patients (**Fig. 2**).[26] This review focuses on the role of opioid therapy and treatment of psychological comorbidities; although other areas of pain management including nonpharmacologic strategies and treatment of medical comorbidities are important, space does not allow for discussion of these additional topics.

OPIOID THERAPY IN THE CONTEXT OF SICKLE CELL DISEASE

After nonpharmacologic strategies are used, opioids are currently the mainstay of treatment of patients with SCD pain. Nonopioid medications likely have a role in SCD pain treatment; however, data supporting their use in SCD are limited. Opioid

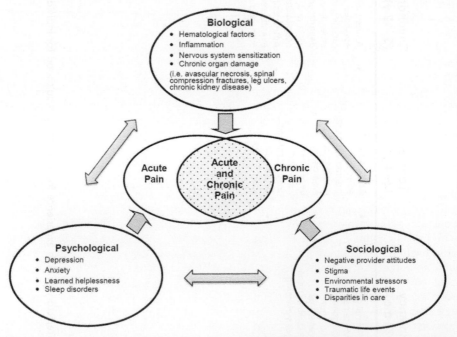

Fig. 2. Biopsychosocial model of pain in individuals with sickle cell disease. Pain management should be delivered in the context of the biopsychosocial model where interactions between biological, psychological, and social influences of pain are addressed.

use in SCD should be anchored by an understanding of the neurobiology of pain and pharmacology of analgesia.

Mechanism of Action and Metabolism of Opioids

Opioids bind to the mu opioid receptors and result in decreased afferent nociceptive input, thereby providing analgesia.[27] Knowledge of opioid metabolism is applicable to the use of codeine in SCD. Individuals with SCD have CYP2D6 polymorphisms associated with low enzyme activity. They do not convert codeine into morphine efficiently, and codeine therefore provides less analgesia in them than it would in patients with high CYP2D6 activity.[28,29] Thus, we do not recommend codeine for routine SCD pain treatment. The US Food and Drug Administration issued a contra-indication to using codeine in children 12 years and younger, and a warning in children 12 to 18 years who are obese, and have obstructive sleep apnea or lung disease.[30] These warnings are based on the risk of individuals being ultrafast co-deine metabolizers, which potentiates the rapid conversion to morphine.[30] **Table 1** outlines pharmacologic properties of selected opioids commonly used in SCD,[31,32] and should be consulted when selecting an opioid for this population. Morphine and hydromorphone are the most common first-line intravenous opioids used in SCD.[31,32]

Understanding the Therapeutic Window of Opioids Is a Fundamental Principle Required to Managing Pain in Sickle Cell Disease

The pharmacologic principle of placing and keeping an individual in the "therapeutic window" should drive the approach to optimal pain control in individuals with SCD. The therapeutic window is defined as a range of opioid doses that maximizes the analgesic effect and minimizes side effects[27,33] **(Fig. 3)**. The amount of opioid required to reach the therapeutic window varies based on renal and hepatic function, the pharmacokinetics and pharmacodynamics of the opioid, individuals' prior pain events and opioid needs, the severity of the pain, and the presence or absence of chronic opioid use.

Once a decision is made to admit an individual for pain management, the choice of opioid, route, frequency, and mode of delivery are integral to achieving adequate pain control. To administer an opioid so the desired effect for the drug level stays in the therapeutic window, there should be incremental titration of the opioid dose until effective analgesia is achieved or dose-limiting side effects occur. Once the therapeutic window is achieved, the optimal approach is to administer a continuous opioid infusion, delivered as part of a patient-controlled analgesia (PCA) regimen that allows for patient-initiated "demand" opioid boluses for anticipated breakthrough pain. Our approach is to give all older children and adults with SCD a continuous opioid infusion at the dose designed to provide relief without use of demand doses on the PCA. The PCA bolus dose is based on the pharmacology of the drug every 20 minutes and at one-sixth of the continuous dose. Thus, an individual with an acute pain episode can obtain relief using the PCA and can increase the dose of an hourly infusion by a maximum of 50% when compared with the continuous infusion. Using this outlined algorithm, we have had no significant untoward events over the last 2 decades. Additional keys to adequate pain management include good nursing care with monitoring for toxicities, having the individual patient be the only person to push the PCA button, and clear guidelines for increasing and decreasing the basal and PCA opioid dose, while keeping patients in their therapeutic windows.

Table 1
Commonly used opioids for the treatment of individuals with pain from sickle cell disease

Drug	Onset of Action Peak Effect	Half-Life	Dose[a]	Metabolism	Dose Adjustment
Intravenous					
Morphine	Onset: 5–10 min Peak effect: 20 min	1.5–4 h	Intermittent bolus dosing Adults and pediatrics: 0.1–0.2 mg/kg q2–4h; max dose 10 mg Basal infusion Patient weight <50 kg: Initial: 0.01 mg/kg/h; dosage range: 0.01–0.04 mg/kg/h Patient weight ≥50 kg: 1–2 mg/h	Liver	Adjust for liver and kidney disease
Hydromorphone	Onset: 5 min Peak effect: 10–20 min	2–3 h	Intermittent bolus dosing Adults: 0.2–1 mg q2–3h prn Pediatrics: <50 kg: 0.015 mg/kg q2–4h prn ≥50 kg: 0.2–0.6 mg q2–4h prn Basal infusion Adults: 0.5–3 mg/h Pediatrics: 0.002–0.005 mg/kg/h	Liver	Adjust for liver and kidney disease
Oral short acting					
Morphine immediate release	Onset: 30 min Peak effect: 1 h	Adults: 2–4 h Children: 1–3 h	Adults: 15 mg q2–4h prn Pediatrics: 0.2–0.5 mg/kg/dose q2–4h prn; initial maximum dose: 15–20 mg (patient weight ≥50 kg can use adult dosing)	Liver	Adjust for liver and kidney disease
Oxycodone	Onset: 10–15 min Peak effect: 0.5–1 h	2–3 h	Adults: 5–15 mg q2–4h prn Pediatrics: 0.1–0.2 mg/kg/dose q4h prn	Liver	Adjust for liver and kidney disease

Oral long acting

Morphine sustained release	Peak effect: 4 h	—	Adults: starting dose is 15 mg q12h Note: Total 24-h morphine requirements can be given in 2 divided doses—q12h or 3 divided doses-q8h Pediatrics: Weight-base dosing: 0.3–0.6 mg/kg/dose q12h Fixed dosing: • 20 to <35 kg: 10–15 mg q8-12h (10-mg tablets not available in the United States) • 35 to <50 kg: 15–30 mg q8-12h • ≥50 kg: 30–45 mg q8-12h	Liver	Adjust for liver and kidney disease
Oxycodone ER (Note: In United States only Oxycontin is available)	Onset: 40–60 min Peak effect: 3–4 h	4.5 h	Adults: starting dose is 10 mg q12h Pediatrics: Children ≥11 y and adolescents: only recommended for children >11 y and taking ≥20 mg of oxycodone or equivalent per day for 2 d before starting oxycodone ER. Starting dose is based on current opioid regimen/ dosing using the following equation: dose of oxycodone ER q12h = (mg/d of current opioid × opioid conversion factor)/2	Liver	Adjust for liver and kidney disease

Abbreviations: ER, extended release; prn, pro re nata (as needed).

a Starting dose. Titrate up to adequate pain relief.

Data from Lexicomp Online®, Clinical Drug Information. Hudson (OH): Lexi-Comp, Inc; 2017.

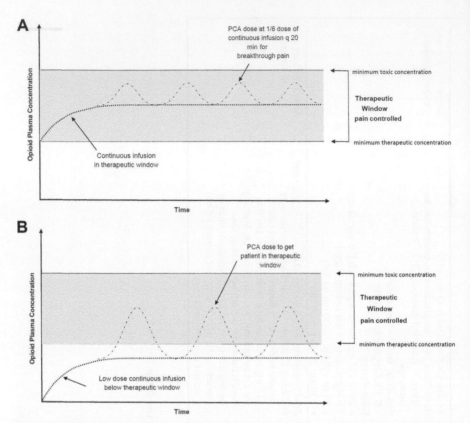

Fig. 3. Different approaches for opioid infusion for inpatient acute pain management in sickle cell disease. (*A*) Continuous opioid infusion with the goal of keeping the individual in the therapeutic window with the addition of breakthrough opioids administered via patient-controlled analgesia (PCA) at one-sixth the dose of the continuous infusion given every 20 minutes. Dose adjustment: If the individual self-administers the PCA dose 3 or more times in 2 consecutive hours, then consider increasing the continuous infusion dose. The new continuous dose should be the equivalence of prior hour's dose (continuous plus cumulative PCA bolus doses). The new PCA dose should be one-sixth of the current continuous dose, given every 20 minutes. (*B*) Low-dose continuous infusion without the goal of infusion being in the therapeutic window. PCA dose is given to put the individual in the therapeutic window. This strategy requires the individual to use the PCA throughout the day and night and to awaken at night to relieve pain. There is no strategy to distinguish breakthrough pain from a persistent increase in pain intensity.

Opioid delivery via PCA in SCD is associated with a decreased duration of hospital stay, decreased total opioid consumption, and greater satisfaction.[34] A randomized controlled trial, the IMPROVE trial (A Randomized Controlled Trial of Patient-Controlled Analgesia for Sickle Cell Painful Episodes), sought to compare 2 PCA dosing regimens (higher demand dose/low constant infusion vs lower demand dose/high constant infusion) on pain control in individuals with SCD. It was, however, terminated early owing to poor accrual.[35] Thus, a variety of PCA dosing approaches exist. One approach is to divide the total initial amount of opioid required to initially achieve adequate pain control by the number of hours over which the drug was administered. This dose becomes the starting inpatient hourly continuous infusion and the demand dose is one-sixth of the hourly basal infusion set with a 20-minute lockout. During the initial management of acute SCD pain, individuals should never be given opioids only as needed. The delay in achieving a therapeutic opioid blood level using only as-needed administration can cause individuals to fall out of the therapeutic window repeatedly and endure undue suffering. When possible, a PCA should be initiated in the acute care setting once a decision is made for admission to decrease the lag time for subsequent opioid doses during transition to the inpatient unit.[34,36] Routine assessment of pain control is required and PCA dose adjustments should be made as needed. Assessment should include pain intensity measures,[14,15] functional ability questionnaires,[20] and other patient-reported outcome measures.[31,37] If additional demand doses are required more than 3 times per hour for 2 hours, the total hourly basal dose should be increased. **Fig. 3** contrasts 2 approaches for opioid administration and how each approach impacts time spent within the therapeutic window.

Individuals with SCD can experience opioid tolerance, in which over time incrementally higher opioid doses are required to reach the therapeutic window. This is likely a result of life-long opioid exposure. There is technically no maximum opioid dose so long as there is careful monitoring for toxicity (ie, somnolence, hypoxia, bradypnea, opioid-induced hypersensitivity, nausea, vomiting, pruritus) and bidirectional communication among all health care providers occurs. The goal is to maintain steady pain control and avoid the peaks and valleys that remove individuals from the therapeutic window, thereby placing them below the minimum effective concentration (suboptimal pain control) or above the minimum toxic concentration (dose-limiting side effects; see **Fig. 3**).

Home-Based Pain Management for Sickle Cell Disease

The majority of SCD pain episodes are managed at home.[4,38] Thus, all individuals should have a personalized home pain management plan. Pain action plans should be established between individuals and providers as part of optimal SCD care.[39] These action plans provide individuals with the autonomy to self-manage their pain, helping them to recognize early phases of pain and optimally treat pain at home. Our action plan follows the World Health Organization's analgesic ladder for pain management.[40] When opioids are required, the same pharmacologic principles of placing and keeping the individual in their therapeutic window should guide home management. At the onset of pain, immediate-release opioids (onset of effect, 20–30 minutes) should be used. If age appropriate, a sustained-release opioid should also be initiated that mimics the continuous intravenous infusion. The combination of long-acting and short-acting opioids provides the optimal approach to keep the individual in the therapeutic window. Pain action plans facilitating home-based management are associated with decreased emergency department visits.[41] **Fig. 4** depicts 2 timelines for receipt of analgesia: a perceived standard approach and an empowered approach using a pain action plan.

PSYCHOSOCIAL ASPECTS OF PAIN IN SICKLE CELL DISEASE

Pain management for SCD should use an interdisciplinary team (potential members: hematologist, psychologist/psychiatrist, nurse, social worker, pain medicine specialist) to address comprehensively all the somatic and psychosocial aspects of the individual's pain. The effectiveness of this model in SCD and non-SCD pain conditions has been demonstrated previously.[42,43]

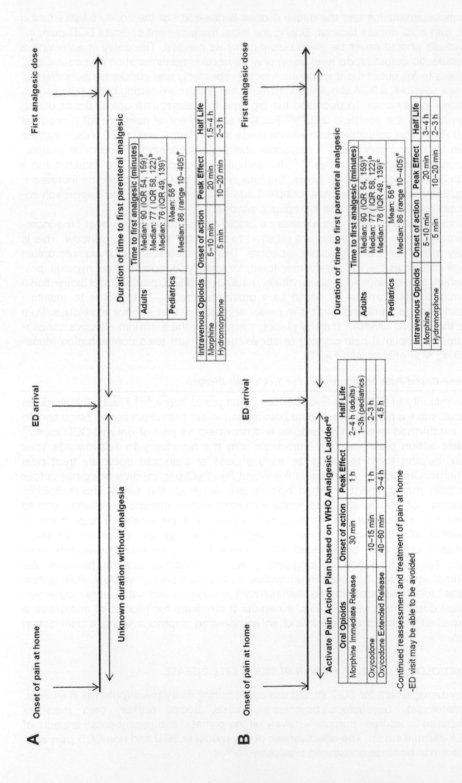

Association Between Psychological Comorbidities and Pain in Sickle Cell Disease

A systematic review showed an estimated prevalence of 26% for depression in individuals with SCD[44] and a higher prevalence when compared with the general African American population.[44] Individuals with SCD and depression experience more pain events.[45,46] In turn, increased SCD pain events are associated with more depression.[47] Adults with depression have a 2.8 times greater relative risk of increased health care use than individuals without depression.[44] The PiSCES study (Pain in Sickle Cell Epidemiology Study) screened 232 individuals for depression and anxiety.[45] Those with depression reported pain on 71% of days compared with 49% for those without depression,[45] and individuals with depression reported greater pain intensity and increased pain interference.[45] Anxiety is also associated with increased pain. Children with SCD and an anxiety disorder had higher admission rates for pain and longer duration of hospital stay.[48] Adults in the PiSCES study with anxiety reported higher mean pain intensity, pain-related distress, and more opioid usage.[45] These data underscore the reciprocal relationship between mental health conditions and SCD pain. The long-term effects of treating depression and anxiety on pain will further delineate this relationship.

Assessment of Psychological Comorbidities

A comprehensive SCD pain assessment should include depression and anxiety screening in the outpatient clinic, using valid self-reported screening tools to identify individuals at risk. Select tools are outlined in **Table 2**; many have been used in individuals with SCD.[44,45] Individuals who have positive screening on self-reported tools require referral to a psychologist/psychiatrist for further evaluation and treatment. In addition to baseline screening, individuals should be screened during episodes of increases in acute pain frequency and opioid needs.

Sleep Disturbance and Pain in Individuals with Sickle Cell Disease

Pain can cause sleep disruption, poor sleep quality, and difficulty with falling and staying asleep.[49,50] This can decrease pain thresholds and impair endogenous pain inhibitory and coping mechanisms, ultimately exacerbating pain.[51,52] A study evaluating sleep quality in 328 adults with SCD using the Pittsburgh Sleep Quality index found a 71% prevalence of sleep disturbances.[46] The individuals with sleep disturbances experienced more days of pain and more frequent acute pain episodes

---

Fig. 4. Potential timelines of pain treatment for an uncomplicated acute pain event. Two potential timelines for the receipt of analgesia are depicted: (*A*) perceived standard approach to acute pain management and (*B*) empowered approach to acute pain management. ED, emergency department; IQR, interquartile range; WHO, World Health Organization. [a] Tanabe P, Myers R, Zosel A, et al. Emergency department management of acute pain episodes in sickle cell disease. Acad Emerg Med 2007;14(5):419–25, [b] Tanabe P, Freiermuth CE, Cline DM, et al. A prospective emergency department quality improvement project to improve the treatment of vasoocclusive crisis in sickle cell disease: lessons learned. Jt Comm J Qual Patient Saf 2017;43(3):116–26, [c] Tanabe P, Hafner JW, Martinovich Z, et al. Adult emergency department patients with sickle cell pain crisis: results from a quality improvement learning collaborative model to improve analgesic management. Acad Emerg Med 2012;19(4):430–8, [d] Kavanagh PL, Sprinz PG, Wolfgang TL, et al. Improving the management of vasoocclusive episodes in the pediatric emergency department. Pediatrics 2015;136(4):e1016–25, [e] Mathias MD, McCavit TL. Timing of opioid administration as a quality indicator for pain crises in sickle cell disease. Pediatrics 2015;135(3):475–82.

Table 2
Select self-reported screening tools for depression and anxiety

Tool	Description
Depression	
BDI-II[57]	• 21 questions • Ages ≥13 y • Assessment of cognitive, affective and somatic symptoms of depression • Questions scored on 0–3 values and summed for total score • Cutoffs indicate minimal, mild, moderate or severe depression (higher scores, more severe depressive symptoms)
Patient Health Questionnaire[58]	• 9 questions • Score 9 of the DSM-IV criteria for depression from 0 (none) to 3 (nearly every day); depressed mood, sleep issues, anhedonia, poor energy, appetite changes, negative self-image, psychomotor retardation/agitation, poor concentration, self-harm • Score summed; higher scores indicate increased depressive symptoms
Center for Epidemiologic Studies-Depression Scale Revised[57]	• 20 questions • Measures frequency of symptoms in 9 groups: sadness, anhedonia, appetite, sleep, thinking/concentration, guilt, fatigue, agitation, suicidal ideation • Scores range from 0-60 with higher scores indicating more depressive symptoms; score ≥16 suggestive of moderate depressive symptoms
Children's Depression Inventory-2[59]	• Modeled after BDI • 24-item questionnaire • Self-reported scales in 5 areas (negative mood, interpersonal problems, ineffectiveness, anhedonia, negative self-esteem)
Center for Epidemiologic Studies Depression Scale for Children[60]	• Ages 6–17 y • 20 self-report items, scored on 0 (not at all) to 3 (a lot) scale • Scores range from 0-60 with higher scores indicating more depressive symptoms; score ≥15 suggestive of depressive symptoms
Anxiety	
Beck Anxiety Inventory[61]	• 21 questions • ≥17 y • Focused primarily on physical symptoms of anxiety (ie, diaphoresis, dizziness) • Scored 0 (not at all) to 3 (severely); higher scores indicate more anxiety (17–29 moderate, 30–63 severe)
State-Trait Anxiety Inventory[62]	• 40 self-report items (20 items for trait anxiety, 20 items for state anxiety) • 6th grade reading level • Items rated on 0 (almost never) to 4 (almost always) scale; higher scores suggest greater anxiety
State-Trait Anxiety Inventory for Children[62]	• 6–14 y • Similar to adult version • 40 self-report items (20 items for trait anxiety, 20 items for state anxiety)

Abbreviations: BDI, Beck Depression Inventory; DSM-IV, Diagnostic and Statistical Manual of Mental Disorders, 4th edition.

requiring health care use.[46] Another study prospectively assessed the impact of sleep on pain in 74 adults with SCD who completed sleep (duration, fragmentation, continuity) and pain diaries for 3 months.[53] Data supported the conclusion that nights with shorter sleep duration, increased fragmentation, and less efficient sleep were associated with greater pain severity on the following days.[53] Continued research in SCD is needed to determine whether interventions to improve sleep can decrease pain.[54,55] However, because the data strongly support this relationship in non-SCD pain-related disorders, a thorough sleep history should be obtained as a part of SCD pain management.[56]

SUMMARY

Acute and chronic pain is the most common complication and cause of health care use in SCD. The pain experience is complex and subjective. Assessment and management of SCD pain should occur in the context of the biopsychosocial model. In SCD, a genetically inherited disease, pain develops over the lifetime of the individual. Thus, this lifelong pain that starts within the first year of life requires comprehensive, interdisciplinary, and compassionate care.

ACKNOWLEDGMENTS

The authors thank Deva Sharma, MD, Djamila Labib Ghafuri, MD, and Melissa Day for their critical review of the article.

REFERENCES

1. Piel FB, Patil AP, Howes RE, et al. Global epidemiology of sickle haemoglobin in neonates: a contemporary geostatistical model-based map and population estimates. Lancet 2013;381(9861):142–51.
2. Brousseau DC, Panepinto JA, Nimmer M, et al. The number of people with sickle-cell disease in the United States: national and state estimates. Am J Hematol 2010;85(1):77–8.
3. Brousseau DC, Owens PL, Mosso AL, et al. Acute care utilization and rehospitalizations for sickle cell disease. JAMA 2010;303(13):1288–94.
4. Smith WR, Penberthy LT, Bovbjerg VE, et al. Daily assessment of pain in adults with sickle cell disease. Ann Intern Med 2008;148(2):94–101.
5. Sil S, Cohen LL, Dampier C. Psychosocial and functional outcomes in youth with chronic sickle cell pain. Clin J Pain 2016;32(6):527–33.
6. Ballas SK, Delengowski A. Pain measurement in hospitalized adults with sickle cell painful episodes. Ann Clin Lab Sci 1993;23(5):358–61.
7. Smith WR, Bauserman RL, Ballas SK, et al. Climatic and geographic temporal patterns of pain in the Multicenter Study of Hydroxyurea. Pain 2009;146(1–2):91–8.
8. Glassberg J, Spivey JF, Strunk R, et al. Painful episodes in children with sickle cell disease and asthma are temporally associated with respiratory symptoms. J Pediatr Hematol Oncol 2006;28(8):481–5.
9. Yoong WC, Tuck SM. Menstrual pattern in women with sickle cell anaemia and its association with sickling crises. J Obstet Gynaecol 2002;22(4):399–401.
10. Resar LM, Oski FA. Cold water exposure and vaso-occlusive crises in sickle cell anemia. J Pediatr 1991;118(3):407–9.
11. Woolf CJ, Salter MW. Neuronal plasticity: increasing the gain in pain. Science 2000;288(5472):1765–9.

12. Treede RD, Rief W, Barke A, et al. A classification of chronic pain for ICD-11. Pain 2015;156(6):1003–7.

13. Dampier C, Palermo TM, Darbari DS, et al. AAPT diagnostic criteria for chronic sickle cell disease pain. J Pain 2017;18(5):490–8.

14. Bieri D, Reeve RA, Champion GD, et al. The faces pain scale for the self-assessment of the severity of pain experienced by children: development, initial validation, and preliminary investigation for ratio scale properties. Pain 1990; 41(2):139–50.

15. Hawker GA, Mian S, Kendzerska T, et al. Measures of adult pain: Visual Analog Scale for Pain (VAS Pain), Numeric Rating Scale for Pain (NRS Pain), McGill Pain Questionnaire (MPQ), Short-Form McGill Pain Questionnaire (SF-MPQ), Chronic Pain Grade Scale (CPGS), Short Form-36 Bodily Pain Scale (SF-36 BPS), and Measure of Intermittent and Constant Osteoarthritis Pain (ICOAP). Arthritis Care Res (Hoboken) 2011;63(Suppl 11):S240–52.

16. Panepinto JA, Torres S, Bendo CB, et al. PedsQL sickle cell disease module: feasibility, reliability, and validity. Pediatr Blood Cancer 2013;60(8):1338–44.

17. Keller SD, Yang M, Treadwell MJ, et al. Patient reports of health outcome for adults living with sickle cell disease: development and testing of the ASCQ-Me item banks. Health Qual Life Outcomes 2014;12:125.

18. Dampier C, Jaeger B, Gross HE, et al. Responsiveness of PROMIS(R) Pediatric Measures to Hospitalizations for Sickle Pain and Subsequent Recovery. Pediatr Blood Cancer 2016;63(6):1038–45.

19. HealthMeasures: pain domains. Available at: http://www.healthmeasures.net/search-view-measures?task=Search.search. Accessed October 1, 2017.

20. Zempsky WT, O'Hara EA, Santanelli JP, et al. Development and validation of the Youth Acute Pain Functional Ability Questionnaire (YAPFAQ). J Pain 2014;15(12): 1319–27.

21. Franck LS, Treadwell M, Jacob E, et al. Assessment of sickle cell pain in children and young adults using the adolescent pediatric pain tool. J Pain Symptom Manage 2002;23(2):114–20.

22. Tan G, Jensen MP, Thornby JI, et al. Validation of the Brief Pain Inventory for chronic nonmalignant pain. J Pain 2004;5(2):133–7.

23. Melzack R. The McGill Pain Questionnaire: major properties and scoring methods. Pain 1975;1(3):277–99.

24. Walco GA, Dampier CD. Pain in children and adolescents with sickle cell disease: a descriptive study. J Pediatr Psychol 1990;15(5):643–58.

25. Wilkie DJ, Molokie R, Boyd-Seal D, et al. Patient-reported outcomes: descriptors of nociceptive and neuropathic pain and barriers to effective pain management in adult outpatients with sickle cell disease. J Natl Med Assoc 2010;102(1):18–27.

26. Taylor LE, Stotts NA, Humphreys J, et al. A biopsychosocial-spiritual model of chronic pain in adults with sickle cell disease. Pain Manag Nurs 2013;14(4): 287–301.

27. Pathan H, Williams J. Basic opioid pharmacology: an update. Br J Pain 2012;6(1): 11–6.

28. Brousseau DC, McCarver DG, Drendel AL, et al. The effect of CYP2D6 polymorphisms on the response to pain treatment for pediatric sickle cell pain crisis. J Pediatr 2007;150(6):623–6.

29. Shord SS, Cavallari LH, Gao W, et al. The pharmacokinetics of codeine and its metabolites in Blacks with sickle cell disease. Eur J Clin Pharmacol 2009;65(7): 651–8.

30. US Food and Drug Administration (FDA). FDA drug safety communication: FDA restricts use of prescription codeine pain and cough medicines and tramadol pain medicines in children; recommends against use in breastfeeding women. Available at: https://www.fda.gov/Drugs/DrugSafety/ucm549679.htm. Accessed October 12, 2017.
31. Brandow AM, Nimmer M, Simmons T, et al. Impact of emergency department care on outcomes of acute pain events in children with sickle cell disease. Am J Hematol 2016;91(12):1175–80.
32. Miller ST, Kim HY, Weiner D, et al. Inpatient management of sickle cell pain: a 'snapshot' of current practice. Am J Hematol 2012;87(3):333–6.
33. Upton RN, Semple TJ, Macintyre PE. Pharmacokinetic optimisation of opioid treatment in acute pain therapy. Clin Pharmacokinet 1997;33(3):225–44.
34. Melzer-Lange MD, Walsh-Kelly CM, Lea G, et al. Patient-controlled analgesia for sickle cell pain crisis in a pediatric emergency department. Pediatr Emerg Care 2004;20(1):2–4.
35. Dampier CD, Smith WR, Wager CG, et al. IMPROVE trial: a randomized controlled trial of patient-controlled analgesia for sickle cell painful episodes: rationale, design challenges, initial experience, and recommendations for future studies. Clin Trials 2013;10(2):319–31.
36. Santos J, Jones S, Wakefield D, et al. Patient controlled analgesia for adults with sickle cell disease awaiting admission from the emergency department. Pain Res Manag 2016;2016:3218186.
37. Brousseau DC, Scott JP, Badaki-Makun O, et al. A multicenter randomized controlled trial of intravenous magnesium for sickle cell pain crisis in children. Blood 2015;126(14):1651–7.
38. Dampier C, Ely E, Brodecki D, et al. Home management of pain in sickle cell disease: a daily diary study in children and adolescents. J Pediatr Hematol Oncol 2002;24(8):643–7.
39. Frei-Jones MJ, DeBaun MR. Personal pain action plans/for children and adolescents with sickle cell disease. In: D'Alonsa S, Grasso K, editors. Acute pain: causes, effects and treatment. Hauppauge (NY): Nova Science Publishers; 2009. p. 213–20.
40. World Health Organization (WHO). WHO's cancer pain ladder for adults. Available at: http://www.who.int/cancer/palliative/painladder/en/. Accessed November 12, 2017.
41. Crosby LE, Simmons K, Kaiser P, et al. Using quality improvement methods to implement an Electronic Medical Record (EMR) supported individualized home pain management plan for children with sickle cell disease. J Clin Outcomes Manag 2014;21(5):210–7.
42. Powell RE, Lovett PB, Crawford A, et al. A multidisciplinary approach to impact acute care utilization in sickle cell disease. Am J Med Qual 2017. 1062860617707262.
43. Brandow AM, Weisman SJ, Panepinto JA. The impact of a multidisciplinary pain management model on sickle cell disease pain hospitalizations. Pediatr Blood Cancer 2011;56(5):789–93.
44. Jonassaint CR, Jones VL, Leong S, et al. A systematic review of the association between depression and health care utilization in children and adults with sickle cell disease. Br J Haematol 2016;174(1):136–47.
45. Levenson JL, McClish DK, Dahman BA, et al. Depression and anxiety in adults with sickle cell disease: the PiSCES project. Psychosom Med 2008;70(2):192–6.
46. Wallen GR, Minniti CP, Krumlauf M, et al. Sleep disturbance, depression and pain in adults with sickle cell disease. BMC Psychiatry 2014;14:207.

47. Edwards CL, Scales MT, Loughlin C, et al. A brief review of the pathophysiology, associated pain, and psychosocial issues in sickle cell disease. Int J Behav Med 2005;12(3):171–9.
48. Myrvik MP, Campbell AD, Davis MM, et al. Impact of psychiatric diagnoses on hospital length of stay in children with sickle cell anemia. Pediatr Blood Cancer 2012;58(2):239–43.
49. Onen SH, Onen F, Courpron P, et al. How pain and analgesics disturb sleep. Clin J Pain 2005;21(5):422–31.
50. Shaver JL. Sleep disturbed by chronic pain in fibromyalgia, irritable bowel, and chronic pelvic pain syndromes. Sleep Med Clin 2008;3:47–60.
51. Onen SH, Alloui A, Gross A, et al. The effects of total sleep deprivation, selective sleep interruption and sleep recovery on pain tolerance thresholds in healthy subjects. J Sleep Res 2001;10(1):35–42.
52. Edwards RR, Grace E, Peterson S, et al. Sleep continuity and architecture: associations with pain-inhibitory processes in patients with temporomandibular joint disorder. Eur J Pain 2009;13(10):1043–7.
53. Moscou-Jackson G, Finan PH, Campbell CM, et al. The effect of sleep continuity on pain in adults with sickle cell disease. J Pain 2015;16(6):587–93.
54. Lerman SF, Finan PH, Smith MT, et al. Psychological interventions that target sleep reduce pain catastrophizing in knee osteoarthritis. Pain 2017;158(11):2189–95.
55. Smith MT, Haythornthwaite JA. How do sleep disturbance and chronic pain interrelate? Insights from the longitudinal and cognitive-behavioral clinical trials literature. Sleep Med Rev 2004;8(2):119–32.
56. Qaseem A, Kansagara D, Forciea MA, et al, Clinical Guidelines Committee of the American College of Physicians. Management of chronic insomnia disorder in adults: a clinical practice guideline from the American College of Physicians. Ann Intern Med 2016;165(2):125–33.
57. Smarr KL, Keefer AL. Measures of depression and depressive symptoms: Beck Depression Inventory-II (BDI-II), Center for Epidemiologic Studies Depression Scale (CES-D), Geriatric Depression Scale (GDS), Hospital Anxiety and Depression Scale (HADS), and Patient Health Questionnaire-9 (PHQ-9). Arthritis Care Res (Hoboken) 2011;63(Suppl 11):S454–66.
58. Kroenke K, Spitzer RL, Williams JB. The PHQ-9: validity of a brief depression severity measure. J Gen Intern Med 2001;16(9):606–13.
59. Saylor CF, Finch AJ Jr, Spirito A, et al. The children's depression inventory: a systematic evaluation of psychometric properties. J Consult Clin Psychol 1984;52(6):955–67.
60. Faulstich ME, Carey MP, Ruggiero L, et al. Assessment of depression in childhood and adolescence: an evaluation of the Center for Epidemiological Studies Depression Scale for Children (CES-DC). Am J Psychiatry 1986;143(8):1024–7.
61. Leyfer OT, Ruberg JL, Woodruff-Borden J. Examination of the utility of the Beck Anxiety Inventory and its factors as a screener for anxiety disorders. J Anxiety Disord 2006;20(4):444–58.
62. Spielberger CD, Gorsuch RL, Lushene R, et al. Manual for the state-trait anxiety inventory. Palo Alto (CA): Consulting Psychologists Press; 1983.

Pain Syndromes and Management in Adult Hematopoietic Stem Cell Transplantation

Joseph D. Ma, PharmD[a],*, Areej R. El-Jawahri, MD[b],
Thomas W. LeBlanc, MD, MA, MHS[c], Eric J. Roeland, MD[d]

KEYWORDS

- Pain • Hematopoietic stem cell transplant • Opioids • Neuropathy

KEY POINTS

- Pain is a significant physical symptom in hematopoietic stem cell transplant (HSCT) patients that can be present across the HSCT spectrum of care.
- Common pain syndromes in HSCT patients include oral mucositis, bone pain, and chemotherapy-induced peripheral neuropathy.
- Unique considerations in HSCT patients require that pain management approaches be individualized.
- Utilization of early palliative care for pain and symptom management is recommended for HSCT patients.

INTRODUCTION

Hematopoietic stem cell transplant (HSCT) is a high-risk procedure focused on the possibility of cure in patients with otherwise incurable benign or malignant disorders. The indications for HSCT, as well as eligibility, vary, often due to patient factors, such as age, performance status, response to prior therapy, and disease status. Disease-specific prognostic factors, such as availability of a suitable graft source and time

Disclosures: J.D. Ma, A.R. El-Jawahri, and E.J. Roeland declare no relevant disclosures. T.W. LeBlanc has received honoraria from Celgene, Pfizer, Helsinn Therapeutics, Medtronic, and Otsuka as well as research funding from Seattle Genetics.
[a] Division of Clinical Pharmacy, UC San Diego Skaggs School of Pharmacy and Pharmaceutical Sciences, 9500 Gilman Drive, MC 0714, La Jolla, CA 92093-0714, USA; [b] Division of Hematology/Oncology, Bone Marrow Transplant, Massachusetts General Hospital, 55 Fruit Street, Boston, MA 02114, USA; [c] Division of Hematologic Malignancies and Cellular Therapy, Duke University School of Medicine, 2424 Erwin Road, Suite 602, Durham, NC 27705, USA; [d] Department of Medicine, UC San Diego Moores Cancer Center, 3855 Health Sciences Drive, MC 0987, La Jolla, CA 92130, USA
* Corresponding author.
E-mail address: jdma@ucsd.edu

Hematol Oncol Clin N Am 32 (2018) 551–567
https://doi.org/10.1016/j.hoc.2018.01.012
0889-8588/18/© 2018 Elsevier Inc. All rights reserved.

to transplant are additional factors for consideration. Autologous HSCT is indicated to treat conditions, including, but not limited to, multiple myeloma, germ cell tumors, and some autoimmune disorders (eg, systemic lupus erythematosus).[1] Allogeneic HSCT is used for patients with acute lymphoblastic leukemia, chronic myeloid leukemia, chronic lymphocytic leukemia, myeloproliferative disorders, myelodysplastic syndromes, and other related diseases.[1] Those with non-Hodgkin lymphoma, Hodgkin disease, and acute myeloid leukemia might receive either an autologous or allogeneic HSCT.[1] According to the Worldwide Network for Blood and Marrow Transplantation, there has been a steady increase from 2006 to 2012 in the number of allogeneic and autologous transplants performed annually.[2] Data from 2012 from 77 countries reported 68,146 HSCTs, with 36,220 autologous and 31,926 allogeneic transplants performed.[2]

Despite the advances made in HSCT and improvements in overall survival, many patients experience physical symptoms and emotional distress that result in significant morbidity and decreased quality of life. In autologous HSCT patients, the incidence of physical symptoms of fatigue, pain, and insomnia can range from 8% to 55%.[3] In allogeneic HSCT patients, 1 study reported an incidence of fatigue, pain, and insomnia ranging from 60% to 80%.[4] Emotional distress is present in approximately 15% to 50% of HSCT patients and peaks prior to and immediately after transplant.[5,6] In a pilot study of 61 patients who received HSCT, one-third of patients reported pain, impaired daily functioning associated with pain, and emotional distress.[7] Although anxiety and depression were associated with functional impairment due to pain (r = 0.33–0.44, $P<.05$), no such associations were observed with pain intensity (r = 0.21–0.27; $P>.05$).[7]

This review summarizes specific pain syndromes and management approaches in adult HSCT patients. General pain assessment in hematology and oncology patients is reviewed in Regina M. Fink and Jeannine M. Brant's article, "Complex Cancer Pain Assessment," in this issue. The HSCT-related pain syndromes that are discussed in this article include procedural pain, growth factor–induced bone pain, oral mucositis, chemotherapy-induced peripheral neuropathy (CIPN), and postherpetic neuralgia. Clinical approaches to the management of pain syndromes are discussed, highlighting relevant issues in adult HSCT patients. Pain management in the pediatric HSCT population is described elsewhere.[8–10]

UNIQUE CONSIDERATIONS IN HEMATOPOIETIC STEM CELL TRANSPLANT PATIENTS

In HSCT patients, the oral route may be limited due to oral mucositis and/or delirium. Commonly used neuropathic pain medications, such as pregabalin, gabapentin, and antidepressants, are exclusively formulated for oral administration. Furthermore, the rectal route of administration is frequently avoided due to concerns about bacterial translocation with rectal manipulation in the setting of neutropenia. Additionally, intestinal GVHD with severe diarrhea may limit drug absorption. Nonopioid adjuvant medications, such as nonsteroidal anti-inflammatory drugs (NSAIDs), may be contraindicated for HSCT patients, due to thrombocytopenia and renal compromise. Drug-drug interactions must be also be assessed, especially when considering methadone for patients receiving concomitant immunomodulatory or anti-infective agents (**Table 1**).

PERITRANSPLANTATION PAIN SYNDROMES
Pain from Bone Marrow Biopsy and Aspiration

Bone marrow biopsy is a required procedure for diagnosis and staging of most hematologic malignancies. Patients typically lay prone or in the lateral decubitus position,

Table 1
Drug-drug interactions between methadone and common therapies used for hematopoietic stem cell transplantation

Drug	Mechanism of Drug-Drug Interaction	Effect of the Interaction	Additional Considerations
Corticosteroids			
Dexamethasone Methylprednisolone	CYP3A substrate overlap between corticosteroids and methadone	Increased methadone plasma concentrations Increased corticosteroid plasma concentrations	Monitor for methadone and corticosteroid side effects if given concurrently
Immunosuppressants			
Tacrolimus Sirolimus Cyclosporine	CYP3A substrate overlap between immunosuppressants and methadone	Increased methadone plasma concentrations Increased immunosuppressant plasma concentrations	Increase monitoring for immunosuppressant side effects Consider therapeutic drug monitoring for immunosuppressants Monitor for methadone side effects
Antifungals			
Fluconazole Posaconazole Voriconazole	CYP3A inhibition by antifungals	Increased methadone plasma concentrations Increased risk for QTc prolongation	Monitor for methadone side effects Perform ECG monitoring Consider alternative opioid, such as morphine Consider alternative therapy, such as micafungin
Anti–Pneumocystis jirovecci			
TMP-SMX Dapsone Pentamadine	CYP3A substrate overlap between dapsone and methadone Minor substrate overlap with other CYPs between pentamadine and methadone	Increased methadone plasma concentrations with TMP-SMX Increased risk for QTc prolongation with TMP-SMX and methadone Increased methadone plasma concentrations with dapsone Increased risk for QTc prolongation with pentamadine and methadone	Perform ECG monitoring Consider alternative therapy, such as atovaquone Consider alternative opioid, such as morphine

Abbreviations: CYP, cytochrome P450; TMP-SMX, trimethoprim-sulfamethoxazole.

and a biopsy of the bone is taken from the posterior-superior iliac crest along with a bone marrow aspirate. Efforts are made to ensure that this procedure is well tolerated, including the use of lidocaine to anesthetize the skin. Many patients struggle, however, with the pain associated with this procedure. The pain associated with the aspirate itself is the most difficult to palliate; this is hypothesized to be due to changes in pressure within the bone architecture on applying suction from the syringe needed to aspirate the marrow cavity. In a study of more than 100 hematologic malignancy patients, more than 65% reported procedural pain, with approximately one-third describing this pain as severe.[11] In this same study, premedication with an oral opioid improved pain scores during marrow aspiration and reduced the number of patients with moderate pain. In contrast to the frequency of bone marrow biopsies, bone marrow harvests are now a less common event, because most hematopoietic stem cells are collected from peripheral blood. For those patients who do undergo a blood cell mobilization, moderate to severe bone pain can be as high as 85%. The median duration of pain was longer for bone marrow donors (14 vs 3 days, $P<.0001$).[12] Multiple aspirations from the anterior and posterior iliac crests are needed to obtain sufficient hematopoietic stem cells from the bone marrow. Iliac crest pain at the donor site is seen in approximately 34% of cases.[13] Severe and prolonged pain is greater in the anterior iliac crest compared with the posterior iliac crest after a marrow harvest.[14] Pain is usually minor in intensity, nociceptive in quality, transient, and localized to the aspiration site (**Table 2**). If pharmacologic interventions are needed, oral acetaminophen is appropriate and often sufficient.

Granulocyte Colony-Stimulating Factor–Associated Bone Pain

Bone pain has been associated with granulocyte colony-stimulating factor (G-CSF) administration during stem cell mobilization.[15] In a meta-analysis, any grade bone pain was reported in 33% to 50% of patients, and severe bone pain (grade 3–4) was less frequently reported, at 3% to 7%.[16] Although a majority of HSCT stem cells are collected from the peripheral blood, stem cell mobilization is another method to collect stem cells. Stem cells are stimulated out of the bone marrow space into the bloodstream so they are available for collection for future reinfusion. The cells are then preserved, frozen, and stored until the time of transplant. G-CSF is used to mobilize hematopoietic stem cells for transplantation. The use of these drugs can cause a deep bone pain, especially in healthy donors and young patients, with the incidence of G-CSF–associated bone pain ranging from 20% to 71%.[17–19] In a retrospective data analysis of 22 clinical trials using pegfilgrastim in patients receiving myelosuppressive chemotherapy (n = 1949), moderate to severe bone pain was seen in 28% of cases.[20]

The mechanism of G-CSF–associated bone pain is unknown. Some investigators hypothesize that it stems from bone marrow expansion due to progenitor and myeloid cell proliferation, resulting in recruitment of monocytes and macrophages. In turn, these cells release proinflammatory cytokines (eg, tumor necrosis factor α and interleukins), resulting in peripheral nerve remodeling and bone pain.[21] Other theorized mechanisms of G-CSF–associated bone pain include histamine production within the bone marrow (causing edema), osteoclast and osteoblast stimulation (resulting in increased bone resorption), and afferent nerve stimulation (sensitizing peripheral nociceptors).[22,23]

The most common regions of G-CSF–induced bone pain are the back, sternum, hips, and legs[12] (see **Table 2**), which can present as nociceptive pain described as deep and achy. Evidence for the treatment of G-CSF–associated bone pain is poor and sparse. The largest study to date evaluated the use of the antihistamine loratadine

Table 2
Pain syndromes in hematopoietic stem cell transplantation

Pain Syndrome	Pain Presentation	Suggested Treatment(s)
Peritransplantation		
Pain from bone marrow aspiration	Quality: superficial or deep somatic nociceptive pain, dullness, achiness, or stabbing Region: localized to aspiration site; iliac crest Radiating: no Timing: temporary	Acetaminophen as needed
Bone pain associated from G-CSF	Quality: deep somatic nociceptive pain, dullness, achiness Inflammatory pain, stiffness, soreness Region: back, hips, legs Radiating: no Timing: intermittent or constant	Unknown Avoid NSAIDs Avoid loratadine
Oral mucositis due to conditioning regimens	Quality: acute nociceptive pain, soreness, burning, dullness, achiness Region: mucosal lining of mouth Radiating: no Timing: constant	Intravenous opioids
Post-transplantation		
Abdominal pain from GVHD	Quality: nociceptive pain, crampiness, tightness Region: abdomen Radiating: no Timing: intermittent or constant	Anticholinergics
CIPN	Quality: neuropathic pain, numbness, tingling, shooting Region: stocking-glove pattern in hands and feet Radiating: yes Timing: constant	Duloxetine 60–120 mg/d, tricyclic antidepressants, gabapentin/pregabalin, methadone
Postherpetic neuralgia	Quality: neuropathic pain, burning, sharpness, stabbing Region: previous areas where shingles infection occurred Radiating: yes Timing: constant	Gabapentin 1600–3600 mg/d, pregabalin, tricyclic antidepressants, duloxetine, methadone

in patients receiving G-CSF after taxane-based chemotherapy. Pegfilgrastim-induced bone pain occurred in 30% of cancer patients.[24] There was no measurable difference in patient-reported bone pain in the loratadine-treated arm. Administration of prophylactic loratadine also did not decrease the incidence of G-CSF–induced bone pain.[24] An additional single-center retrospective cohort study evaluating dual histamine therapy with loratadine and famotidine reported a lack of efficacy in the palliation of bone pain.[25] Prevention strategies are limited to the non-HSCT setting, with the best data supporting the use of NSAIDs. In a randomized, placebo-controlled study in patients with nonmyeloid cancer, naproxen, 500 mg twice a day for 5 days to 8 days, after pegfilgrastim administration was effective in reducing the severity and incidence of bone pain.[26] Although naproxen seems effective for prevention, the risk of NSAID-induced platelet dysfunction and nephrotoxicity may limit NSAID use for HSCT patients.

Consequently, pain management approaches are challenging in this situation. There is a suggestion that opioids or G-CSF dose reduction are an alternative, but caution is warranted given a lack of evidence.[27,28]

Oral Mucositis

Conditioning regimens are used to eradicate malignant cells, and, for an allogeneic HSCT, the conditioning regimen also suppresses the recipient's immune system, to better prepare the recipient's immune systems to accept a foreign one, thereby reducing graft rejection. One consequence of the conditioning regimen is the development of painful oral mucositis. The incidence and severity of mucositis vary based on the conditioning regimen. In acute myeloid leukemia, patients who receive high-dose idarubicin and busulfan (n = 40) have an incidence of mucositis of 98%, with 82% experiencing severe mucositis.[29] In non-Hodgkin lymphoma or Hodgkin disease, mucositis occurred in 75% of patients receiving carmustine, etoposide, cytarabine, and melphalan (BEAM) for a conditioning regimen.[30] In patients with central nervous system (CNS) involvement by non-Hodgkin lymphoma, severe mucositis was 73% for conditioning with thiotepa, busulfan, and cyclophosphamide.[31] A lower incidence of mucositis (5%–23%) has been reported with melphalan, 100 mg/m^2 and 200 mg/m^2, for multiple myeloma patients.[32,33] High-dose myeloablative conditioning regimens plus total-body irradiation have reported mucositis incidence rates of greater than 50%.[34] The development of mucositis encompasses 5 stages: initiation, the primary damage response via cellular messaging and signaling, amplification, ulceration, and healing.[35,36]

In HSCT patients, severe mucositis pain can present as an acute, nociceptive pain that is sore, burning, dull, and achy (see **Table 2**).[37] According to the World Health Organization handbook, mucositis can range from grade 0 (none or normal) through 4 (life threatening).[38] Mucositis onset in autologous HSCTs is approximately 2 to 10 days, whereas for allogeneic HSCTs it is approximately 4 days to 16 days.[39] Epithelial sloughing, mucosal inflammation, and ulceration are believed to be the mechanisms associated with mucositis pain.[40] Mucosal erythema occurs 4 days to 5 days after conditioning, with the accompanying painful ulcerations occurring a few days later. This generally lasts approximately 1 week and resolves several weeks after conditioning. In contrast, radiation-induced mucositis begins at a cumulative dose of approximately 10 Gy and is characterized by painful oral ulcerations occurring at a cumulative dose of 30 Gy. Symptoms improve at least 2 weeks after radiation completion.[35]

Given the severity of the pain, intravenous opioids are used to treat acute mucositis pain, with morphine commonly used in HSCT patients.[29,41,42] The rationale for intravenous opioids is both the challenge of oral opioid administration and the favorable intravenous pharmacokinetic profile. Intravenous opioids have an onset of action at 5 minutes to 10 minutes and a greater peak effect compared with oral opioids.[43] Doses can be rapidly titrated and repeated with subsequent dose adjustments over a short period of time.

Patient-controlled analgesia is one method for intravenous opioid administration. Patient-controlled analgesia regimens must specify a demand or breakthrough dose (ie, a dose given on demand when patient requests), a lockout period, a maximum hour limit, and, when applicable, a continuous or basal infusion rate. Patient-controlled analgesia demand doses vary based on individual opioid tolerance, drug-drug interactions, and kidney function. For an opioid-naïve patient, some investigators have suggested a morphine demand dose of 1 mg to 2 mg with a lockout interval of 10 minutes.[44] In contrast, for opioid-tolerant patients, the demand dose should be approximately 50% of the continuous infusion rate with a lockout interval of 8 minutes to 10 minutes.[45] A scenario, coined *chasing the pain*, may occur if a lockout interval exceeds 10 minutes, whereby repeated demand doses do not achieve sustainable morphine plasma concentrations needed to provide pain relief. These are suggested starting demand doses for morphine patient-controlled analgesia and may not be applicable in all patients. Initial intravenous bolus opioid doses are another option to help determine an appropriate demand dose.

During this dose-finding period, frequent pain assessment is performed after each bolus dose, with a doubling of the dose if the pain remains severe and continual dose increases of 50% to 100%, as appropriate, until pain has improved.[46] Not all patients need a continuous infusion in addition to the bolus dosing, but for those who do, base the continuous infusion rate for a morphine patient-controlled analgesia on the most recent opioid consumption pattern (eg, mg of opioid/d). If a patient has been taking around-the-clock oral opioids, convert the patient's current 24-hour oral opioid dose into an approximate intravenous equianalgesic dose per hour.[43] End-organ damage and any potential drug-drug interactions should always be considered when starting an intravenous opioid.

Professional organizations recommend bland rinses (eg, 0.9% saline, sodium bicarbonate) and topical anesthetics for management of minor to moderate mucositis pain.[42,47] For treatment of minor (grade 1) mucositis pain, topical anesthetics (eg, magic mouthwash) are preferred. When using a topical anesthetic-based rinse, these drugs typically have a low acid dissociation constant and may cause burning in open sores in the mouth.[48] Patients should be educated that these drugs may burn before numbing the areas of pain and be instructed that there is a maximum dose of anesthetic-based rinses due to concerns of cardiac arrhythmias and methemoglobinemia.[49] For moderate (grade 2) pain, some investigators have suggested topical morphine or topical ketamine.[50,51] Regarding preventative oral mucositis strategies, the effectiveness of therapies and detailed reviews of current modalities and those under investigation are published elsewhere.[52–54]

POST-TRANSPLANT PAIN SYNDROMES
Graft-Versus-Host Disease

Despite improvements in transplant medicine, graft-versus-host disease (GVHD) remains a common complication of allogeneic HSCT. Donor T lymphocytes recognize the host antigens as foreign, thus inducing an immune response against the immunocompromised host. Acute GVHD is mediated by donor T cells that are coinfused with the stem cell graft and likely involves intricate interactions between cellular and cytokine components of the immune system. The main risk factor for acquiring GVHD is the amount of HLA disparity between the host and donor HLA complex (matched unrelated donors and haploidentical matches). Other risk factors for developing GVHD include increased age, prior pregnancy, prior transfusions, gender mismatch (female to male), and intensity of the conditioning regimen (ablative vs nonmyeloablative).

GVHD has been traditionally defined by the time of onset but is now defined by clinical and pathologic features. The 2 main categories of GVHD are acute and chronic. Acute GVHD appears from time of engraftment to a range in time from as early as 10 days to 100 days post-HSCT. Chronic GVHD has traditionally been assigned to occurring after 100 days post-HSCT. Some patients, however, may present with acute symptoms at a late onset (termed, *late-onset acute GVHD*). Alternatively, some HSCT recipients may present earlier with chronic type features. Therefore, these 2 diseases are best classified by clinical presentation versus time of onset.[55] When considering pharmacologic approaches to the palliation of pain in this setting, key considerations to assess are available route(s) of administration, potential for drug-drug interactions, and absorption properties of the drug. For example, intestinal GVHD is characterized by diarrhea measured in volumes of liters per day that can have a significant impact the absorption of drugs.

Acute GVHD is associated with 15% to 40% mortality and is the major cause of morbidity postallogeneic HSCT. The timing of the onset of acute GVHD is also an important prognostic factor, where early onset (prior to day 14) is associated with worse prognosis. To effectively treat GVHD, a timely and accurate diagnosis must be made. An acute GVHD diagnosis is based on clinical presentation and a tissue diagnosis (**Table 3**). The management and outcome of acute GVHD are based on the staging and overall grading of the various organs involved, because GVHD can affect organs in isolation or in combination with other organs.

Pain can occur with acute and chronic GVHD. A detailed review of chronic GVHD complications is discussed elsewhere.[56] Pain associated with acute GVHD depends on the organ involved. Given that the mechanism of toxicity is mediated by an immune response, most treatment strategies use corticosteroids and immunosuppressants. When symptoms do not respond to corticosteroids, additional immunosuppressant

Table 3
Acute graft-versus-host disease

Organ	Symptoms	Histologic Grading	Organ Staging
Acute GVHD[55]			
Skin	Maculopapular or diffuse erythematous rash. May progress to desquamation	Grade1: epidermal basal cell vacuolization Grade 2: epidermal basal cell death or apoptosis with lymphoid infiltration and satellitosis Grade 3: bulla formation Grade 4: ulceration/separation of epidermal/dermal junction	0: no rash 1: <25% BSA 2: >25%–50% BSA 3: generalized erythroderma, vesicular eruption, or desquamation >50% 4: generalized exfoliative dermatitis, ulcerative dermatitis, or bulla
Liver	Elevated serum bilirubin, ± transaminases, prolonged PT/PTT	Cholestatic changes predominate with bile duct atypia and degeneration	0: total bilirubin <2× upper limit of normal 1: 2×–3× upper limit of normal 2: 3.1×–6× upper limit of normal 3: 6.1×–15× upper limit of normal 4: >15× upper limit of normal
Intestinal tract	Diarrhea, abdominal pain, nausea/vomiting, abdominal pain, ileus	Crypt cell necrosis; crypt dropout with diffuse loss of epithelium	0: ≤500 mL/d of diarrhea 1: 500–1000 mL/d 2: 1000–1500 mL/d 3: >1500 mL/d 4: severe abdominal pain with or without ileus, or stool with frank blood or melena

Abbreviations: BSA, body surface area; PT, prothrombin time; PTT, partial thromboplastin time.

agents are used (eg, mycophenolate mofetil, basiliximab, pentostatin, etanercept, and infliximab). Extracorporeal photophoresis is also an option, whereby this process down-regulates activated T-cells with the goal to treat and/or control GVHD in patients who are not responding to corticosteroids. This technique is contraindicated in patients with severe cardiovascular or renal impairment. If it is believed that if a patient's GVHD is resistant to corticosteroids, then they should be tapered off as tolerated.

Skin GVHD is often the initial organ to manifest GVHD and can be painful.[57] Acute cutaneous GVHD is characterized by a maculopapular rash that involves the palms and soles and, as the disease progresses, the upper trunk, neck, cheeks, and ears. A differential diagnosis of drug reaction and/or viral infection should be considered and skin biopsies are frequently used to confirm the diagnosis of acute GVHD.[58] Systemic therapy with corticosteroids is typically required for the management of acute GVHD along with the addition of high-potency topical corticosteroids. Once initiated, the duration of treatment is usually for a minimum of 6 weeks, depending on the grade and extent of skin involvement. Additionally, immunosuppressants, such as cyclosporine, are used for 3 months to 4 months (related donor) or 6 months (unrelated donor) after HSCT. Patients should perform skin care, including regular use of emollients on intact skin. If present, pruritus is best managed with topical and systemic antihistamines. Second-generation antihistamines are preferred to diphenhydramine to minimize sedation and anticholinergic side effects.[59]

The liver and gastrointestinal system are also involved in acute GVHD. Generally, liver GVHD does not cause an acute pain but can be accompanied by intense pruritus associated with hyperbilirubinemia. For the pruritus, consider agents, such as cholestyramine or ursodiol, in addition to second-generation antihistamines. Intestinal GVHD can cause severe, crampy abdominal pain in the setting of diarrhea. In addition to systemic corticosteroids, budesonide, 3 mg 3 times daily, can be used; however, the data on this approach are limited and prospective randomized trials lacking.[60] Intravenous opioids may have some benefit in select patients but do not palliate the underlying etiology of the pain (smooth muscle contraction). Anticholinergic antispasmodic drugs (**Table 4**) like dicyclomine may be needed as an adjuvant for the crampy abdominal pain that is frequent in patients with intestinal GVHD. Glycopyrrolate, the only quaternary anticholinergic, has reduced penetration across the blood-brain

Table 4
Commonly used anticholinergic antispasmodic drugs

Drug	Dosage	Adverse Effects
Atropine	0.4–0.6 mg SC, IM, IV every 3–4 h routinely or as needed	Anticholinergic side effects CNS and cardiac excitation Photophobia Palpitations, tachycardia Constipation Difficulty urinating
Belladonna and opium	1 suppository (16.2 mg belladonna and 30/60 mg opium) every 6 h as needed	Anticholinergic side effects Photophobia Constipation Difficulty urinating Somnolence
Dicyclomine	10–20 mg po three to four times daily	Anticholinergic side effects
Glycopyrrolate	0.1–0.4 mg IM, IV every 4–6 h as needed	Anticholinergic side effects

Abbreviations: IM, interamuscular; IV, intravenous; SC, subcutaneous.

barrier and a decreased incidence of unwanted centrally mediated side effects, like delirium. A list of anticholinergic antispasmodic drugs for crampy abdominal pain are included in **Table 4**. Given the incidence of ileus in the setting of intestinal GVHD, opioids and anticholinergics must be used with caution and with close monitoring.

Chemotherapy-Induced Peripheral Neuropathy

Peripheral neuropathy is an adverse effect from several cytotoxic chemotherapeutic, targeted, and immunomodulatory agents. The incidence of CIPN is particularly notable in multiple myeloma patients receiving proteasome inhibitors and immunomodulators (**Table 5**). In patients who receive bortezomib, CIPN was observed in 35% of patients with relapsed and refractory multiple myeloma.[61–63] Grades 1 and 2 peripheral neuropathy were most prevalent (eg, $\geq$20% of patients), whereas grades 3 and 4 occurred at rates of 13% and 0.4%, respectively.[63] Higher incidences of 15% and 7% of grades 3 and 4 peripheral neuropathy respectively, have been reported in a retrospective analysis of relapsed and refractory multiple myeloma patients, presumably related to more prolonged or repeated exposure to neuropathy-inducing therapies.[64]

The predominant theory of bortezomib-induced peripheral neuropathy is that bortezomib contributes to neurofilament and juxtanuclear cytoplasmic deposits in the dorsal root ganglia neurons.[65–67] Bortezomib-associated CIPN is also related to the route of administration. More CIPN occurs with the intravenous administration versus the subcutaneous, which may be related to peak levels of drug.[68]

Immunomodulatory agents are also known to cause CIPN. A down-regulation of tumor necrosis factor α, resulting in wallerian degeneration, and the influence of systematic inflammatory disorders (eg, leukocytostatic vasculitis) have been proposed as mechanisms.[69,70] Pomalidomide is associated with an overall incidence of peripheral neuropathy of approximately 38%.[71–73] In comparison to bortezomib, the incidence of grades 3 and 4 peripheral neuropathy is lower with pomalidomide. In a phase 2 study of patients with relapsed and refractory multiple myeloma, no cases of grades 3 or 4 peripheral neuropathy were observed.[72] Additional, supportive evidence of the low incidence (eg, $\leq$1%) of grades 3 and 4 neuropathy was observed in a randomized, open-label, phase 3 study.[73]

CIPN presents with signs and symptoms of neuropathic pain. These include numbness, tingling, stabbing, radiating, and shooting pain in the hands and/or feet in a stocking-glove pattern (see **Table 2**). Patient risk factors for the development of CIPN include diabetes, smoking history, heavy alcohol use history, decreased renal function, and presence of baseline neuropathy symptoms.[64,74,75] Depending

Table 5	
Chemotherapies and targeted therapies associated with neuropathy	
Drug Class	**Drug Examples**
Proteasome inhibitors	Bortezomib, carfilzomib
Immunomodulatory agents	Thalidomide, lenalidomide, pomalidomide
Platinum agents	Cisplatin, carboplatin, oxaliplatin
Taxanes	Paclitaxel, docetaxel, cabazitaxel
Epothilones	Ixabepilone
Plant alkaloids	Vinblastine, vincristine, vinorelbine, etoposide
Nontaxane microtubule inhibitor	Eribulin

on individual risk factors and cumulative treatment exposure, CIPN can be continuous and can occur within the first month of chemotherapy, after 6 months of completing chemotherapy, or beyond 1 year after completion of therapy.[76] Optimal CIPN management includes early and regular monitoring with neurologic evaluations, consideration for dose modification or treatment discontinuation, and nonpharmacologic and pharmacologic therapy considerations.

Empiric nonpharmacologic approaches should be considered for all patients experiencing not only CIPN but also any neuropathic pain in the hands and feet. Patients should protect both hands and feet and wear loose-fitting but protective shoes along with cotton socks and padded slippers. Patients should keep feet uncovered in bed, because bedding that presses down on toes may be uncomfortable. Moderate walking is recommended to maintain blood circulation in feet along with massage.[66] Patients should avoid products that cause drying of the skin, such as prolonged contact with hot water and use of hand gels.

Pharmacologic management of CIPN is based on limited evidence. Various medications have been used, including tricyclic antidepressants, selective serotonin reuptake inhibitors, noradrenaline/serotonin reuptake inhibitors, neuroleptics, anticonvulsants, opioids, topical drugs, and muscle relaxants, but almost all agents that decrease neuropathic pain from other causes do not help patients with CIPN. A detailed review of current therapies for neuropathic pain from other causes is available[77-79] (see also Mellar P. Davis' article, "Cancer-Related Neuropathic Pain: Review and Selective Topics," in this issue, for a discussion of mechanism and treatment of non-CIPN neuropathic pain syndromes).

The oral anticonvulsant duloxetine is the only medication with moderate evidence recommended to treat CIPN.[80] This recommendation is based on a randomized, double-blind, placebo-controlled crossover study in 231 patients with at least a grade 1 severity of CIPN and a pain intensity score of greater than or equal to 4.[81] The duloxetine dose was titrated up to 60 mg daily with a total treatment duration of 5 weeks. The mean difference in pain score was 0.73 (95% CI, 0.26–1.2) between duloxetine and placebo. A larger mean decrease in average pain scores was observed during duloxetine treatment compared with placebo (1.06 vs 0.34; $P<.005$).[81] The 2014 American Society of Clinical Oncology guidelines state that tricyclic antidepressants and gabapentin are options to consider even with minimal evidence supporting their use.[80] Sparse low-quality evidence exists regarding efficacy for these medications in other noncancer, neuropathic pain syndromes.

If nonopioid adjuvants or current opioid therapy is providing insufficient neuropathic pain relief, another option is to switch to a different opioid (ie, opioid rotation). Methadone is sometimes used in this setting. Methadone is discussed in Mary Lynn McPherson and colleagues' article, "Methadone: Maximizing Safety and Efficacy for Pain Control in Patients with Cancer," in this issue.

Postherpetic Neuralgia

HSCT patients are at high risk for opportunistic infections, such as herpes zoster, caused by reactivation of varicella-zoster virus and often resulting in severe pain and postherpetic neuralgia. In a mixed population of autologous and allogeneic HSCT patients, reactivation of varicella-zoster ranged from 16% to 37%, with the onset occurring 4.5 months to 8.3 months post-transplant.[82-84] Postherpetic neuralgia incidence has varied across studies. In patients receiving a nonmyeloablative conditioning regimen, postherpetic neuralgia occurred at a rate of 25% in 1 study,[84] but a higher incidence has been reported elsewhere in HSCT patients.[82,83] In allogeneic HSCT patients, increased postherpetic neuralgia risk has also been associated with age and male gender.[82] In addition, varicella-zoster reactivation is associated with some myeloma therapies often used pretransplant or post-transplant, including bortezomib.[85]

Postherpetic neuralgia can present as burning, numb, tingling, sharp, stabbing, and achy. Allodynia, pain that occurs out of proportion to normal touch, can also be present. The pain is generally located in the same nerve distribution (dermatome) area where a previous zoster infection occurred. There are no specific treatment guidelines for postherpetic neuralgia in HSCT. In the context of noncancer postherpetic neuralgia, a recent review of 37 studies in 5914 adults suggests that gabapentin, 1800 mg/d to 3600 mg/d, can provide pain relief to some patients with postherpetic neuralgia.[79] Consequently, with the lack of conclusive evidence, treatment options remain empiric and based on evidence from other neuropathic pain syndromes. Pharmacologic approaches for postherpetic neuralgia are similar to those previously described in Mellar P. Davis' article, "Cancer-Related Neuropathic Pain: Review and Selective Topics," in this issue.

FUTURE DIRECTIONS AND SUMMARY

Chimeric antigen receptor T cell–based therapy will become another strategy to treat B-cell malignancies in addition to HSCT.[86] Select patients who can tolerate this highly toxic approach will also experience multiple new symptoms resembling those of HSCT without the associated GVHD. To effectively palliate patients with these hematologic malignancies undergoing toxic but potentially curative strategies, new and effective tools need to be developed. Nonoral routes of administration will also be required to ensure adequate drug delivery and absorption in the setting of mucositis and diarrhea.

As pharmacologic approaches are individually tailored in the care of hematologic malignancy patients, individualizing supportive care strategies also will be needed. Given the growing evidence of the many benefits of early, concurrent palliative care among patients with serious illness, the authors anticipate that future approaches to pain management in HSCT patients will include the integration of specialist palliative care.[87] Similar to solid tumor patients demonstrating different palliative care needs depending on cancer type and other patient variables,[88,89] the authors anticipate that hematologic malignancy patients will have unique needs depending on the type of malignancy, stage of disease, and/or treatment regimen. Future palliative care research combined with education on the role of palliative care and meaningful access to palliative care specialists will likely be an area of collaborative research.

HSCT is a high-risk procedure with treatment goals focusing on a potential cure. Concurrent with the goal for a cure, patients experience high symptom burden. Pain is a significant physical symptom that can be observed across the spectrum of HSCT care. Specific pain syndromes in HSCT patients include procedural pain, G-CSF–induced bone pain, oral mucositis, skin and abdominal pain in the setting of acute GVHD, CIPN, and postherpetic neuralgia. Management varies based on the type of HSCT-specific pain syndrome.

REFERENCES

1. Cutler C, Antin JH. An overview of hematopoietic stem cell transplantation. Clin Chest Med 2005;26(4):517–27, v.
2. Niederwieser D, Baldomero H, Szer J, et al. Hematopoietic stem cell transplantation activity worldwide in 2012 and a SWOT analysis of the Worldwide Network for Blood and Marrow Transplantation Group including the global survey. Bone Marrow Transplant 2016;51(6):778–85.

3. Anderson KO, Giralt SA, Mendoza TR, et al. Symptom burden in patients under-going autologous stem-cell transplantation. Bone Marrow Transplant 2007; 39(12):759–66.

4. Bevans MF, Mitchell SA, Marden S. The symptom experience in the first 100 days following allogeneic hematopoietic stem cell transplantation (HSCT). Support Care Cancer 2008;16(11):1243–54.

5. Hjermstad MJ, Knobel H, Brinch L, et al. A prospective study of health-related quality of life, fatigue, anxiety and depression 3-5 years after stem cell transplantation. Bone Marrow Transplant 2004;34(3):257–66.

6. Sherman AC, Simonton S, Latif U, et al. Changes in quality-of-life and psychosocial adjustment among multiple myeloma patients treated with high-dose melphalan and autologous stem cell transplantation. Biol Blood Marrow Transplant 2009;15(1):12–20.

7. Sherman AC, Coleman EA, Griffith K, et al. Use of a supportive care team for screening and preemptive intervention among multiple myeloma patients receiving stem cell transplantation. Support Care Cancer 2003;11(9):568–74.

8. Golianu B, Krane EJ, Galloway KS, et al. Pediatric acute pain management. Pediatr Clin North Am 2000;47(3):559–87.

9. Niscola P, Romani C, Cartoni C, et al. Epidemiology of pain in hospital haematological setting: an Italian survey. Leuk Res 2008;32(1):197–8.

10. Vasquenza K, Ruble K, Chen A, et al. Pain management for children during bone marrow and stem cell transplantation. Pain Manag Nurs 2015;16(3):156–62.

11. Vanhelleputte P, Nijs K, Delforge M, et al. Pain during bone marrow aspiration: prevalence and prevention. J Pain Symptom Manage 2003;26(3):860–6.

12. Karlsson L, Quinlan D, Guo D, et al. Mobilized blood cells vs bone marrow harvest: experience compared in 171 donors with particular reference to pain and fatigue. Bone Marrow Transplant 2004;33(7):709–13.

13. Heary RF, Schlenk RP, Sacchieri TA, et al. Persistent iliac crest donor site pain: independent outcome assessment. Neurosurgery 2002;50(3):510–6 [discussion: 516–7].

14. Ahlmann E, Patzakis M, Roidis N, et al. Comparison of anterior and posterior iliac crest bone grafts in terms of harvest-site morbidity and functional outcomes. J Bone Joint Surg Am 2002;84-A(5):716–20.

15. Lieschke GJ, Burgess AW. Granulocyte colony-stimulating factor and granulocyte-macrophage colony-stimulating factor (1). N Engl J Med 1992;327(1):28 35.

16. Gregory S, Schwartzberg L, Mo M, et al. Evaluation of reported bone pain in cancer patients receiving chemotherapy in pegfilgrastim clinical trials: a retrospective analysis. Commun Oncol 2010;7(7):297–308. Available at: http://www.mdedge.com/sites/default/files/jso-archives/Elsevier/co/journal/articles/0707297.pdf. Accessed February 23, 2018.

17. Crawford J, Ozer H, Stoller R, et al. Reduction by granulocyte colony-stimulating factor of fever and neutropenia induced by chemotherapy in patients with small-cell lung cancer. N Engl J Med 1991;325(3):164–70.

18. Heil G, Hoelzer D, Sanz MA, et al. A randomized, double-blind, placebo-controlled, phase III study of filgrastim in remission induction and consolidation therapy for adults with de novo acute myeloid leukemia. The International Acute Myeloid Leukemia Study Group. Blood 1997;90(12):4710–8.

19. Vogel CL, Wojtukiewicz MZ, Carroll RR, et al. First and subsequent cycle use of pegfilgrastim prevents febrile neutropenia in patients with breast cancer: a multi-center, double-blind, placebo-controlled phase III study. J Clin Oncol 2005;23(6): 1178–84.

20. Xu H, Gong Q, Vogl FD, et al. Risk factors for bone pain among patients with cancer receiving myelosuppressive chemotherapy and pegfilgrastim. Support Care Cancer 2016;24(2):723–30.

21. Bennett A. The role of biochemical mediators in peripheral nociception and bone pain. Cancer Surv 1988;7(1):55–67.

22. Moore DC, Pellegrino AE. Pegfilgrastim-induced bone pain: a review on incidence, risk factors, and evidence-based management. Ann Pharmacother 2017;51(9):797–803.

23. Lambertini M, Del Mastro L, Bellodi A, et al. The five "Ws" for bone pain due to the administration of granulocyte-colony stimulating factors (G-CSFs). Crit Rev Oncol Hematol 2014;89(1):112–28.

24. Moukharskaya J, Abrams DM, Ashikaga T, et al. Randomized phase II study of loratadine for the prevention of bone pain caused by pegfilgrastim. Support Care Cancer 2016;24(7):3085–93.

25. Gavioli E, Abrams M. Prevention of granulocyte-colony stimulating factor (G-CSF) induced bone pain using double histamine blockade. Support Care Cancer 2017;25(3):817–22.

26. Kirshner JJ, Heckler CE, Janelsins MC, et al. Prevention of pegfilgrastim-induced bone pain: a phase III double-blind placebo-controlled randomized clinical trial of the university of rochester cancer center clinical community oncology program research base. J Clin Oncol 2012;30(16):1974–9.

27. Kirshner J, Hickock J, Hofman M. Pegfilgrastim-induced bone pain: incidence, risk factors, and management in a community practice. Community Oncology 2007;4:455–9. Available at: http://www.mdedge.com/sites/default/files/jso-archives/Elsevier/co/journal/articles/0407455.pdf. Accessed February 23, 2018.

28. Iacovelli L, Harms R, Mo M. Effects of a reduced dose of pegfilgrastim on the incidence of febrile neutropenia and bone pain: a retrospective analysis. J Hematol Oncol Pharm 2012;2(3). Available at: http://jhoponline.com/jhop-issue-archive/2012-issues/september-vol-2-no-3/15150-effects-of-a-reduced-dose-of-pegfilgrastim-on-the-incidence-of-febrile-neutropenia-and-bone-pain-a-retrospective-analysis. Accessed February 23, 2018.

29. Ferrara F, Palmieri S, De Simone M, et al. High-dose idarubicin and busulphan as conditioning to autologous stem cell transplantation in adult patients with acute myeloid leukaemia. Br J Haematol 2005;128(2):234–41.

30. Wang EH, Chen YA, Corringham S, et al. High-dose CEB vs BEAM with autologous stem cell transplant in lymphoma. Bone Marrow Transplant 2004;34(7):581–7.

31. Cote GM, Hochberg EP, Muzikansky A, et al. Autologous stem cell transplantation with thiotepa, busulfan, and cyclophosphamide (TBC) conditioning in patients with CNS involvement by non-Hodgkin lymphoma. Biol Blood Marrow Transplant 2012;18(1):76–83.

32. Palumbo A, Bringhen S, Bertola A, et al. Multiple myeloma: comparison of two dose-intensive melphalan regimens (100 vs 200 mg/m(2)). Leukemia 2004;18(1):133–8.

33. Palumbo A, Bringhen S, Petrucci MT, et al. Intermediate-dose melphalan improves survival of myeloma patients aged 50 to 70: results of a randomized controlled trial. Blood 2004;104(10):3052–7.

34. Sonis ST, Elting LS, Keefe D, et al. Perspectives on cancer therapy-induced mucosal injury: pathogenesis, measurement, epidemiology, and consequences for patients. Cancer 2004;100(9 Suppl):1995–2025.

35. Scully C, Sonis S, Diz PD. Oral mucositis. Oral Dis 2006;12(3):229–41.

36. Sonis ST. The pathobiology of mucositis. Nat Rev Cancer 2004;4(4):277–84.
37. McGuire DB, Yeager KA, Dudley WN, et al. Acute oral pain and mucositis in bone marrow transplant and leukemia patients: data from a pilot study. Cancer Nurs 1998;21(6):385–93.
38. Organization WH. WHO handbook for reporting results of cancer treatment. 1979. Available at: http://apps.who.int/iris/bitstream/10665/37200/1/WHO_OFFSET_48. pdf. Accessed October 12, 2017.
39. El-Jawahri A, Traeger L, Kuzmuk K, et al. Physical and psychological symptom burden and prognostic understanding during hospitalization for hematopoietic stem cell transplantation. Biol Blood Marrow Transplant 2014;20:S193.
40. Harris DJ. Cancer treatment-induced mucositis pain: strategies for assessment and management. Ther Clin Risk Manag 2006;2(3):251–8.
41. Coda BA, O'Sullivan B, Donaldson G, et al. Comparative efficacy of patient-controlled administration of morphine, hydromorphone, or sufentanil for the treatment of oral mucositis pain following bone marrow transplantation. Pain 1997;72(3):333–46.
42. Lalla RV, Bowen J, Barasch A, et al. MASCC/ISOO clinical practice guidelines for the management of mucositis secondary to cancer therapy. Cancer 2014; 120(10):1453–61.
43. Portenoy RK, Ahmed E. Principles of opioid use in cancer pain. J Clin Oncol 2014;32(16):1662–70.
44. Grass JA. Patient-controlled analgesia. Anesth Analg 2005;101(5 Suppl):S44–61.
45. Prommer E. Fast facts and concepts #92. Patient controlled analgesia in palliative care. Available at: https://www.mypcnow.org/blank-ypz41. Accessed September 15, 2017.
46. Weissman DE. Fast facts and concepts #20. Opioid dose escalation. Available at: https://www.mypcnow.org/blank-it0kw. Accessed September 15, 2017.
47. Bensinger W, Schubert M, Ang KK, et al. NCCN Task Force Report. prevention and management of mucositis in cancer care. J Natl Compr Canc Netw 2008; 6(Suppl 1):S1–21 [quiz: S22–4].
48. Chan A, Ignoffo RJ. Survey of topical oral solutions for the treatment of chemo-induced oral mucositis. J Oncol Pharm Pract 2005;11(4):139–43.
49. Karim A, Ahmed S, Siddiqui R, et al. Methemoglobinemia complicating topical lidocaine used during endoscopic procedures. Am J Med 2001;111(2):150–3.
50. Shillingburg A, Kanate AS, Hamadani M, et al. Treatment of severe mucositis pain with oral ketamine mouthwash. Support Care Cancer 2017;25(7):2215–9.
51. Vayne-Bossert P, Escher M, de Vautibault CG, et al. Effect of topical morphine (mouthwash) on oral pain due to chemotherapy- and/or radiotherapy-induced mucositis: a randomized double-blinded study. J Palliat Med 2010;13(2):125–8.
52. Cinausero M, Aprile G, Ermacora P, et al. New Frontiers in the Pathobiology and Treatment of Cancer Regimen-Related Mucosal Injury. Front Pharmacol 2017;8: 354.
53. Gholizadeh N, Mehdipoor M, Sajadi H, et al. Palifermin and chlorhexidine mouth-washes in prevention of chemotherapy-induced mucositis in children with acute lymphocytic leukemia: a randomized controlled trial. J Dent (Shiraz) 2016;17(4): 343–7.
54. Wu JC, Beale KK, Ma JD. Evaluation of current and upcoming therapies in oral mucositis prevention. Future Oncol 2010;6(11):1751–70.
55. Przepiorka D, Weisdorf D, Martin P, et al. 1994 Consensus Conference on acute GVHD grading. Bone Marrow Transplant 1995;15(6):825–8.

56. Dignan FL, Amrolia P, Clark A, et al. Diagnosis and management of chronic graft-versus-host disease. Br J Haematol 2012;158(1):46–61.
57. Vogelsang GB, Hess AD, Santos GW. Acute graft-versus-host disease: clinical characteristics in the cyclosporine era. Medicine 1988;67(3):163–74.
58. Zhou Y, Barnett MJ, Rivers JK. Clinical significance of skin biopsies in the diagnosis and management of graft-vs-host disease in early postallogeneic bone marrow transplantation. Arch Dermatol 2000;136(6):717–21.
59. Wong-Sefdan I, Ale-Ali A, DeMoore PA, et al. Implementing inpatient, evidence-based, antihistamine-transfusion premedication guidelines at a single academic US hospital. J Community Support Oncol 2014;12(2):56–64.
60. Bertz H, Afting M, Kreisel W, et al. Feasibility and response to budesonide as topical corticosteroid therapy for acute intestinal GVHD. Bone Marrow Transplant 1999;24(11):1185–9.
61. Gupta S, Pagliuca A, Devereux S, et al. Life-threatening motor neurotoxicity in association with bortezomib. Haematologica 2006;91(7):1001.
62. Richardson PG, Barlogie B, Berenson J, et al. A phase 2 study of bortezomib in relapsed, refractory myeloma. N Engl J Med 2003;348(26):2609–17.
63. Richardson PG, Briemberg H, Jagannath S, et al. Frequency, characteristics, and reversibility of peripheral neuropathy during treatment of advanced multiple myeloma with bortezomib. J Clin Oncol 2006;24(19):3113–20.
64. Badros A, Goloubeva O, Dalal JS, et al. Neurotoxicity of bortezomib therapy in multiple myeloma: a single-center experience and review of the literature. Cancer 2007;110(5):1042–9.
65. Csizmadia V, Raczynski A, Csizmadia E, et al. Effect of an experimental proteasome inhibitor on the cytoskeleton, cytosolic protein turnover, and induction in the neuronal cells in vitro. Neurotoxicology 2008;29(2):232–43.
66. Mohty B, El-Cheikh J, Yakoub-Agha I, et al. Peripheral neuropathy and new treatments for multiple myeloma: background and practical recommendations. Haematologica 2010;95(2):311–9.
67. Richardson PG, Delforge M, Beksac M, et al. Management of treatment-emergent peripheral neuropathy in multiple myeloma. Leukemia 2012;26(4):595–608.
68. Moreau P, Pylypenko H, Grosicki S, et al. Subcutaneous versus intravenous administration of bortezomib in patients with relapsed multiple myeloma: a randomised, phase 3, non-inferiority study. Lancet Oncol 2011;12(5):431–40.
69. Chaudhry V, Cornblath DR, Corse A, et al. Thalidomide-induced neuropathy. Neurology 2002;59(12):1872–5.
70. Yildirim ND, Ayer M, Kucukkaya RD, et al. Leukocytoclastic vasculitis due to thalidomide in multiple myeloma. Jpn J Clin Oncol 2007;37(9):704–7.
71. Lacy MQ, Hayman SR, Gertz MA, et al. Pomalidomide (CC4047) plus low-dose dexamethasone as therapy for relapsed multiple myeloma. J Clin Oncol 2009; 27(30):5008–14.
72. Richardson PG, Siegel DS, Vij R, et al. Pomalidomide alone or in combination with low-dose dexamethasone in relapsed and refractory multiple myeloma: a randomized phase 2 study. Blood 2014;123(12):1826–32.
73. San Miguel J, Weisel K, Moreau P, et al. Pomalidomide plus low-dose dexamethasone versus high-dose dexamethasone alone for patients with relapsed and refractory multiple myeloma (MM-003): a randomised, open-label, phase 3 trial. Lancet Oncol 2013;14(11):1055–66.
74. Dimopoulos MA, Mateos MV, Richardson PG, et al. Risk factors for, and reversibility of, peripheral neuropathy associated with bortezomib-melphalan-prednisone in

newly diagnosed patients with multiple myeloma: subanalysis of the phase 3 VISTA study. Eur J Haematol 2011;86(1):23–31.

75. Kawakami K, Tunoda T, Takiguchi T, et al. Factors exacerbating peripheral neuropathy induced by paclitaxel plus carboplatin in non-small cell lung cancer. Oncol Res 2012;20(4):179–85.

76. Trivedi MS, Hershman DL, Crew KD. Management of chemotherapy-induced peripheral neuropathy. Am J Hematol Oncol 2015;11(1):4–10.

77. Cooper TE, Derry S, Wiffen PJ, et al. Gabapentin for fibromyalgia pain in adults. Cochrane Database Syst Rev 2017;(1):CD012188.

78. Derry S, Wiffen PJ, Aldington D, et al. Nortriptyline for neuropathic pain in adults. Cochrane Database Syst Rev 2015;(1):CD011209.

79. Wiffen PJ, Derry S, Bell RF, et al. Gabapentin for chronic neuropathic pain in adults. Cochrane Database Syst Rev 2017;(6):CD007938.

80. Hershman DL, Lacchetti C, Dworkin RH, et al. Prevention and management of chemotherapy-induced peripheral neuropathy in survivors of adult cancers: American Society of Clinical Oncology clinical practice guideline. J Clin Oncol 2014;32(18):1941–67.

81. Smith EM, Pang H, Cirrincione C, et al. Effect of duloxetine on pain, function, and quality of life among patients with chemotherapy-induced painful peripheral neuropathy: a randomized clinical trial. JAMA 2013;309(13):1359–67.

82. Onozawa M, Hashino S, Haseyama Y, et al. Incidence and risk of postherpetic neuralgia after varicella zoster virus infection in hematopoietic cell transplantation recipients: Hokkaido Hematology Study Group. Biol Blood Marrow Transplant 2009;15(6):724–9.

83. Rogers JE, Cumpston A, Newton M, et al. Onset and complications of varicella zoster reactivation in the autologous hematopoietic cell transplant population. Transpl Infect Dis 2011;13(5):480–4.

84. Su SH, Martel-Laferriere V, Labbe AC, et al. High incidence of herpes zoster in nonmyeloablative hematopoietic stem cell transplantation. Biol Blood Marrow Transplant 2011;17(7):1012–7.

85. Chanan-Khan A, Sonneveld P, Schuster MW, et al. Analysis of herpes zoster events among bortezomib-treated patients in the phase III APEX study. J Clin Oncol 2008;26(29):4784–90.

86. Jackson HJ, Rafiq S, Brentjens RJ. Driving CAR T-cells forward. Nat Rev Clin Oncol 2016;13(6):370–83.

87. El-Jawahri A, LeBlanc T, VanDusen H, et al. Effect of inpatient palliative care on quality of life 2 weeks after hematopoietic stem cell transplantation: a randomized clinical trial. JAMA 2016;316(20):2094–103.

88. Nipp RD, Greer JA, El-Jawahri A, et al. Age and gender moderate the impact of early palliative care in metastatic non-small cell lung cancer. Oncologist 2016; 21(1):119–26.

89. Greer JA, El-Jawahri A, Pirl WF, et al. Randomized trial of early integrated palliative and oncology care. Palliative Care in Oncology Symposium. San Francisco, CA, September 9-10, 2016.

Printed and bound by CPI Group (UK) Ltd, Croydon, CR0 4YY

07/10/2024

01040506-0002